EYE MOVEMENTS AND PSYCHOLOGICAL FUNCTIONS: INTERNATIONAL VIEWS

EYE MOVEMENTS AND PSYCHOLOGICAL FUNCTIONS: INTERNATIONAL VIEWS

edited by

RUDOLF GRONER
CHRISTINE MENZ
University of Bern, Switzerland

DENNIS F. FISHER
RICHARD A. MONTY
U.S. Army Human Engineering Laboratory

LEA LAWRENCE ERLBAUM ASSOCIATES, PUBLISHERS
1983   Hillsdale, New Jersey   London

Lawrence Erlbaum Associates, Inc., Publishers
365 Broadway
Hillsdale, New Jersey 07642

Library of Congress Cataloging in Publication Data
Main entry under title:

Eye movements and psychological functions.

  Bibliography: p.
  Includes indexes.
  1. Eye—Movements—Psychological aspects. 2. Visual
perception. I. Groner, Rudolf. [DNLM: 1. Eye movements
—Congresses. 2. Mental processes—Congresses.
3. Visual perception—Congresses. WW 400 E969 1981]
BF241.E895 1983   612'.846   83-9017
ISBN 0-89859-281-X

Printed in the United States of America
10 9 8 7 6 5 4 3 2 1

Participants

(*denotes Contributor)

* **Sven Ingmar Andersson,** University of Lund and St. Lars Hospital, Sweden
* **Paola Avanzini,** University of Pavia, Italy
* **B. Diane Barnette,** Human Engineering Laboratory, Aberdeen Proving Ground, MD, USA
  B. Biehl, University of Mannheim, German Federal Republic
  Walter F. Bischof, University of Bern, Switzerland
* **Didier Bouis,** Fraunhofer Institut, Karlsruhe, German Federal Republic
  Henk J. Breimer, Kath. Hogeschool, Tilburg, Netherlands
* **Francis Breitenbach,** Human Engineering Laboratory, Aberdeen Proving Ground, MD, USA
* **Angelo Buizza,** University of Pavia, Italy
* **Carlo Cabiati,** University of Pavia, Itlay
  Amos S. Cohen, Swiss Federal Institute of Technology, Zürich, Switzerland
* **Peter Coles,** University of Geneva, Switzerland
* **Trevor Crawford,** University of Durham, Great Britain
  Reinhard Daugs, Free University of Berlin, German Federal Republic
  Patrick Davous, Centre Hospitalier Sainte-Anne, Paris, France
  Ernst G. De Langen, University of Munich, German Federal Republic
* **Robert W. Ditchburn,** University of Reading, Great Britain
* **J. Fassl,** Akademie der Wissenschaften, Berlin, German Democratic Republic
* **John M. Findlay,** University of Durham, Great Britain
  Hans-Ueli Fisch, University of Bern, Switzerland
  Hardi Fischer, Swiss Federal Institute of Technology, Zürich, Switzerland
* **Dennis F. Fisher,** Human Engineering Laboratory, Aberdeen Proving Ground, MD, USA
  d'Arcais, G. B. Flores, University of Leiden and Max-Planck Institute, Nijmegen, Netherland
  Peter Fries, University of Lund, Sweden
* **Alistair G. Gale,** Queens Medical Center, Nottingham, Great Britain
* **Niels Galley,** University of Köln, German Federal Republic
* **Marina Groner,** Universities of Bern and Basel, Switzerland
* **Rudolf Groner,** University of Bern, Switzerland
  Annelies Heinisch, University of Würzburg, German Federal Republic
* **Dieter Heller,** University of Bayreuth, German Federal Republic
  Friederich W. Hesse, Rheinisch-Westfällische Technische Hochschule Aachen,
  German Federal Republic
  René Hirsig, Swiss Federal Institute of Technology, Zürich, Switzerland

W. F. Hoyt, University of California, San Francisco, USA
Ulf Hörberg, University of Uppsala, Sweden
* **Walter Huber,** Rheinisch-Westfällische Technische Hochschule Aachen,
    German Federal Republic
* **H. B. Ishak,** University of Köln, German Federal Republic
Arthur Jacobs, University of Würzburg, German Federal Republic
* **Zoi Kapoula,** Université René Descartes, Paris, France
* **Robert Karsh,** Human Engineering Laboratory, Aberdeen Proving Ground, MD, USA
* **Jean-Louis Kaufmann,** University of Geneva, Switzerland
Lothar Kehrer, University of Bielefeld, German Federal Republic
Alan F. Kennedy, University of Dundee, Scotland, Great Britain
G. Klaas, Max-Planck Institute, Nijmegen, Netherlands
G. Kleindienst, University of Mannheim, German Federal Republic
* **Axel Korn,** Fraunhofer Institut für Informations- und Datenverarbeitung, Karlsruhe,
    German Federal Republic
* **Werner Krause,** Akademie der Wissenschaften, Berlin, German Democratic Republic
Denny Kunak, Swiss Federal Institute of Technology, Zurich, Switzerland
Uta Lass, Rheinisch-Westfällische Technische Hochschule Aachen, German Federal Republic
* **Ariane Lévy-Schoen,** Université René Descartes, Paris, France
Per Lövsund, National Swedish Road and Traffic Research Institute, Linköping, Sweden
* **Gerd Lüer,** Rheinisch-Westfällische Technische Hochschule, Aachen,
    German Federal Republic
G. Magenes, University of Pavia, Italy
E. D. Megaw, University of Birmingham, Great Britain
O. Meienberg, University of Bern, Switzerland
* **Christine Menz,** University of Bern, Switzerland
Pierre Messerli, University of Geneva, Switzerland
Wolfgang Möckel, University of Oldenburg, German Federal Republic
* **Hermann Müller,** University of Würzburg, German Federal Republic
Dieter Nattkemper, University of Bielefeld, German Federal Republic
Michel Neboit, O.N.S.E.R. Monthéry, France
Karl-Ernst Neeb, University of Giessen, German Federal Republic
Birger Nygaard, Statens Väg-och Trafikinstitut, Linköping, Sweden
* **Mauro Pastomerlo,** University of Pavia, Italy
Franck Perronet, Bron, France
John Perry, University of London, Great Britain
Helen Petrie, University of Melbourne, Parkville, Victoria, Australia
* **Wolfgang Prinz,** University of Bielefeld, German Federal Republic
J. Richardson, University of Paris, France
J. G. M. Rovers, Kath. Hogeschool, Tilburg, Netherlands
A. + E. Safran, Hospital Cantonal, Geneva, Switzerland
K. Schaffer, University of Munich, German Federal Republic
* **Roberto Schmid,** University of Pavia, Italy
H. W. Schroiff, Rheinisch-Westfällische Technische Hochschule, Aachen,
    German Federal Republic
* **Wilfried Schumacher,** Fraunhofer Institut Karlsruhe, German Federal Republic
* **Wayne Shebilske,** University of Virginia, Charlottesville, USA
Lawrence Stark, University of California, San Francisco, USA
Bruno Steurer, Swiss Federal Institute of Technology, Zürich, Switzerland
François Stoll, University of Zürich, Switzerland
Michel Tisserand, INRS, Vandoevre, France
Harry Van der Vlugt, Kath. Hogeschool, Tilburg, Netherlands

M. N. Verbaten, University of Utrecht, Netherlands
Wietske Vonk, Max-Planck-Institute, Nijmegen, Netherlands
* **Gerhardt Vossius,** University of Karlsruhe, German Federal Republic
A. H. Wertheim, Institute for Perception, Soesterberg, Netherlands
Peter Whalley, The Open University, Milton Keynes, Great Britain
* **Heino Widdel,** Forschungsinstitut für Anthropotechnik, Wachtberg-Werthofen,
        German Federal Republic
* **M. Widera-Bernsen,** University of Köln, German Federal Republic
Peter Winterhoff, University of Mannheim, German Federal Republic
Peter Wittenburg, Max-Planck-Institute, Nijmegen, Netherlands
* **Brian S. Worthington,** Queen's Medical Center, Nottingham, Great Britain
Othmar Würmle, University of Zürich, Switzerland
* **F. Wysotzki,** Akademie der Wissenschaften, Berlin, German Democratic Republic
G. d'Yedewalle, University of Leuven, Belgium
Daniela Zambarbieri, University of Pavia, Italy
W. H. Zangemeister, University of Hamburg, German Federal Republic

Contents

Preface

This volume represents the edited proceedings of the first conference organized by the European Group for Eye Movement Research with the theme "Eye Movements: Current Research and Methodology." The conference was held at the Department of Psychology, University of Bern, Switzerland, on September 16–19, 1981.

The origin of the European Group for Eye Movement Research goes back to symposia held at the Annual Workshops for Experimental Psychology in Germany, Erlangen, 1973, and Giessen, 1974. These were organized by the first editor of this volume and attended by about twenty participants from Germany, Austria, and Switzerland. The next meeting took place in Heidelberg, Germany, 1979, also organized by the first editor in collaboration with Henk Breimer, Tilburg, Netherlands. Heidelberg was the first place where all presentations and discussions were in English, due to the addition of participants from Holland, England, and France. Here it was also decided that a European Group for Eye Movement should be founded with the purpose of maintaining an address list informing recipients about ongoing research and equipment in use, and to organize regular meetings in different countries.

The conference in Bern was organized by the first two editors and supported by the Swiss National Science Foundation. It took place in a lively atmosphere. Although it was not the primary intention of the conference to have the proceedings published, there was a general wish to bring together the contributions in a volume which should preferably be contained in the series on eye movements and psychological processes published by Lawrence Erlbaum Associates.

The contributors sent their manuscripts to the first two editors who took care of a preliminary editing in contact with the authors and then forwarded the manuscripts to the second two editors at Aberdeen Proving Ground in the United States. It was also the task of the first two editors to organize the book into the four sections as it stands now. This division appeared most natural with respect to the topics covered by the contributions. We are most grateful to the session chairpersons of the conference who were willing to write short introductions to the respective sections of this volume, especially to Professor Robert Ditchburn who also provided a number of most valuable suggestions.

RUDOLF GRONER
CHRISTINE MENZ
Bern, Switzerland

When Rudy and Christine approached us about co-editing a volume on eye movements largely represented by Europeans, we had first thoughts of refusal. After all, we had recently published the proceedings of "The Last Whole Earth Eye Movement Conference" from 1980—what more could be said so soon? We nevertheless agreed to do the project, and as you will read, much more could be said. Our primary task as editors was to scrutinize for scientific credibility and attend to grammer without Americanizing the respective contributions—we hope we have met the challenge. This volume then is intended to serve as an additional complement to R. A. Monty and J. W. Senders (Eds.), *Eye movements and psychological processes* (1976), J. W. Senders, D. F. Fisher, and R. A. Monty (Eds.), *Eye movements and the higher psychological functions* (1978) and D. F. Fisher, R. A. Monty, and J. W. Senders, *Eye movements: Cognition and visual perception* (1981), all published by Lawrence Erlbaum Associates. Not only did one of us get to experience the lively atmosphere of the conference, but also the wonders of the Swiss and their country.

DENNIS F. FISHER
RICHARD A. MONTY
Aberdeen Proving Ground, MD, USA

ACKNOWLEDGMENTS

We all wish to thank the Swiss National Science Foundation for supporting the preparation and realization of the conference. We are also grateful to Franziska S. Walder for her help in many conference organizational details and to B. Diane Barnette who now has become a participant as well as volume organizer. Many thanks go to Charlotte Apostolou, Karin Fricker, and Christine Walter in Bern and to Dannette Holland at Aberdeen Proving Ground for their extensive secretarial help. To Dr. John Weisz, Director of the U.S. Army Human Engineering Laboratory, Aberdeen Proving Ground, goes special recognition for his continued support of our efforts in the study of eye movements and collaboration on international projects like those represented in this volume.

EYE MOVEMENTS AND PSYCHOLOGICAL FUNCTIONS: INTERNATIONAL VIEWS

▌ METHODS

INTRODUCTION

It was not my intention in this introduction to be particularly controversial, or perverse, but in thinking about the questions implied by the papers presented in this section, I felt an irresistible urge to be both! The perversity arises because, although I have worked with many different techniques for recording eye movements over the past ten years, from the least to some of the most sophisticated, I cannot say that I am an expert on technical matters. So, I do not try to do the job, admirably performed by the authors in this section, of discussing technical advances to render eye movement recording more accurate and reliable. Instead, I try to take a broader view and to situate current methodological concerns within what might loosely be called an epistemological perspective.

My first remark is that the papers presented in this section almost all focus on the problems of *analyzing* data furnished in abundance by measuring systems of greater or lesser intrinsic precision. This is a notable change in focus with respect to efforts of the past twenty years, when psychologists and physiologists joined with electronics engineers in an attempt to achieve optimal accuracy and subject comfort at the recording stage.

Back in those giddy days when eye movements seemed to some the key to the soul, psychologically interesting questions about attention, scanning, and so on were tackled by cinematographic recording of the eye on a few subjects for a few minutes, followed by months or years of manual, frame-by-frame analysis.

Physiologically interesting questions about oculo-motor parameters—the biomechanical characteristics of saccades, pursuit and fixations for example—required the subject to be bolted into immobility. Yet some of the most interesting data were furnished by these studies and still form the basis of much current research. I am thinking of Buswell's studies on reading and picture perception in the thirties, of Mackworth's studies in the sixties and of Yarbus' work, also in the sixties, on oculomotor parameters.

To my mind, the technological boom of the seventies has been of great value to our understanding of the neurophysiology and biomechanics of eye movements. The use of oculomotor-contingent studies has revealed invaluable, if still controversial data regarding saccade refractory times, saccadic supression, pre-programming and oculomotor control. Such studies are often only possible with high-precision, fast, on-line measurement techniques and sophisticated algorithms based upon reliable knowledge about, for example, saccade velocities and accelerations which, themselves, may be used to trigger stimulus events.

In the psychological domain I am not so certain that such precision is always necessary; efforts towards natural situations and subject mobility are more impor-tant concerns. I feel that sometimes the investment of time and, of course, money in high-tech apparatus discourages us from tackling experimental questions in a simple way. I am thinking here of experiments carried out by Pailhouse using EOG and an alert experimenter who intervened to blank out the stimulus every time the polygraph pen showed three saccades, or passed a cer-tain amplitude criterion. It would have been possible to carry out the same experiment automatically, but it would have demanded on-line saccade-detecting routines, very careful calibration, sampling rates of at least 100hz, and fast input-output times. In short, a lot of worry without guarantee of improved data reliability.

If the past decade or so has seen a blossoming of varied techniques for recording eye movements with an increasing part of the calculations carried out by computer, this has brought its own problems in its wake. Recording eye movements (or fixations, as the case may be) is now relatively easy and, depending on the system, is comfortable enough to permit studies with infants, children, automobile drivers, airplane pilots and quality-control inspectors. Usually, the most comfortable systems permit the analysis of fixations only, being based upon video recording and sample rates of 50 or 60Hz.

Fifteen years ago this would have meant, for a ten-minute recording with one subject, about 30,000 frames of video to be analyzed manually. Nowadays it might mean 30,000 data points to be analyzed by *a suitable computer program*. Here is the first problem discussed in the following papers: What exactly constitutes a suitable analysis program?

The suitability of the program must in part be defined by the objectives of the experiment. Two of the papers in this section (Buizza & Avanzini; Cabiati et al.) are concerned with eye *movements*—pursuit or saccadic—and describe programs that operate on high-frequency sampled data using look-up tables containing velocity and acceleration thresholds. The remaining three papers are more concerned with *fixations* and their partitioning from data points belonging to eye movement, blinks, or noise. Karsh and Breitenbach's paper demonstrates most forcefully an experience that others may have encountered.

Changing the values of analysis parameters (e.g. minimum fixation duration) can have a dramatic effect on the appearance of the plotted data. Schuhmacher and Korn's paper presents a useful means of digitizing the plethora of analog data furnished by the seductive, but often problematic head-mounted eye camera.

Heller's paper, as well as presenting information useful to those who employ EOG recording, also attempts to define the *precision* of the system and asks how this may be related to psychological measures. This is an extremely important question and one that is also tackled by Schumacher and Korn, as well as by the expanding literature on the "periphery."

Some years ago, using an infra-red retinal reflection oculometer, my colleagues and I (Coles, Sigman & Chessell, 1977; Sigman & Coles, 1980) at Oxford University launched an ambitious project to study the development of oculomotor scanning in infants, children, and adults. We produced probably millions of data points and set about analyzing these data, essentially to determine the succession and loci of fixations with respect to the stimuli. Apart from the problems of identifying what constituted a fixation, another problem arose. How does one *represent* a fixation in a two-dimensional, analog plot? Does one use a single point, a number, a disk of a certain size . . .? A single point seems to overestimate the possible precision of the recording system and drastically to misrepresent the perceptual process. In a single fixation the entire stimulus may be represented on the retina and, depending on the task, the spatial and temporal frequency characteristics of the stimuli, the age or level of cognitive elaboration of the subject with respect to the task, the field of useful vision may vary from $1°$ to a zone of diameter as large as $60°$ or more. It is also not clear that a single fixation yields any psychologically useful information, but rather that the succession of fixations is what is important. The assimilation of a fixation to a point corresponding to the center of the fovea is often an implicit a priori of the psychologist's use of eye movement recording (where has the subject looked to solve the problem?), but often leads to interpretive problems when as often happens subjects locate relevant information without having fixated it directly. In such cases, a very precise recording system reduces the uncertainty introduced by the measurement process but still only defines the center of gravity of a little-understood attentional process.

Despite these cautionary remarks it is a welcome sign that researchers are seeking to broadcast and to share the hard-won possibilities of efficient and accurate data analysis. This also implies an urge to create some procedural, hardware and software standards in a domain that, until recently, has often obliged researchers to construct their own apparatus and to write their own specialized software, frequently and unwillingly repeating parallel efforts elswhere.

Peter R. Coles

I.1 Computer Analysis of Smooth Pursuit Eye Movements

Angelo Buizza and Paola Avanzini
Instituto di Informatica e Sistemistica
Università di Pavia
Italy

The oculomotor control system can be considered as a multi-input, one-output system. Each input corresponds to a sensory channel (visual, vestibular, auditory, proprioceptive . . .) able to provide the central nervous system (CNS) with information that can be used to control eye movement. The output is eye rotation in the orbit. According to the input that is considered and to the modality of stimulation, different types of eye movement can be evoked. That is—for visual input—smooth pursuit, saccadic, or nystagmic eye movements can be elicited, depending on whether the subject is presented with a small target moving in a continuous or in a discontinuous way, or with a moving visual scene.

Each input-output pathway of the oculomotor control system is made by a number of neural circuits. Some circuits are specific to the input considered, others are shared among several inputs depending on the type of eye movement being evoked, and the remaining circuits belong to common input-output pathways for all types of eye movements. One approach to the differential analysis of the CNS could be that of comparing the oculomotor responses evoked by appropriate stimulations of the various sensory channels either separately or differently combined. As a matter of fact, thanks to the recent progress in oculomotor research (Bach-y-Rita, Collins, & Hyde, 1971; Dichgans & Bizzi, 1972; Lennerstrand, Bach-y-Rita, & Collins, 1975; Baker & Berthoz, 1977; Carpenter, 1977; Becker & Fuchs, 1981), most of the nervous centers and neural pathways subserving the different oculomotor responses have been identified and described. Moreover it has been reported by many authors that important pathological situations (e.g., vestibular, cerebellar, brainstem, and cortical pathologies) induce significant modifications in one or more oculomotor responses (Lennerstrand, Bach-y-Rita, & Collins, 1975; Kommerell, 1978; Schmid & Zambarbieri, 1981). Then it is not surprising that eye movement analysis has been accepted as an important diagnostic and research tool not only in neurology, but also in other medical fields, such as ophthalmology and otolaryngology, and in psychology. At present, tests of ocular motility are performed routinely in many clinics.

When eye movement analyses are made for diagnostic purposes, complex patterns of eye movements should be considered and/or subtle pathological modifications should be recognized. In these cases, simple eye inspection of the records is completely inadequate. Computer based systems for automatic or interactive analysis of eye movements offer the possibility of processing a tremendous amount of data in a rigorous quantitative way. In the last ten years, several programs have been proposed for the analysis of either nystagmic (Herberts, Abrahamsson, Einarsson, Hofmann, & Linder, 1968; Tole & Young, 1971; Schilder, Pasik, & Pasik, 1973; Allum, Tole, & Weiss, 1975; Anzaldi & Mira, 1975; Sills, Honrubia, & Kumley, 1975; Buizza, Schmid, Zanibelli, Mira, & Semplici, 1978; Huygen, 1979; Ni, 1980) or saccadic eye movements (Sills et al., 1975; Baloh, Sills, Kumley, & Honrubia, 1975; Baloh, Kumley, & Honrubia, 1976; Michaels & Tole, 1977; Dick, 1978; Cabiati & Pastormerlo, 1979) whereas only few attempts have been made toward computer analysis of smooth pursuit eye movements. It is not clear whether this lack of interest is the consequence or one of the causes of the fact that smooth pursuit has so far received little attention in comparison with other types of eye movements. Actually, the computation of functional parameters describing smooth pursuit is exposed to gross errors unless precise recording techniques are used and accurate quantitative analysis is made.

Smooth pursuit eye movements (SPEM) can be elicited by asking the subject to track a small target moving slowly in the line of sight. Due to the static and dynamic limitations of the smooth pursuit control system (SPCS), correcting saccades are frequently required to foveate the target when target velocity exceeds 50–60 deg/sec or in pathological situations. The result is a typical pattern of the tracking in which periods of smooth pursuit are interrupted by correcting saccades in the same direction. For a given experimental situation, the duration of the smooth components and the number and frequency of saccades depend on the subjects' psychophysical conditions. The evaluation of these parameters can therefore provide a first, although incomplete, estimation of the SPCS function. A more complete and correct appreciation of SPCS performances can be obtained only after removing the saccadic contribution to eye tracking. The removal of saccades actually represents the major problem in the analysis of SPEM. It has been approached either in the frequency or in the time domain.

A frequency domain analysis was proposed by Wolfe, Engelken, Olson, and Allen (1978). Eye positions during the tracking of targets moving sinusoidally in the horizontal plane (frequencies 0.2 to 1.6 Hz, peak velocities 12–100 deg/sec) were recorded, and the auto-power spectrum $G_x(f)$ of the input (stimulus), the auto-power spectrum $G_y(f)$ of the output (eye position), and the input-output cross-power spectrum $G_{xy}(f)$ were computed. Then "the oculomotor system gain, phase and spectral purity" were calculated as:

$$\text{Gain} = G_{xy}(f) \,/\, G_x(f) \Big|_{f=f_s}$$

$$\text{Phase} = \text{Arctan} \left(\text{Im } G_{xy}(f) \,/\, \text{Re } G_{xy}(f) \right)_{f=f_s}$$

$$\text{Spectral Purity} = G_y(f) \Big|_{f=f_s} \,/\, \sum_{f_s/8}^{32\,f_s} G_y(f) \tag{1}$$

where f_s is the stimulus frequency. These parameters were computed for each eye separately.

For sinusoidal target motion, the spectral purity as defined above is equal to 1 only if no saccades are present in eye tracking and the smooth eye movement is perfectly sinusoidal (linear mode). The spectral purity progressively decreases as the importance of the saccadic components increases. This parameter can thus provide an estimate of the relative contributions of the saccadic and the smooth pursuit systems to the tracking. For example a spectral purity of 0.9 would indicate that 90% of the output power spectrum is produced by "linear tracking," the remaining 10% results from "nonlinear tracking" and from noise. Unfortunately, the remaining two parameters that have been suggested for a quantification of SPCS performances (i.e., the gain and phase shift given by Equation 1) are meaningful only in the case of linearity, that is only if the spectral purity is equal to 1. Otherwise they can hardly be interpreted and, in any case, they depend on the behavior of the overall oculomotor system and not of the SPCS alone. As a matter of fact, saccades are present in eye tracking when SPCS is behaving nonlinearly, due to intrinsic limitations or to the presence of pathological situations. Thus linear systems analysis cannot be applied when the spectral purity is different from 1. The gain and the phase shift given by Equation 1 will normally refer to the describing function of the overall oculomotor system, and only a rough indirect estimate of SPCS performances can normally be obtained from these parameters.

The difficulty in separating the contribution of the SPCS from that of the saccadic system is a general limitation of any analysis made in the frequency domain. Since the main components of SPEM power spectrum are concentrated at low frequency (up to a few hertz) whereas saccades are thought to introduce only high frequency spectral components, one could be tempted to isolate SPEM by an appropriate low-pass filtering of the oculographic signal. Unfortunately this is not possible since the two spectra are overlapping at the low frequencies. The following example emphasizes the inadequacy of low-pass filtering by considering the extreme case of pure saccadic tracking. Let us suppose the subject (e.g., a cerebellar patient) is tracking the sinusoidal motion of the target only by saccades. Since eyes are making a staircase approximation of a sinusoidal pattern, the output power spectrum still presents a peak at the frequency of target motion. However, in this case the low frequency components of the spectrum have nothing to do with smooth pursuit; they depend only on the saccadic system.

A more accurate and meaningful quantification of the characteristics of the smooth pursuit control system can be obtained through a time domain analysis.

The classical procedure for removing saccadic contribution in the time domain is shown in Fig. 1. Since saccades are much faster than smooth pur-

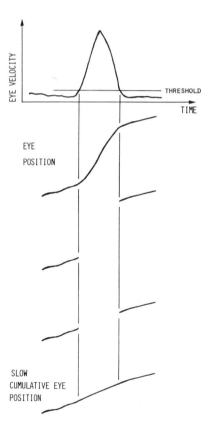

FIG. 1. Construction of the slow cumulative eye position. The presence of saccades is recognized by means of a velocity test; then the saccadic contribution is removed from the diagram of eye position and smooth components are connected to each other by using some function which extrapolates the smooth component preceding the saccade.

suit, their presence in eye tracking can be revealed by a velocity test comparing eye velocity with an appropriate threshold. The saccadic contribution to eye displacement is then removed and the smooth components are put together filling the gap by some curve which extrapolates the eye movement preceding the saccade. The resulting diagram of eye position is referred to as "slow cumulative eye position" and it is normally accepted as representing the eye displacement due to the smooth pursuit control system alone.

For its simplicity, this method was first used for manual processing of the tracings (Merrill & Stark, 1963). Then it was implemented in a computer program for SPEM analysis (Bahill, Iandolo, & Troost, 1980). However, it has not been adequately stressed that the choice of the extrapolating curve is extremely critical. Figure 2 shows how the construction of the slow cumulative eye position may be influenced by the choice of the extrapolating curve. Since the errors that can be so introduced add to each other, it is easy to predict that a repeated use of an uncorrect extrapolation will give rise to gross approximations. The amplitude of the slow cumulative eye position is normally used to estimate the SPCS input-output gain. Then significant errors in the computation of this parameter can sometimes be expected.

What is the extrapolation that minimizes these errors? An answer could be given only if the behavior of the smooth pursuit system during a saccadic event were known. This is not the case at the present, and extrapolation is normally done by a straight line with a slope equal to the average slope of the eye position diagram immediately before the saccade. This is equivalent to a double assumption. First, smooth pursuit and saccades add linearly. Second, smooth pursuit velocity remains constant during the saccade, with a value equal to that assumed just before the saccade. There is some experimental evidence for excluding linear addition (Jürgens & Becker, 1975). Moreover constant eye velocity can reasonably be assumed only at steady state during the tracking of a target moving at constant velocity. It cannot be accepted for other patterns of target motion, or during transients. To give a measure of the errors that can be introduced by linear extrapolation, let us consider the tracking of a sinusoidal target motion at 1 Hz. For each saccade to be removed, assuming for it a duration of 100 msec, an error of 1% to 10% can be introduced in the evaluation of the peak-to-peak amplitude of the slow cumulative eye position. Obviously, smaller errors correspond to saccades occurring when eye acceleration is minimal. A further source of significant errors can be the computation of eye velocity before the saccades.

The reconstruction of SPCS output in time domain is much more reliable if it is made by operating on the diagram of eye velocity instead of that of eye position. Actually, both eye velocity before and after the saccades are

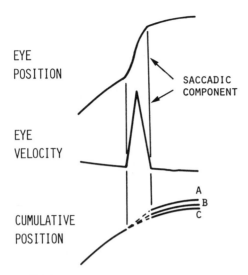

EYE
POSITION

SACCADIC
COMPONENT

EYE
VELOCITY

CUMULATIVE
POSITION

A
B
C

FIG. 2.   Different choices of the extrapolating function result in different shapes of the slow cumulative eye position. In the lower trace the effects of the following extrapolating functions are schematized: (A) Straight line with a slope equal to the mean slope of the smooth component preceding the saccade; (B) Straight line tangent to the same smooth component in its end point; (C) Function identified through a hypothetical best fitting procedure.

available. Then an interpolation and not an extrapolation is needed, and possible errors do not accumulate. In addition eye velocity appears to be a more significant parameter than eye position to describe the characteristics of the smooth pursuit control system which is actually considered as a "velocity servomechanism." Its static and dynamic characteristics are concerned with eye velocity more than with eye position.

The preceding considerations led us to develop a program for the analysis of smooth pursuit eye movements working in time domain and making reference to eye velocity. The program has been conceived to be interactive, since our experience was that interactive programs are much more reliable than fully automatic programs, and runs off-line. Eye position is measured by conventional DC electro-oculography or by infrared oculography and recorded on an analogue magnetic tape together with stimulus profile. Analogue data are then low-pass filtered with a selectable cut-off frequency and digitized at a sampling rate of 250 Hz. This frequency is highly redundant if the dynamic characteristics of the smooth pursuit control system are considered, but it is needed to ensure an accurate estimation of the refractory time of the responses and to isolate saccades with enough precision. A major concern is the cut-off frequency of the analogue filters and, according to Shannon's (1948) theorem, it is useless to exceed 125 Hz. With this value, a faithful reproduction of saccade profiles is guaranted (Bahill, Clark, & Stark, 1975), but the power supply noise (50 or 60 Hz) cannot be rejected. As a matter of fact, cut-off frequencies as low as 30–40 Hz do not jeopardize the successive procedure for saccade recognition and can produce a good improvement of the signal to noise ratio.

After analogue to digital conversion, samples are stored in the computer mass-memory from where they are recalled during the analysis. Programs for the analysis are written partially in Assembler and partially in FORTRAN IV and implemented on a general purpose minicomputer (Laben 70) with 16K 16 bit words. A graphic display (Tektronix 4010) allows man–machine interaction giving the operator the possibility of controlling and correcting the analysis.

The program performing the analysis has a tree structure. It is divided into four subsystems, each one controlling a particular function: data acquisition and retrieval, calibration of the records, analysis, and presentation of the results. After data acquisition, the first step is the construction of the calibration curve relating the output voltage of the recording chain to the corresponding eye deviation. To this purpose, the program presents the eye movement recorded during calibration (Fig. 3A), which was obtained by asking the subject to move his eyes from the central position to appropriate reference points placed in front of him. The operator communicates the amplitudes of eye rotations (e.g. 15° and 30° to the left in Fig. 3A) and indicates the level of the corresponding eye position signal by using the hair-cursors of the graphic display. The picture in Fig. 3A was taken while the operator was placing the cursors at the level corresponding to 30° left. As shown in the list on the left side of the picture, a level of − 86 was measured for the eye rotation of 15° left. At the end of this interactive procedure the program computes and displays the "calibration curve" (Fig. 3B: eye rotation in abscissa, voltage level in ordinate). The calibration curve will later be used to convert recorded signals into the corresponding eye deviation in degrees.

The eye movement recorded during tracking is then displayed (Fig. 4A). Due to the way in which data were stored, pieces of record of 1.1 sec are presented. Eye position (Fig. 4A, upper trace) is presented together with eye velocity computed numerically (middle trace) and with target velocity (lower trace, constant velocity). In order to reduce the effects of noise on the computation of eye velocity, eye position is smoothed before derivation. Both smoothing and derivation are performed according to the methods proposed by Savitzky and Golay (1964) and based on least squares interpolations. Windows of eleven points (44 msec) and a quadratic interpolating function are used.

The operator can now decide whether to ask the program to make the analysis or to skip on. If the analysis is requested, the program recognizes the saccades and marks their beginning and end points by asterisks (Fig. 4B). Then the program removes saccades from the diagram of eye velocity and displays the corrected curve (Fig. 4C). The latency of the response is also computed by measuring the interval between the beginning of the stimulation and the starting of the eye rotation.

The procedure used to recognize and remove saccades is schematically il-

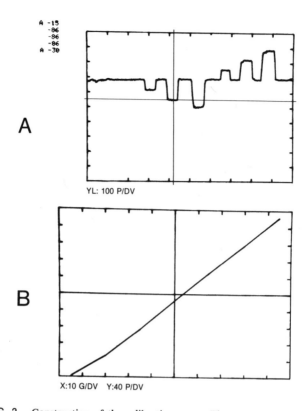

A -15
-86
-86
-86
A -38

YL: 100 P/DV

X:10 G/DV   Y:40 P/DV

FIG. 3. Construction of the calibration curve. The program displays the
eye movement recorded during the calibration and the operator communicates the amplitudes of eye rotations and indicates the corresponding
signal levels by using the display hair-cursors. (A). On the basis of these
values the program builds the calibration curve (B) relating eye deviation
(abscissa) to the amplitude of the recorded signal (ordinate). Writings at the
bottom of each square give the relevant scale factors. YL: 100 P/DV gives the
ordinate sale in A, it means that 100 units of a computer internal scale are
contained between two tics (one division); 1 unit correspond to 1 A/D con-
verter output level, or 2,45 mV. X:10 G/DV indicates an abscissa scale in B
of 10 deg/division. Y:40 P/DV indicates an ordinate scale in B of 98
mV/division (see above). Abscissa (time) scale in A is of 2 sec/division.

lustrated in Fig. 5. The three diagrams give from the top to the bottom: eye
position (P), eye velocity (V), and eye acceleration (A) before, during, and
after the saccade. Saccades are detected by comparing eye velocity with a
threshold value that is set quite high in order to reduce noise sensitivity.
Once a saccade has been found, the program computes the values of eye acceleration backwards from the instant T_1 and forwards from the instant T_2,
making T_1 and T_2 the upward and downward crossing points of the eye
velocity diagram with the threshold. The instants T_B and T_E, at which eye acceleration becomes smaller than a given threshold, are then found. These instants are assumed as the starting and end points of the saccade, respective-

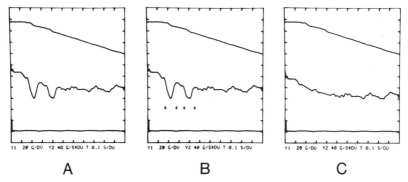

FIG. 4.   Saccade recognition and removal. In each panel top trace gives eye position, middle trace gives real (A and B) or corrected (C) eye velocity, and bottom trace gives stimulus velocity. A piece of record is presented to the operator on the graphic display (A). On the operator request, the program identifies saccades and marks their extremes by asterisks (B), and finally it removes them from eye velocity diagram (C). Scale factors are 20 deg/division (Y1: 20 G/DV) for eye position; 40 deg sec^{-1}/division (Y2: 40 G/S*DV) for eye velocity; 60 deg sec^{-1}/division (not displayed here) for target velocity; 0,1 sec/division (T: 0.1 S/DV) for time (abscissa) scale.

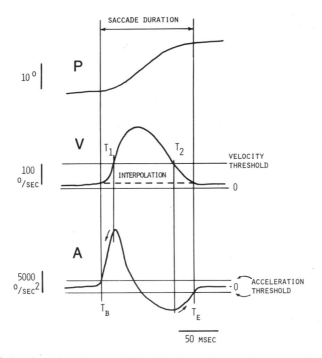

FIG. 5.   Procedure for saccade identification and removal. P: eye position, V: eye velocity, A: eye acceleration. Saccade is identified by means of a test on eye velocity, then saccade duration is evaluated by means of a test on eye acceleration, and finally saccade is removed from eye velocity diagram by means of a linear interpolation between $V(T_B)$ and $V(T_E)$.

15

ly. Finally, the program removes the saccadic component by giving eye velocity the values corresponding to a linear interpolation between eye velocity in T_B and eye velocity in T_E.

After the saccades have been removed, the operator has to decide whether to accept the results of computer analysis or to ask the computer to repeat this procedure with different program parameters. Typically, new values for the different thresholds used to identify saccades could be reassigned by the operator. When the analysis is considered to be correct, the program samples and stores the values of corrected eye velocity at regular intervals of 40 msec. A new piece of record is then presented and so on.

When the entire record has been analyzed, the pattern of eye velocity obtained from the data stored at the end of each piece of analysis is displayed. If several responses obtained in the same experimental condition are present in the same record, eye velocity averaged over the all responses is presented. An example is given in Fig. 6. The smooth pursuit eye velocity averaged over 25 trials performed in the same experimental condition as considered in Fig. 5 is shown.

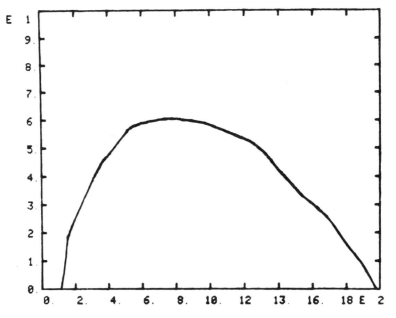

FIG. 6.   Smooth pursuit eye velocity diagram resulting from a computer analysis. The curve represents smooth pursuit eye velocity averaged over 25 trials in which a subject followed a spot moving at constant linear velocity on a linear screen, from 45 deg left to 45 deg right. Maximal angular velocity of the target was 60 deg/sec and was reached when the spot crossed the subject's medial plane. Abscissa (time) and ordinate (eye velocity) scales are 200 msec/division and 10 deg $\sec^{-1}$/division, respectively.

The program is now being tested not only to assess its ability to analyze tracings recorded under different experimental conditions, but also to find the best analogue or digital filtering and to improve interactivity.

ACKNOWLEDGMENTS

This work has been supported by a grant from HUSPI Project. We gratefully thank Prof. Roberto Schmid from the University of Pavia for continuous assistance and for critically reviewing the manuscript.

I.2 Computer Analysis of Saccadic Eye Movements

Carlo Cabiati, Mauro Pastormerlo,
Roberto Schmid and Daniela Zambarbieri
Instituto di Informatica e Sistemistica
Università di Pavia
Italy

Saccades are fast eye movements that are normally used to drive the eyes from one point of fixation to another as quickly as possible. Their characteristics have been largely investigated both in different species of animals (Fuchs, 1967; Collewijn, 1970; Stryker & Blakemore, 1972; Easter, 1975; Evinger & Fuchs, 1978), and in humans, either normal (Hyde, 1959; Westheimer, 1954; Robinson, 1964; Becker & Fuchs, 1969; Fuchs, 1971; Becker, 1972; Boghen, Troost, Daroff, Dell'Osso, & Birkett, 1974; Körner, 1975; Henriksson, Pyykkö, Schalen, & Wennmo, 1980) or suffering from various types of neurological disorders (Starr, 1967; Newman, Gay, Stroud, & Brooks, 1970; De Jong & Melvill Jones, 1971; Troost, Weber, & Daroff, 1972; Kirkham & Kamin, 1974; Perenin & Prablanc, 1974; Troost, Weber, & Daroff, 1974; Baloh, Konrad, Sills, & Honrubia, 1975; Zee, Optican, Cook, Robinson, & King-Engel, 1976; Baloh, Yee, & Honrubia, 1978; Henriksson, Hindfelt, Pyykkö, & Schalen, 1981).

Saccades are stereotyped eye movements that can be described by few parameters, namely their amplitude, duration and peak velocity (Fig. 1). In the case of saccades evoked by the presentation of targets, a fourth parameter can be introduced, the saccade latency defined as the time between stimulus presentation and beginning of eye movement.

For the example shown in Fig. 1, it has been assumed that the final eye position is reached through a primary saccade that falls short of target position, followed by a corrective secondary saccade. The latency of corrective saccades can be defined as the time between the end of the primary saccade and the beginning of the corrective saccade.

Duration and peak velocity of saccades are related to their amplitude in a

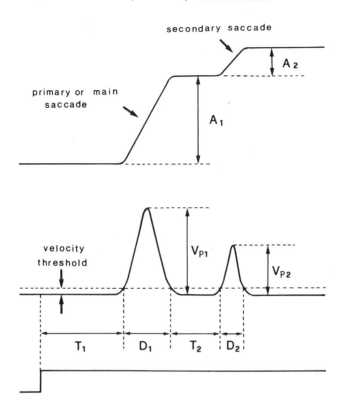

FIG. 1.   Definition of saccade parameters. Upper trace: eye position; middle trace: eye velocity; lower trace: target position. A: amplitude; D: duration, Vp: peak velocity; T: latency.

characteristic way. The relationship between duration and amplitude is linear for saccades driving the eyes from the central position up to 40° right or left. A 5° normal human saccade lasts about 30–40 msec with each additional degree increase in magnitude requiring about another 2–3 msec (Robinson, 1964; Cook, 1965; Baloh et al., 1975a). A linear relationship between duration and amplitude is found also for saccades from one hemisphere to the other up to a 80° deg amplitude (Hyde, 1954; Baloh et al., 1975b). The amplitude-peak velocity characteristic is linear only up to an amplitude of 20°, then eye peak velocity saturates (Fuchs, 1971). Significant variations in saccade parameters have been observed in many pathological situations of the central nervous system, with a high specificity with respect to the site and the extension of the lesion. Saccade analysis can therefore be used for neurological diagnosis.

Since hand computation of saccade parameters is a formidable task that can introduce many inaccuracies, some computer programs for saccade analysis have been developed in the last ten years (Baloh et al., 1975b; Baloh, Kumley, & Honrubia, 1976; Dick, 1978).

The aim of this paper is to decide a new program that is available in two versions; an interactive one (SACCAD 1) and a semi-automatic one (SAC-CAD 2). The first version is more suitable for research purposes or when noisy records need to be analyzed. The second version can be conveniently used for clinical routine when a great number of saccades need to be examined.

THE PROGRAM SACCAD 1

The program is implemented on a general purpose minicomputer (LABEN 70) with 16K 16 bit words. A graphic output is provided by a TEKTRONIX 4010 display that allows man-machine interaction. The subroutines for the analysis of saccades are written in FORTRAN IV, whereas the subroutines for data acquisition and for the control of the graphic display are written in ASSEMBLER. Eye movement measured by electro-oculography (EOG) or by infrared oculography is recorded on an analogue magnetic tape, together with a signal giving target position. Recorded data are low-pass filtered with a cut-off frequency of 125 Hz and then converted at a sampling frequency of 250 Hz.

The choice of filtering and sampling parameters is a critical point in the analysis of saccadic eye movements. The filter cut-off frequency should be as low as possible in order to reject most of the noise superposed on the signal, but high enough to preserve the frequency spectrum of the signal. Thus, the filter cut-off frequency must be selected in relation to the type of eye movement that will be analyzed. Smooth pursuit eye movements can be conveniently filtered at 20–30 Hz without introducing any significant distortion. On the contrary, the same filtering applied to saccadic eye movements leads to an apparent longer duration and a smaller peak velocity of saccades (Bahill, Clark, & Stark, 1975; Schmid, 1981). On the other hand, since the presence of noise below 100 Hz (in particular the power supply noise) can hardly be avoided in EOG clinical recording, errors can be introduced in an evaluation of saccade parameters unless this noise is attenuated by an appropriate filtering. It has been shown that the modifications of saccade parameters occurring in many pathological situations can still be appreciated even after low-pass filtering at 15 Hz (Henriksson et al., 1980).

As far as the sampling frequency is concerned, although a frequency two times greater than the cut-off frequency of the preceding analog filter is enough to preserve information, it is worth keeping the sampling frequency as high as possible, without overloading the memory. In fact, aliasing noise can be avoided even if the slope of the analog filter is not very high, and time discretization in the computation of durations will be reduced.

The solution, adopted in our system, was to use a sampling frequency giving a time discretization of 4 msec, to place the analog filter cut-off frequency at half the sampling frequency, to reject the aliasing noise and to attenuate the low frequency noise superposed on the EOG signal by an appropriate smoothing of the sampled data. The program has a tree structure. From the main program, whose flow chart is given in Fig. 2, it is possible to reach a number of subsystems, each of them oriented to a particular function.

The *subsystem AC* makes the search of the desired file of data on the digital tape and presents an identification card of both subject and test on the display.

The *subsystem TR* performs the analysis of the calibration signals in

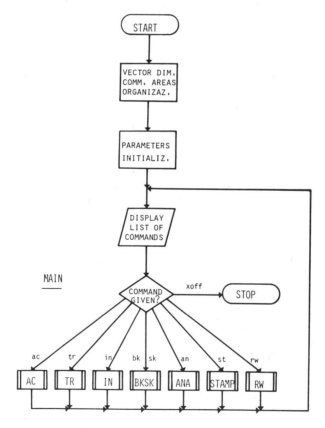

FIG. 2.   Flow chart of the main program.

order to compute the relationship between eye movement and recorded signal. Each test of ocular motility is actually preceded by the calibration of eye movements, during which the subject is asked to fixate a number of visual targets placed at different positions in front of him. The subsystem TR presents the eye movement, recorded during calibration, on the display (Fig. 3). For each position of the target, the operator communicates the amplitude of eye rotation and indicates the level of the corresponding electro-oculographic signal by using the horizontal hair cursor of the graphic display. The program reads this level and stores it with the relevant amplitude of eye rotation. At the end of this interactive procedure, the diagram relating the amplitude of the recorded signal to the amplitude of eye movement is presented on the display (Fig. 4). The program then uses this calibration curve to convert the amplitude of the recorded signal to the position of the eyes.

The *subsystem IN* allows the operator to assign numerical values to the parameters used by the program to recognize the occurrence of saccades.

The *subsystem BKSK* is designed to run back and forth on the digital tape. The analysis of some parts of the file can thus be repeated or some other parts can be skipped over.

The *subsystem ANA* performs the analysis of the desired file of data by examining successive records of 1 sec. Its flow chart is given in Fig. 5a, b, c, and d. The first record giving both EOG signal and target position is presented on the display. If no step change in target position is present, the operator demands for the next record. Otherwise, the operator places the vertical hair cursor at the instant of target jump and the position in the record of this instant is stored. Starting from the first sample, the program makes a smoothing of the EOG singal, but the routine for seeking the evoked saccade is activated (ANALYSIS ON) only when a minimum time (TMIN) from target jump is elapsed. The EOG signal is differentiated, and eye velocity (EV) is compared with a threshold value (VT1). When the threshold is exceeded, a series of tests are run. In order to exclude short time artifacts like spikes produced by eye blinks, an eye movement is not accepted as a saccade if eye deviation (EDEV) does not remain greater than an assigned value (INCR) for at least 20 msec from eye velocity threshold overpassing. The choice of 20 msec makes this test insensitive to the power supply noise, which has a frequency of 50 Hz (period of 20 msec).

Peak eye velocity (PEV) is then computed and tested to see whether it lies within a given range. The lower bound (VT2) and the upper bound (VT3) for peak velocity can either be assigned by the operator or computed by the subsystem ANA in relation to eye deviation from the instant of velocity threshold overcoming and the time of peak velocity. This latter test has been introduced to exclude some artifacts that could have escaped the previous test since their duration was greater than 20 msec. If both tests are passed

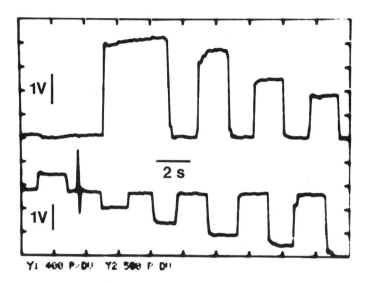

FIG. 3.   Calibration procedure. The two traces presented at the computer display give eye movement during calibration. The time scale for abscissa is the same for the two traces (2 sec/division). The ordinate scale for each trace is chosen by the computer in relation to the maximum amplitude of the signal in the piece of record presented on the display. The scale factors for the upper (Y1) and the lower (Y2) trace are presented at the bottom of the figure using computer units (1 P/DV = 2,45 mV/division). The physical units reported on the picture have been drawn by hand.

successfully, the analyzed eye movement is accepted as a saccade. Its termination is determined by means of a further velocity test performed during the deceleration phase (EV ≤ VT4). Saccade parameters are then computed, the latency as the time between the target jump and the overpassing of the first velocity threshold, the duration as the time between the instants at which the velocity thresholds VT1 and VT4 are passed, and the amplitude as the eye deviation between the same two instants. Peak eye velocity was already computed.

The symmetry of the examined saccade is quantified by the ratio between the durations of the acceleration and deceleration phases. The beginning and the end of the saccade are marked by vertical bars on the displayed record and saccade parameters are presented (Fig. 6). Afterward the program stands by. The operator now has to decide whether to accept these results or to ask the program to repeat the analysis. In the former case, the operator provides agreement. The results are stored, and the program goes on looking for the existence of corrective saccades until a maximum time (TMAX) from the instant of target jump is elapsed. If the analysis should be repeated, the operator will change some parameters of the analysis by using the subsystem IN for re-assignment. To conclude the description of the subsystem ANA, it is worth giving some details about the algorithms used to smooth input data and to compute eye velocity.

Since input data are obtained by sampling a continuous signal at a constant frequency, both smoothing and differentiation can be obtained by using an algorithm for discrete convolution. The current value $\hat{y}_j$ of the relevant variable (eye position or velocity) can be computed as

$$\hat{y}_j = \frac{1}{n} \sum_{-m}^{m} c_i y_{j-i} \tag{1}$$

where $c_m, \ldots, c_o, \ldots, c_m$ are the convolution factors, y_{j-i} is the input data at the sampling instant $j - i$, n is a normalizing factor and $2m$ is the width of the window used for convolution. By an appropriate choice of the factors c_i, it can be obtained that $\hat{y}_j$ given by Equation 1 represents the central point of a minimum square best fit curve of a given order (Savitsky & Golay, 1964). In terms of filtering, $\hat{y}_j$ can be interpreted as the output at time j of a digital filter with a finite impulse response given by the series $c_{-m}, \ldots, c_o, \ldots, c_m$.

Smoothing was done by using a window of 6 sampling intervals and giving the convolution factors the values of $c_o = 7$, $c_{-1} = c_1 = 6$, $c_{-2} = c_{-2} =$

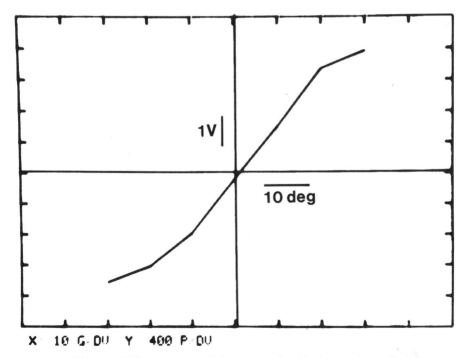

X 10 G DU   Y   400 P DU

FIG. 4.   Calibration curve relating eye rotation (abscissa) to the amplitude of the recorded signal (ordinate).

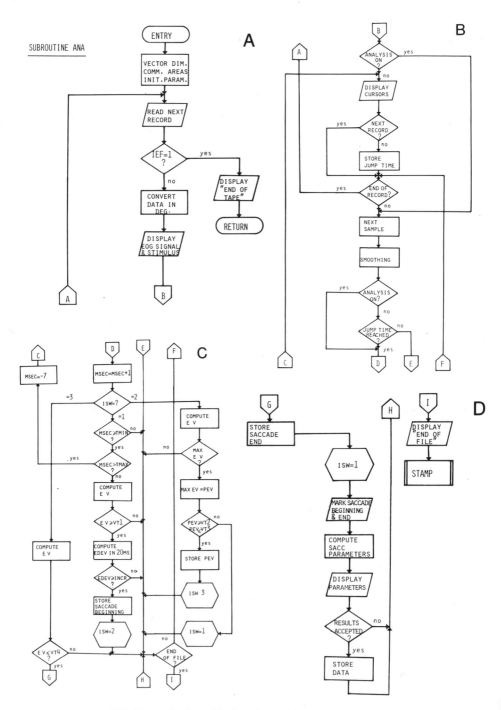

FIG. 5. A, B, C, and D flow chart of the subsystem ANA.

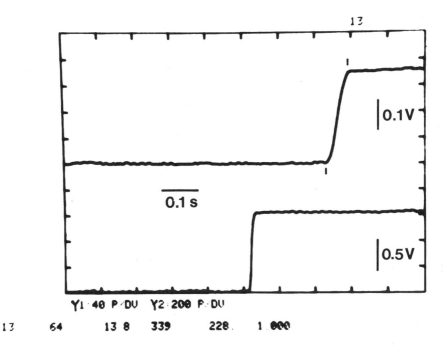

FIG. 6.   Example of saccade analysis. Upper trace: eye position; lower trace: target position. At the bottom: saccade parameters as computed by the program. From left to right: serial number of examined saccade, duration in msec, amplitude in deg, peak velocity in deg/sec, latency in msec and symmetry coefficient.

3 and $c_{-3} = c_3 = -2$. Each input sample y_j was so replaced by the central point $\hat{y}_{j-3}, \ldots , y_j, \ldots , y_{j+3}$.

This operation was equivalent to a low-pass filtering of the frequency components of the input signal whose period was shorter than about two times the width of the convolution window. At the used sampling frequency of 250 Hz, the width of the window as 24 msec. Then signal components with a frequency greater than about 30 Hz become to be attenuated. The aliasing noise as well as the power supply noise are completely rejected.

In order to detect the beginning of a saccadic eye movement and to compute saccade peak velocity, smoothed eye position data were differentiated by using Equation 1 with $m = 3$ and $c_{-3} = -3, c_{-2} = -2, c_{-1} = -1, c_0 = 0, c_1 = 1, c_2 = 2$ and $c_3 = 3$. The same algorithm with a more narrow window (4 sampling intervals corresponding to 16 msec) was used during the deceleration phase to detect the end of the saccadic movement. The opportunity of reducing the width of the convolution window was suggested by the difficulties encountered in detecting the end of overshooting saccades. When a 24 msec window was used, the end of overshooting saccades was usually placed beyond the point of overshooting. Saccade duration was then overestimated. The overshoot could be excluded by increasing the velocity threshold, but the end of the saccade was then placed in front of the overshoot point and saccade duration was underestimated. The precision in computing saccade duration was significantly improved when the width of the window was reduced to 16 msec.

At the end of the analysis, the *subsystem STAMP* is called to print the identification record, the values given to the program parameters and the results of the analysis (latency, amplitude, duration, peak velocity, and symmetry coefficient of each saccade). The results of the analysis are also punched on a paper tape that can later be used as input to a separate program for the presentation of the results on the graphic display in the form of diagrams. Saccade duration and peak velocity can be plotted versus amplitude, and experimental data can be fitted by using regression functions, either linear or nonlinear. The histogram of saccade latency and that of saccade symmetry coefficient can also be presented.

THE PROGRAM SACCAD 2

The program SACCAD 2 represents an intermediate step between the interactive system previously described and a next program for on-line analysis to be implemented on a microprocessor.

Although saccade analysis is made in a completely automatic way, the program still works on data stored on a digital tape, and all the preliminary operations (from tape positioning to the analysis of the calibration signals) are still made under the operator control.

SACCAD 2 is therefore a semi-automatic system for off-line analysis. The automatic procedure is started once the operator has answered the following questions presented on the display: How long is the record that should be analyzed? Should the stored standard values of the analysis parameters be modified? If modifications are required, a reassignment can be done by calling the subroutine IN, which operates as in SACCAD 1 system.

Afterwards, the program continues to analyze the target position signal. Step changes in target position are detected by comparing the difference between two successive samples with a given threshold value. When a change in target position is found, the same subroutine for seeking the corresponding evoked saccadic response as that used in SACCAD 1 system is started.

When the analysis of the selected record has been completed, the latency, amplitude, duration, peak velocity and coefficient of symmetry of each examined saccade are presented on the display. The operator then decides whether to accept these results or to repeat the analysis after a reassignment of the parameters of the analysis. If the results are accepted they are printed and punched.

CONCLUSIONS

Two systems for off-line computer analysis of saccadic eye movements have been presented. The SACCAD 1 system is characterized by a high level of interactivity, whereas the SACCAD 2 system performs saccade analysis in a completely automatic way. Only some preliminary operations and the processing of the calibration signals require man-machine interaction.

The SACCAD 2 system is faster and easier to be used than the SACCAD 1 system, but it could be less acurate in the computation of single saccade characteristics. As a matter of fact, the SACCAD 1 system gives the operator the possibility of controlling the analysis of each saccade and to repeat this analysis whether necessary. In the SACCAD 2 system, such a control can be done only on the complete set of saccades present in the examined record. Thus, the program SACCAD 2 is preferred when a large number of saccades has to be processed, and the average values of saccade parameters rather than the characteristics of single saccades must be examined.

A peculiar feature of the routines used in SACCAD 2 system for seeking saccades and for computing their parameters is that they are fast enough to run on-line on a microprocessor system. Since smoothing is made on 7 input samples and differentiation is made on 5 or 7 smoothed samples, by means of two buffers of 7 positions the analysis can be made on-line with a delay of less than 30 msec with respect to real time. Moreover, a small amount of memory is needed to store the coordinates of the beginning and the end of saccades and the value of their peak velocity. All saccade parameters can then be computed from these stored data. The next step in our program will be that of implementing a system derived from SACCAD 2 on a microprocessor.

ACKNOWLEDGMENT

This work was supported by CNR, Roma, Italy.

Automatic Evaluation of Eye or Head Movements for Visual Information Selection

I.3

W. Schumacher and A. Korn
Fraunhofer-Institut fur Informations- und Datenverarbeitund
Federal Republic of Germany

One means of increasing the efficiency of military combat reconnaissance is the use of remotely piloted vehicles (RPV) equipped with electro-optical sensors, whose image data are signaled to a ground station. The TV operator then must interpret the transmitted data on-line. Viewing time is physically determined by the flight parameters and the optical parameters of the sensor (Mutschler, 1979). Because the on-line evaluation places high demands on the TV operator, it is felt that knowledge of the strategies used in target acquisition may give some clues for improvements of data presentation.

The limited capability of the human visual system allows only a small fraction of the optical information to be processed in any individual glimpse, especially if the recognition of small detail is necessary for target acquisition. Therefore, it is possible to transmit a small picture corresponding to the area around the observer's fixation point to reduce the bandwith of the data transmission without loss of relevant information (Erickson, 1964.)

There have been several works on the determination of the search strategies (e.g. Megaw & Richardson, 1979; Krendel & Wodinsky, 1960; Farrel & Anderson, 1975) and on the determination of the size of field of view for a single fixation (e.g. Engel, 1971, 1977; Saida & Ikeda, 1979). This area around the fixation point from which usable information can be extracted depends on the task, the kind of target and background objects, and the picture quality. It is referred to as the conspicuity area, and is described as the retinal field in which targets can be detected in a given background during brief presentation (Engel, 1971).

The aim of the described experiment is to determine the size of conspicuity areas and the search strategies when subjects are searching for a vehicle in a natural scene. A special apparatus for an automatic evaluation of eye movements measured by corneal reflection was employed. The main emphasis of this chapter is on the methodical aspects of the measurement of eye movements and on experiments with a variable field of view. The problem investigated is how much of the field of view is needed at each fixation pause to get similar detection performance as in the case of a non-restricted visual field.

For the investigation of the search strategies, the NAC Eye-mark-recorder was employed. This recorder is suitable for mobile use. We have developed a fully automatic evaluation process reducing data reduction time.

Method.   The following sections describe the device and some of the evaluation methods. The manual evaluation of the records of the NAC Eye-Mark-System is very time consuming. In semi-automatic evaluation methods, the storage of the results is by digital computer, but it is necessary to enter the coordinates of each fixation point manually. In the following section we present a device for analyzing a video signal and the generation of different patterns for the fully automatic evaluation of the NAC Eye-Mark-Recorder and for running experiments dealing with the useful visual field of view. Furthermore a Sensorsystem for "Automation and Measurement" is presented, which can be applied for the simultaneous measurement of the eye and head movements.

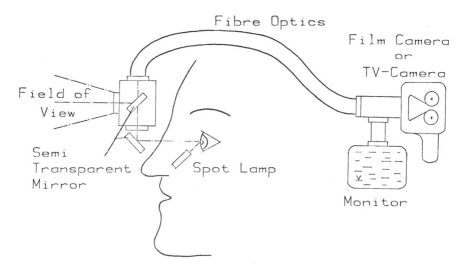

FIG. 1.   Operation Analysis of NAC Eye-Mark-Recorder.

DESCRIPTION OF THE NAC EYE-MARK-RECORDER

The unit (Fig. 1) is fitted with two optical channels having separate image-forming systems. Channel 1 transmits the optical information of the observer's visual field. Channel 2 transmits the corneal reflection, that is the virtual, reflected image of a spot lamp. The position of the corneal reflection is changed by fixation movement (e.g. saccades) of the eye. The output of both channels is mixed. After an appropriate adjustment, the position of the marking arrow will, ideally, coincide with the position of the fixation point of the eye. The composite image is transmitted via fiber optics to a film or TV camera.

REVIEW OF SOME SEMI-AUTOMATIC METHODS OF THE REGISTRATIONS WITH THE NAC EYE-MARK-RECORDER

The manual evaluation of the recorded eye movements is very time consuming and is feasible only for small data sets. In a semi-automatic process, the visual field to be checked is divided into separate fields, each field being represented by a key. By each touch of the keys, voltages are applied to the digital computer. The image showing the eye movements is displayed on a TV monitor by a video recorder, which is operated in slow motion. The TV monitor is subdivided in several fields. When the corneal reflection appears in one of the fields, the corresponding key is actuated. The different positions of the touched keys and the time course are stored in a computer for further processing steps (Schick & Radke, 1981).

Brigham (1979) recorded eye movements on film that were subsequently projected on a digitizer tableau. The evaluation is performed by feeding the position of the corneal reflection into a computer with the aid of the pen of the digitizer tableau.

METHOD OF FULLY AUTOMATIC EVALUATION OF THE EYE AND/OR HEAD MOVEMENTS

The semi-automatic methods of evaluating the eye movements—as described before—facilitate evaluation work in that the storage of the results and the time course are taken over by a digital computer. It is, however, still necessary to feed in the coordinates of the eye movements manually via push button keys, by a potentiometer, or a pen.

Measurement of Eye of Head Movements. In the fully automatic evaluation of the eye movements, the marking arrow of the Eye-Mark-

Recorder is registered by a commercial TV camera. The output of the TV camera is fed into an electronic device where the x–y coordinates of the corneal reflection are extracted out of the video signal if the contrast of the corresponding light spot is sufficiently high. In other words, the light spot that corresponds to the corneal reflection must have a higher intensity than any other point in the displayed image. The electronic device also contains a function generator that generates a square of adjustable size, the corneal reflection being the center of the square.

The scheme of the electronic device, which is called Video-Analyzer (Sung, 1980), is shown in Fig. 2. Inputs from a TV camera, a videorecorder, a lightpen, a joystick, and a computer are established. Outputs for different purposes are established, namely oscilloscope, monitor, plotter, and computer. It is possible to carry along windows of different sizes in order to carry out experiments about the useful visual field of view (Fig. 3). The region inside or outside the window can be cut out according to the experimental conditions. A division of the TV pictures into grid panels of different sizes is also possible. Luminosity can be adjusted, and a contrast reversal of black-on-white, or white-on-black can be achieved.

For the calibration of this equipment the coordinates of the fixation points were subjected to a transformation:

$$x_/ = (x - x_M)\, A,$$

$$y_/ = (y - y_M)\, B$$

with x, y the measured coordinates of the eye position, and $x_/$, $y_/$ is the fixation point in an equally spaced grid. The coordinates x_M, y_M give the measured eye position when the eye fixates the center of the monitor. A and B are constants for the adjustment.

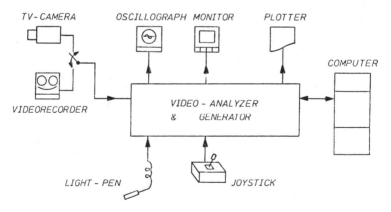

FIG. 2.   Device for analyzing a video signal and the generation of different patterns.

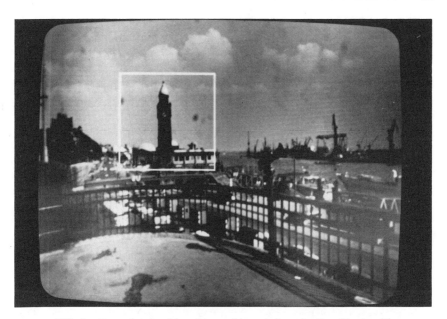

FIG. 3. Example of a video picture with a window of adjustable size. The region inside or outside the window can be cut out according to the experimental conditions.

The scheme of the experimental arrangement for measurement of head movements is shown in Fig. 4. A light source emitting a parallel light beam is closely connected with a flexible ring around the subjects head. The beam is projected on a diffusing screen. The position of the corresponding light spot is measured by a TV camera and fed into the Video-Analyzer. The amplitudes of the x-, y-signals, i.e., the output of the Video-Analyzer, are proportional to the rotation angles of the head around a vertical and a horizontal axis for the small visual angles under consideration.

MEASUREMENT OF EYE AND HEAD MOVEMENT

A more complex system than the Video-Analyzer is the "Sensorsystem for Automation and Measurement" (S.A.M.) described by Geibelmann and Tropf (1982). S.A.M. consists of a number of hardware and software modules that perform an extremely fast analysis of binary images. In general, the S.A.M.-configuration can be applied to visual inspection, optical measurements, and workpiece recognition. The S.A.M. can be applied to simultaneous measurement of eye and head movements in order to obtain the eye position relative to the background automatically. For this purpose

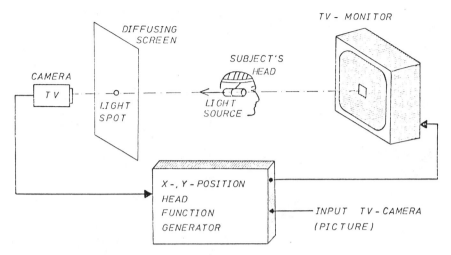

FIG.4.   Schematic view of the apparatus to restrict visual field size and to change the position by head movements.

some marks with different forms may be fixed in the background. The S.A.M.-system is able to compute the coordinates of the corneal reflection relative to the features of the background and the simultaneous measurement of eye and head movements is undergoing tests.

Apparatus.   The experiments were carried out with the Video-Analyzer, in order to investigate the visual search strategies and the useful visual field of view of the TV operator in reconnaissance mission tasks.

The complete experimental apparatus is given by Fig. 4 and Fig. 5.

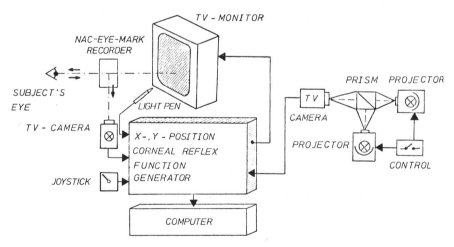

FIG. 5.   Schematic view of the experimental arrangement.

The slides were either scenes or a neutral pause picture. They were scanned by a TV camera and presented on a standard 625–line TV monitor with 30 cm screen size. The position of the detected targets was signaled with the aid of a light pen using a TV camera for the registration of eye movements. The coordinates of the eye position were picked up by the Video-Analyzer, fed into a computer and stored there together with the target position. In the experiments related to the determination of the useful visual field of view, the picture on the TV monitor appeared to the subject only within a small square whose position coincided exactly with his visual axis when eye movements are used to change the position of the window.

Static scenes were taken as slides from a 1:87 terrain model with four summer sceneries, i.e. forest, meadow, field, village. A scene consisted of one of these sceneries and covered a ground area of 130 × 130 m^2 at a simulated altitude of 300 meters with vertical aspect angle. The slides were taken from diffusely illuminated scenes. The targets were military vehicles of 4 types: 2 different types of tanks and 2 different types of trucks.

The subjects were 10 untrained male school boys and college students, and 6 military observers.

Results

To analyze the eye movement behavior, the scanpath has been recorded for each subject, each picture, and each visual field size. In Fig. 6 the record of

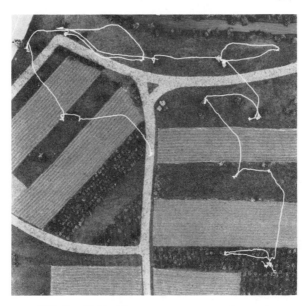

FIG. 6.   Field with eye movement traces (see text).

eye movements with a $x-$, $y-$ plotter is superposed on the picture of a field. Here the visual field size of $18° \times 24°$ was not restricted. The starting point for all presentations was the center of the picture. The target in Fig. 6 is a tank in the lower right corner, which has been detected after 6 sec. The reason for this rather long detection time is the low contrast and the position in the picture periphery. The search pattern clearly indicates that visual conspicuities like trees and bushes are mainly the goal of saccadic movements.

In addition to the analysis of the scanpath, a statistical evaluation of eye movement patterns has been performed, namely:

— mean duration of fixations in a selected field,
— frequency distribution of fixations as a function of the picture co-ordinates,
— distribution of fixation duration as a function of picture coordinates,
— transition probability from one point to another point in the image,
— frequency distribution of the fixation amplitudes,
— time course of fixation amplitude.

In Fig. 7a an example of the scanpath of eye movements is recorded for a village scene. The scene is subdivided into a 5×5 grid. The numbers at the scanpath indicate the search time in sec. The targets are in the field elements (3,5) and (3,2). Fig. 7b shows the 2-dimensional frequency distribution of fixations. Forty percent of the field elements are scanned by the subject.

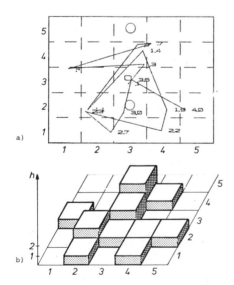

FIG. 7. Example of a scanpath of eye movement (7a) and the 2-dimensional frequency distribution of fixations (7b).

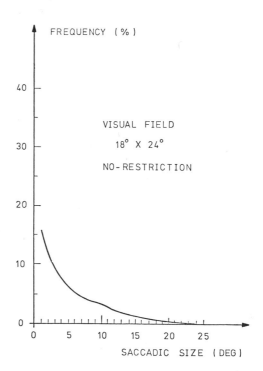

FIG. 8. Distribution of the relative frequency of saccading eye movement sizes.

The frequency distribution of the saccadic sizes for a non-restricted visual field size is shown in Fig. 8. Twenty percent of all saccadic sizes are larger than 10°. The median is about 5°. Such distributions yield a very crude estimation of the size of conspicuity areas. This is in agreement with the result of Bahill, Adler, and Stark (1975).

It is interesting to note that observers who are trained and skilled in air-to-ground reconnaissance tasks have an average saccadic amplitude that is significantly lower compared to less experienced subjects. The difference of the medians amounts to 1°. Differences were also revealed in the saccadic amplitude from the last fixation before detection. For the last saccade before target fixation, the amplitudes range 6° to 10° (Fig. 9).

Figure 10 shows two examples of eye movement records for two different visual field sizes. Here a tank must be detected in an open field. For a 2.25° × 3° visual field size in Fig. 10a, the detection time was 100 sec. For a 4.5° × 6° visual field size, the same scenery, and the same subject, the detection time was 16 sec. The corresponding scanpath is shown in Fig. 10b. Since peripheral information has been reduced, the subject must choose a systematic scanpath. Otherwise the orientation in the scene is very hard.

A systematic search can be performed easier by head or hand movements.

Fixation amplitude (degrees)

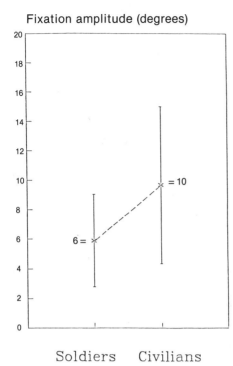

FIG. 9. Average saccadic sizes from the last fixation before detection of trained observers (soldiers) and less experienced subjects (civilians).

Soldiers   Civilians

Figure 10c shows an example for the shift of the visual field by head movements. Here a systematic path for the 3° visual field size is perceptible. Nevertheless, the subject couldn't find the target in 120 sec, i.e., a tank in a village. In 10d, head movements are shown for a non-restricted search in the same scene. The detection time was 28 sec. This record shows very clearly that head movements can be very large during a search in natural scenes in spite of the relatively small display size of 24° visual angle. Figure 11 shows the detection time as a function of the visual field size for different modes of control. The large variability of the detection time can be explained by the very different types of sceneries and differences between the detection performance of the subjects. Detection time decreases with increasing visual field size. The average detection times for the 3° visual field size and non-restricted search differ by a factor of about ten. No significant dependency upon the mode of control could be found. In other words, if a visual search is performed with a restricted visual field that can be shifted by eye, head, or hand movements, the mechanism of motor control doesn't play a significant role for the detection performance (Korn, 1981).

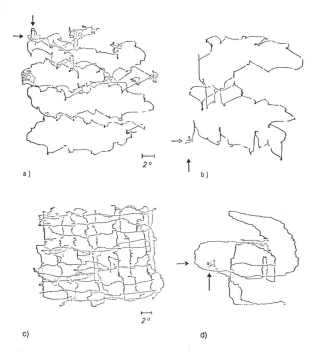

FIG. 10.   Scanpath of eye movements recorded for (a) 3° visual field size, (b) 6° visual field size. Records of head movements recorded for (c) 3° visual field size, (d) 6° visual field size.

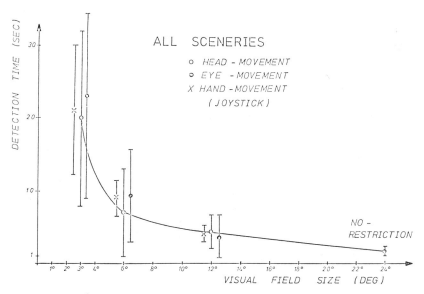

FIG. 11.   Detection time as a function of the visual field size for different modes of control.

CONCLUSION

The application of the Video-Analyzer for the fully automatic evaluation of eye movements registered by the NAC Eye-Mark-Recorder indicates that the main drawback, namely the complicated and time consuming evaluation can be largely eliminated. For the method to be effective it is necessary that the contrast of the corneal reflection be sufficiently high.

The experiments with the registration of the eye movements by the NAC Eye-Mark-Recorder were carried out with a fixed head. For a natural search process, the head should be movable and therefore eye *and* head movement must be registered, in order to obtain more suitable material for models of the search strategy.

ACKNOWLEDGMENT

This research was supported by the German Federal Ministry of Defense. The authors want to thank Mrs. Waltraud Nowatzke-Quast and Mrs. Renate Grob for the careful conduction of the experiments.

I.4 Problems of On-line Processing of EOG-Data in Reading

Dieter Heller
Universität Bayreuth
German Federal Republic

INTRODUCTION

Eye movement monitoring is partly physics not only with regard to its techniques but also with regard to its self awareness. Considering this, the high variance of data occurring in eye movement investigations is astonishing. Apparently an important element of basic psychological research in this field is insufficiently considered: the calibration of measuring instruments with regard to the experimental question. In psychological experiments this includes not only the apparatus but also the experimental set-up as a whole. The use of such a procedure is to learn more about the sources of data variance, which are extremely heterogeneous especially in eye movement research in reading. One source certainly is the oculomotoric process as such. But from a methodological point of view, the real problematic variance results from apparatus, procedures, identification programs, or from insufficiently trained or instructed subjects (the variance resulting from a reader's reading intention, from the way in which a text is read, or from reading skill is higher than even the worst apparatus can produce).

Precautions actually taken to handle this problem are as well heterogeneous and consist mainly in: (1), formulating very restricted hypothetical models and looking at their proof as a result; (2), enlarging the number of subjects; (3), doing macro-analysis of reading behavior; and (4), revising the model of the retina.

The latter certainly is necessary in so far as the physiological and anatomical structure of the retina is not necessarily of psychological relevance—otherwise there would be no need of Fechner's law. Some considerations and results on this matter already have been discussed (Heller, 1982). There are data indicating that under certain conditions the area of highest acuity is less nearly than 1½ degrees of visual angle on the fovea, for example, when following return sweeps from one line to the next, small corrective saccades of 30'–60' are observed, or when dyslectic children need up to 20 saccades to identify (read ?) a single short word. Other facts, however, emphasized by Findlay (1981a), point toward a larger area of special clarity of perception within the retina from which information can be drawn. This fits with our results because in bisection experiments of lines we have found that lines up to about 7° of visual angle (= 6 cm) could be bisected in a single gaze; that is, without any noticeable saccade to the end of the lines (Heller, Moos, & Stahl, 1980).

The real problem concerning the fovea seems to be finding a psychological measure that conforms to the physical measure of fovea diameter (as an ordinate in a psychophysical experiment); this could be, for example, the measured difficulty of a visual identification task. Certainly such experiments would lead to a reduction of variance and this should be the proper beginning of psychological research in this field.

From what I have said earlier it follows that from covariation of insufficiently calibrated experimental devices with the described different other sources of variance either no knowledge or much knowledge can be obtained. Therefore, one should first attempt to come to uniform, or at least comparable, experimental procedures and calibration studies. The following calibration of an electro-oculographical experimental set-up for registration of eye movement in reading (including the question of sampling rate and identification program) should be understood as an attempt to contribute to the resolution of this problem.

The Registration System. The hardware configuration consists of modified amplifiers from ZAK–Instruments and a Kontron microcomputer (Z 80 A processor, 4 MHz clock rate, Altos Platine, 64 K dyn. RAM, CP/M operating system) with two 8–inch floppy disks. With this system, input voltages of ± IV can be digitalized up to 500 values per sec into integers between − 128 and 127. The values were first held in the RAM–memory because the floppy-disk is not quick enough to store the values immediately. For this purpose there is about 30K bits of RAM memory. On this account the time for a single reading trial is limited depending on the sampling rate (5 min for a sampling rate of 100/s). Usually there are no problems with this restriction because the text that we can present in a single reading trial is never longer than about 150 words. During the replacement of the text the data of the eye-movement function were stored from the RAM–memory on the floppy-disk.

Our usual experimental set-up with a reading distance of 31 cm and a length of the lines between 10 cm and 15 cm causes maximal angles of rotation of the eye from 18.48° to 27.72°. The registration system therefore has a theoretical precision for eye-movement measurement for a 10 cm line of $\frac{18.48°}{256} = .07219°$ and for a 15cm line of $\frac{27.72°}{256} = .1083°$. In other words, even when only half of the measuring range of the amplifiers is used, the theoretical precision of the registration is between a fifth and a seventh of a degree.

The texts were attached to the subject's head with a balsa wood framework. The weight of this framework is 85 grams; i.e., it is lighter than a usual pair of spectacles (Heller, 1976).

DATA AND SOURCES OF ITS VARIATION

The registration system yields in the most extreme case the differences shown in Fig. 1. The real difference in the quality of registration could be seen only on the plotted part where each digitalized value has its own dot. Besides electrical noise, the source of this variation could be such bioelectrical events as, for example, muscle activity, skin conductance changes, and cortical activity (which interfere with EOG because voltage changes are scalar quantities), as well as microsaccades and tremors of the eye. (According to Ditchburn, 1973, the amplitude of the tremor is between 20″ and 40″ with a frequency of 80–150 Hz; drifts and microsaccades range between 3′ and 6′—in 50% of the cases.)

Observations repeatedly made under different experimental conditions convinced us that bioelectrical influences as well as micromovements of the eyes depend very much on subjects' actual and habitual activation level, and that applies also to eyelid blink-rate. To reduce subjects' uncertainty and degree of tension, we always conducted a buffer-experiment on a previous day that was in all details identical with the main experiment excluding the reading texts.

THE FIXATION AND SACCADE IDENTIFICATION PROGRAM

Looking at the data more closely, however, the computerized identification of the eye-movement parameters is a stratified problem. With a first on-line registration-system (consisting of a modified Lafayette datagraph and a Nova 1210 computer, Heller, 1976; Algayer & Heller, 1978), the data reduction was done on the basis of numerical differentiation of the graph of the

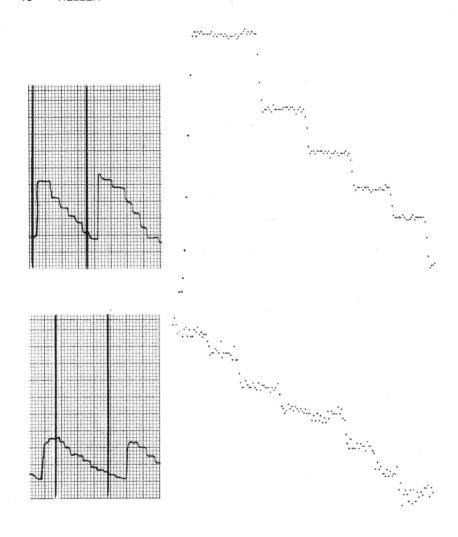

eye-movement function to determine the relative extrema. A similar method to the one we used was recently described by Oster & Stern (1980). Their program calculates the absolute difference in amplitude for four consecutive 10 msec samples and stores these values with their associated signs. If two of these three values are greater than ¼ of the saccade amplitude criterion and have the same sign (the third value could be zero or must have the same sign), the saccade initiation is identified. Our own experience with this actually fashionable method shows that it is susceptible to any kind of noise resulting from electrical events as well as from micromovements of the eyes. Moreover, this identification program is inflexible to alternations in the sampling rate.

For this reason we have developed another identification routine that guards more against noise and is primarily directed toward the fixations. The two criteria with which the program works are a chosen suppression rate for differences in amplitude between two consecutive values and a minimal fixation duration:

First phase: Starting from the first value, each consecutive value is inspected if it is the same or differs no more than a definite percentage from the previous value. As long as the consecutive values differ no more than the choiced percentage they get the same worth as the first value. In this way one reaches a number of intervals with identical values.

In the second phase, the mean is calculated from the original values of each interval (fixations).

In the third phase, the suppression of differences, as in the first phase, is repeated because the calculation of the means from the original values could produce a reduction of the initial suppression percentage.

In the final phase, the shortest intervals were interpreted into saccade duration. This fixation and saccade indentification program has two critical points: the choice for the suppression rate and for the shortest intervals which were added to the saccades as their duration.

Our first experiments should give empirical support to the decision about these values.

CALIBRATION STUDY

In the following calibration study we are working with different sampling rates (from 50/sec to 500/sec), with different suppression rates (1%, 2%, and 3%) and finally with a longer and a shorter fixation duration. The question is how the eye-movement parameters change under the different conditions. The subject has to shift his gaze between points as shown in Fig. 2. The fixation duration was given with a metronome.

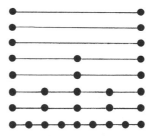

FIG. 2. Calibration points for eye-movement recording originally marked with greek and latin letters, with figures and other signs. The maximal distance between the dots range from 10 to 15 cm.

The Identification of Fixations and Saccades

The minimal duration of fixation in reading, for instance, Salthouse & Ellis (1980) have found is about 190 msec, but they also had some subjects with a mean fixation duration of 150 msec. Including our own results regarding the latency of corrective saccades (Heller, 1982; Fröschl, Heller, & Müller, 1980), which we found to be between 120 and 140 msec with a standard deviation of 20 msec, it is plausible to begin with a minimal fixation duration of 80 msec.

Table 1 gives a survey of the shortest intervals that were found by the program under the condition of different suppression and sampling rates, (up to 250/sec, whereby each sampling rate represents its own experimental trial).

It can be seen that with this time criterion, saccades and fixations easily can be divided. From a sampling rate of 100/sec there are in all trials only two values between 60 msec and 80 msec. From a suppression rate of 2%, correspondence between the program identified and the visually identified saccades and fixations is complete. (Nevertheless, a visual control of each identification trial is advisable in any case.)

TABLE 1

The Number of the Shortest intervals which were found
under Different Conditions of Suppression rates and Sampling Rates

50 *value/sec*				100 *value/sec*				150 *value/sec*				200 *value/sec*				250 *value/sec*			
suppression rate msec	1%	2%	3%	msec	1%	2%	3%	msec	1%	2%	3%	msec	1%	2%	3%	msec	1%	2%	3%
																4	345	237	170
												5	325	225	180	8	46	52	66
								6.6	260	190	150	10	30	51	32	12	10	14	9
				10	183	137	107	13.3	14	29	36	15	7	12	18	16	5	0	1
20	99	74	66	20	22	14	11	20	3	3	3	20	0	0	1	20	2	0	1
																24	1	0	0
												25	0	0	0	28	3	1	0
								26.6	1	2	0	30	1	0	1	32	2	0	0
				30	2	7	9	33.3	2	0	1	35	2	1	0	36	0	1	0
40	6	4	1	40	1	1	2	40	1	1	0	40	0	0	0	40	1	1	1
																44	0	0	0
												45	0	0	0	48	1	0	0
								46.6	1	0	1	50	0	0	0	52	0	1	0
				50	2	2	0	53.3	0	0	0	55	0	0	0	56	0	0	0
60	0	3	2	60	0	1	1	60	0	0	0	60	0	0	0	60	0	0	0
																64	0	0	0
												65	0	0	0	68	0	1	0
								66.6	1	0	0	70	0	0	0	72	0	0	0
				70	0	0	0	73.3	0	0	0	75	0	0	0	76	0	0	0
80	0	0	0	80	0	0	0	80	0	0	0	80	0	0	0	80	0	0	0

TABLE 2
The Effect of the Suppression Rates upon the Measured Size of
Saccades in Two Experimental Trials with a Shorter and a Longer
Fixation Duration (sampling rate 50/s)

suppression rate		1%	2%	3%
longer	1/1 reg.	172.3 = 27.9°	172.1 = 27.9°	171.6 = 27.9°
	1/1 prog.	167.3 = 27.1°	166.7 = 27.0°	165.7 = 27.0°
fix.	1/2 prog.	86.3 = 14.0°	86.3 = 14.0°	86.0 = 14.0°
	1/4 prog.	43.0 = 7.0°	43.0 = 7.0°	43.0 = 7.0°
dura-				
tion	1/1 prog./reg.	171.2 = 27.7°	171.0 = 27.7°	170.4 = 27.7°
shorter	1/1 reg.	167.7 = 27.9°	167.9 = 27.9°	167.7 = 27.9°
	1/1 prog.	161.3 = 26.9°	161.7 = 26.9°	161.3 = 26.9°
fix.	1/2 prog.	84.8 = 14.1°	84.8 = 14.1°	84.8 = 14.1°
	1/4 prog.	42.0 = 7.0°	42.0 = 7.0°	42.0 = 7.0°
dura-				
tion	1/1 prog./reg.	166.6 = 27.7°	166.8 = 27.7°	166.6 = 27.7°

On the Relation Between Saccade Size and Suppression Rate

In this connection the variation of saccade size depending on the suppression rate is observed. Again there are three suppression rates (1%, 2%, 3%) and a longer and a shorter fixation duration given to the subject in two different experimental trials with 138 beats per min and 88 beats per min from a metronome. (The observed fixation duration is $\overline{X}$ = 435 ms s = 63 ms and $\overline{X}$ = 685 ms s = 126 ms.)

The upper part of Table 2 shows the trial with the longer fixation duration. The absolute differences of the raw scores in the upper and the lower part of the table indicate only that there were two trials in which the amplification was not identical. Although this example from a sampling rate of 50/s is the worst case, all observed variations are below the degree of resolution that is in this case about .16°. This signifies that the identified saccade size does not depend on the suppression rate nor on the sampling rate (between 50/s and 250/s).

The Variation of the Fixation Duration Depending on the Suppression and the Sampling Rate

The sampling rate in this experiment is 500, 250, 166, 125, 100, and 50/s. This is realized with different recording channels, each of them with a different sampling rate, so that each measurement is comparable with the others. The fixation duration is given the subject with a metronome, in this experiment 144 beats per min (that is an interval of about 400 ms between each beat).

Table 3 shows the effect of the different suppression and sampling rates on the fixation duration. The upper part of Table 3 shows the fixation durations which were identified only by the identification program. The lower part represents the manually identified fixation durations.

The main effect is that with an increasing suppression rate the fixation duration also increases. There are two reasons for this: (1) With a low suppression rate, it is possible that a drifting fixation will be divided by the program into two fixations (which is to be corrected manually); (2) With an increasing suppression rate, a little part of the beginning of the saccade is added to the fixation. But because of the sinusoidal course of saccades in time (that is, that the velocity of the saccade rises smoothly, reaches a maximum, and then falls smoothly to zero), a problem exists in determining the end of a fixation in each identification modality.

Much more surprising is another observation that can be made as regards the measurement error for fixation duration depending on the sampling

TABLE 3

Means and Standard Deviations of Fixation Durations Depending on Different Sampling Rates and Suppression Rates (2 – 5 values = 1% – 3%). The Lower Part is Visually Identified.

			50	100	125	166	250	500	$\bar{x}$
	sampling rate								
suppression rate	2 value 1%	$\bar{x}$	317.0	371.9	364.1	377.6	374.4	362.3	361.2
		s	63.6	73.4	84.8	74.0	60.9	87.0	
	3 value 2%	$\bar{x}$	392.9	391.0	390.7	391.5	391.4	390.6	391.3
		s	49.1	50.3	51.7	51.5	50.0	49.5	
	5 value 3%	$\bar{x}$	401.3	399.7	397.9	396.4	397.7	398.5	398.6
		s	52.0	52.6	51.8	50.5	49.6	49.0	
	sampling rate		50	100	125	166	250	500	$\bar{x}$
suppression rate	2 value 1%	$\bar{x}$	380.8	376.4	389.8	379.7	380.2	376.4	380.5
		s	52.8	52.1	54.7	48.9	52.7	52.9	
	3 value 2%	$\bar{x}$	386.2	385.5	392.4	384.0	386.7	381.2	386.0
		s	47.3	52.5	55.0	50.2	53.2	51.9	
	5 value 3%	$\bar{x}$	389.4	393.2	400.7	388.3	392.8	389.4	392.3
		s	50.9	54.7	54.5	50.3	52.5	52.2	

rate. Following Oster & Stern (1980) the measurement error depends directly on the sampling rate, i.e., 20 ms for 50/s and 2 ms for 500/s.

With good reasons it could also be assumed that finding a fixation with one value each 20 ms causes an error of 20 ms at the beginning and at the end of a fixation, and therefore the measurement error for a sampling rate of 50/s might be 40 ms.

In fact, however, if one looks at the third or fourth row of the upper part of Table 3, one sees that there is nearly no variation of the main fixation duration nor the standard deviation depending on the sampling rate. That is, in the range betwen 50/s and 500/s, there is no difference in the measurement error of fixation duration depending on the sampling rate.

The Accuracy of Localization with EOG-Registration

Certainly the EOG is not what Groner (Groner, Kaufman, Bischof, & Hirsbrunner, 1974) calls "lokalisationstreu" (localization-true). One always needs an assumption about the starting point of the eye movement. But in reading this could reasonably be the beginning of the line. If such a point exists the accuracy is assumed to be between 1.5 ° (Shackel, 1967) and 1 ° (Oster & Stern, 1980).

From the first experiments with different trials for each sampling rate it is possible to compare the distances between the points with the measured saccade size. Table 4 shows these values, the confidence intervals, and the coefficient of variation.

Table 4 shows that we can reassure a previous finding (Heller, 1982): The relative precision of the saccades increase with their size, as the coefficient of variation demonstrates.

This is true even though one takes into consideration that the theoretical measurement error of about .15 ° in this recording is of a heavier weight for the smaller saccades. Accounting for this, we have calculated a theoretical coefficient of variation and subtracted it from the observed (last row of Table 4). Nevertheless the result is the same.

But back again to the question of the accuracy of the EOG: The maximum difference in Table 4 between the measured saccade size and the real distance of the points is .16 °. The observed variation can serve as an estimation of the measurement error, it ranges between .98 ° and .32 °. Following this the accuracy in the horizontal plane seems to be higher than it is assumed for example by Oster & Stern (1980). But the main problem of measurement error in EOG probably is that it increases with each consecutive fixation point. This demands a stochastical model that predicts the addition of partial measurement errors to a total measurement error.

As a first approximation of the measurement error, it could be assumed

TABLE 4
Means and Standard Deviation of the Saccade Size for Different
Distances, the Coefficients of Variation and the Confidence intervals

real distance	27.72°	13.86°	6.93°	3.44°
n	100	40	80	80
observed saccade size $\bar{x}$	27.62°	14.02°	7.02°	3.47°
confidence interval				
upper bound	27.35°	13.77°	7.15°	3.56°
$\alpha = .01$ lower bound	27.89°	14.27°	6.89°	3.38°
s	.98°	.58°	.41°	.35°
confidence interval				
upper bound	1.20°	.81°	.51°	.40°
$\alpha = .01$ lower bound	.83°	.45°	.34°	.27°
observed variation coefficient	3.55%	4.14%	5.84%	9.17%
theor. variation coefficient for an error of .15° (assumption of uniform distribution)	.31%	.63%	1.25%	2.52%
corr. variation coefficient	3.24%	3.51%	4.59%	6.65%

that all errors are independent and normally distributed with expected value
$\mu = 0$ and a standard deviation σ_i (as for example Groner, 1974, p. XVI).
From this it follows, according to a well known proposition of probability
theory that the total measurement error (me_t) per line which is read with n
equidistant saccades will be $me_t = \sqrt{n}\, \sigma_i$. The resulting values are shown in
Table 5.

The differences between the observed standard deviation of the largest
saccade and the value of row 3, Table 5 (max. .16°) are not big
enough—considering the confidence intervals from Table 4 to reject the
assumed model. But further experiments should be done to determine the
functional relation between saccade size and related standard deviation.

TABLE 5
Measurement error for n equidistant saccades

real distance	27.72°	13.86°	6.93°	3.44°
n	1	2	4	8
observed s	.98°	.58°	.41°	.32°
$\sqrt{n}\sigma_i$		.82°	.82°	.91°

I.5 Looking at Looking: The Amorphous Fixation Measure

Robert Karsh and Francis W. Breitenbach
U.S. Army Human Engineering Laboratory
Aberdeen Proving Ground, Maryland

In the study of cognitive and perceptual processes, exactly where an eye is fixating at any instant and the time history of fixations are among the most commonly used measures of eye movement behavior. Conceptually, a fixation is simply the intersaccade time during which the eye is relatively stationary. However, isolating a fixation from a stream of raw eye-movement data requires using a data partitioning scheme that can be quite complex depending on specific parameters of the instrumentation, the subject, the task the subject is performing, and the temporal and spatial thresholds used in the fixation criteria.

A large variety of eye movement recording instruments in use today (Young & Sheena, 1975) as well as many possible approaches to the partitioning of raw eye movement data, make it imperative for researchers to document in detail their specific fixation criteria so that more meaningful cross-comparisons can be made between studies using eye-movement behavior as a dependent variable.

This chapter describes an eye movement recording device presently in use and the construction of a computer algorithm which defines a fixation. Also, to underline the importance of researchers reporting their fixation criteria, examples are provided of how subtle changes in some fixation criteria may dramatically affect the processed fixation data output.

It is well known that different tasks like reading, search, or picture recognition produce different fixation patterns. However, the test environment may also affect eye-movement behavior, a fact that is often overlooked. For example, the eye movement recording device presently in use at the Human Engineering Laboratory (HEL) is a rather unique system in that the subject's head is not required to be constrained (Monty, 1975) and, more significantly, neither the device nor the experimenter are visually apparent to the subject. Further, there is no indication given to the subjects that their eyes are being monitored. Even the calibration tasks given each new subject are integrated into the same context as the test tasks. Such covert procedures produce more candid and, it is believed, more natural subject behavior than systems that constrain the subject. During a concept formation task for example, subjects frequently look away from the viewing screen while mentally processing information. Such behavior as well as eye blinks, gross head movements caused by sneezing or coughing, natural manifestations of the experimenter-task-subject interaction like laughing, and other factors like highlight loss and video noise are all accounted for in a fixation algorithm originally developed by Lambert (Lambert, Monty, & Hall, 1974) and presently being used at the HEL.

To provide a context for discussing the construction of the fixation algorithm, the HEL eye-movement recording device (oculometer) is briefly described. (A detailed description of an earlier version of this system may be found in Lambert, Monty, & Hall, 1974.) Whether it is tracking a stationary model of an eye or a moving human eye, the optical tracking system is continually relaying information to a TV camera and feeding control information to a computer processor. The processor feeds back information to servo-motors that maintain an image of the eye in the center of the field-of-view of the camera which composes a picture of the eye 60 times per second. Information from each picture is computer analyzed in real-time and displayed graphically on a CRT computer terminal. Raw data is also stored on magnetic tape for any future off-line processing.

SOME PARAMETERS OF THE RAW DATA

One video field (1/60th sec), contains a fixed image of the entire eye. In the vicinity of the pupil, a corneal reflection (highlight) of a fixed point-source of light is used as a spatial reference point. The point of regard of the eye is computed from the relative position of the center of the pupil and the highlight. The location of the point, called a "data point," is given by its vertical and horizontal distance (x and y coordinates) from the center of the subject's viewing screen.

Video recording devices are limited to a sampling rate of 60 per second, which is too slow to measure either the short voluntary eye jumps (saccades) between fixations or the more rapid involuntary eye movements that occur during a fixation. Other recording devices are more suitable for measuring eye *motion* per se (Young & Sheena, 1975), but our interest is in measuring fixation positions and their time history. As such, the sampling rate will affect the accuracy of determining exactly when a fixation begins and ends.

All video recording systems have residual noise caused by electronic jitter. This may be seen when a stationary artificial glass eye is placed in front of the instrument. The system "tracks" it and generates a stream of data points or eye position coordinates that are not mutually identical. The dispersion of such a cluster of points is essentially a normal distribution about a mean. Theoretically, if a closed boundary were drawn about the mean to include the majority of the points, the size of that area would in a sense, represent the minimum residual noise of the system and would describe its maximum resolution. This implies that any two data points that fall within that size boundary or "window of resolution" must be considered as one point whose position is given by the mean of the data points' positions. This concept of spatial resolution is used as a basic criterion in determining whether a given dispersion of collected data points is to be considered as a single population of points whose centroid may be used to define eye fixation position. The minimal size of this area of dispersion relative to the viewing screen is given by the viewing angle subtending approximately one degree.

THE FIXATION ALGORITHM

The first step in constructing the fixation is a selection procedure that determines whether each consecutive video field contains sufficient information to compute a data point. If a highlight is present there is a resultant data point (which may be either inside or outside the subject's viewing screen area) and the video field is considered usable. Some fields will contain insufficient information to compute a data point if for example, the subject blinks, thus occluding the necessary highlight. If the subject makes gross head movements or simply looks away from the viewing screen, the tracking device will momentarily lose track of the eye, requiring the operator to manually override the system to bring the image of the eye back into the camera's field-of-view. Video fields occurring during such situations are designated unusable. The number of unusable fields and their specific causes are temporarily stored in memory.

Next, a sorting procedure plots each data point on an *x-y* coordinate system (actually a memory matrix) equivalent to the viewing screen area. This procedure continues until a total of six successive data points (serially following one another, but not necessarily contained within six consecutive fields) have been plotted. One contingency may abort this procedure: If after plotting any one of the first five data points, a string of 20 consecutively occurring unusable fields is encountered, all data points plotted up to that time are removed from the plot and the fields containing them are temporarily filed with the rest of the unusable fields. The sorting procedure is then restarted. As soon as six data points have been successfully plotted, further decision making takes place.

The centroid of the cluster of points is computed first. Then, the "dispersion" (in the descriptive sense) of those points about their centroid is compared with the dispersion as given by the window of resolution. If it is less than or equal to the window (the maximum acceptable dispersion), the *onset* of a fixation is established. If the dispersion is greater than the window, an additional sorting procedure begins.

During this procedure, the point most distant from the centroid is removed from the cluster plot and its field temporarily stored in the file of unusable fields. The next occurring data point is then obtained and plotted with the remaining five points to form a new cluster of six points. This new cluster is then subjected to the same test as before, and so on, until the condition of minimal dispersion is met.

In the continuing description of the procedure it may be helpful to visualize the window of resolution as an overlay on the viewing screen. The window will always be placed so that its center coincides with the current mean position of the ongoing fixation cluster. When the *onset* of a fixation is established, data points continue to be selected, each new point's position falling either inside or outside of the window. If it falls inside, its position is added to the cluster, a new cluster mean is computed and the center of the window is repositioned over it. If the point falls outside, its field is temporarily filed away. If, during this continuing selection process, a string of 20 consecutively occurring unusable fields is encountered, the selection process is terminated, the ongoing fixation is considered ended and is output and the program returns to the initial selection procedure to establish the onset of the next fixation. Otherwise, the point-by-point selection and testing process continues until two successively occurring data points are selected whose positions *and their mean spatial position* all fall outside the window of resolution. If two successive points fall outside but their mean spatial position falls inside, the mean is simply added to the cluster, thus updating it. However, if both points and their mean fall outside the window, the point-by-point test with the ongoing cluster is temporarily suspended. Then, using this pair as the first two points, the construction of a totally new cluster of six points is begun, applying all the criteria used before to establish the onset of a fixation. When the new cluster of six points is established, its mean will fall either inside or outside of the window over the previous cluster mean. If it falls inside the window, it is said to be unresolvable from that cluster, and is therefore considered a continuation of the previous fixation. The mean of all points included in both clusters then becomes the new mean of the ongoing fixation, the window is repositioned over it and the process of selecting and testing each new point against the mean is restarted. However, if the two means were resolvable, i.e., the new mean fell outside the window over the previous cluster, then the first fixation is ended and outputted, the new cluster becoming the *onset* of a new fixation.

At this point a recordkeeping procedure deals with all unusable fields that have been temporarily filed away. All fields that occurred after the last usable field that made up a fixation and prior to the first usable field that belonged to a new fixation are labeled as lost data. (Lost data can only occur between fixations.) The fields temporarily filed as unusable but that occurred between the usable fields within a fixation are converted into a time value where each field represents the passage of 16.7 msec. The total number of fields (both usable and unusable) that make up a fixation, multiplied by 16.7 is the duration time of that fixation. The position of a fixation at any point in time is, of course, given by the mean of the most recently collected cluster of data points.

In summary then, a fixation may be operationally defined as a cluster of a minimum of six data points (or a minimum duration of 100 msec) whose deviation from their centroid cannot exceed the maximum resolution of the measuring instrument. The position of a fixation or a "point" of gaze is then an area of uncertainty about a mean position whose area boundaries are probabilistic in nature. Because the residual area of resolution of the measuring instrument is probabilistic as well, the definition of a "point" becomes in a sense, an arbitrary one.

THE CRITICALNESS OF CRITERIA

The partitioning of raw eye movement data into meaningful fixations is the first and most important step in data reduction. There are many steps within the algorithm just described where decisions may critically affect the data output in terms of fixation frequency, duration, time history, and location. Some of the steps are shown in Fig. 1.

One critical step concerns the number of data points used to establish the onset of a fixation (Note A in Fig. 1). Any quantity of points could have been required. The eye-movement literature, however, suggests that the minimal duration of a fixation is about 100 msec (see Flagg, 1977; Young & Sheena, 1975), so for the present algorithm, six data points are used. If two, four, or eight points were used instead, the total number of fixations obtained during the course of a test session would be significantly altered. Figure 2 illustrates how using different values for this criterion affect one subject's representative scan path, superimposed on a matrix of numbers that the subject had viewed. Each inflection of a path is a fixation point (as defined by the criterion). The lines connecting them merely indicate the

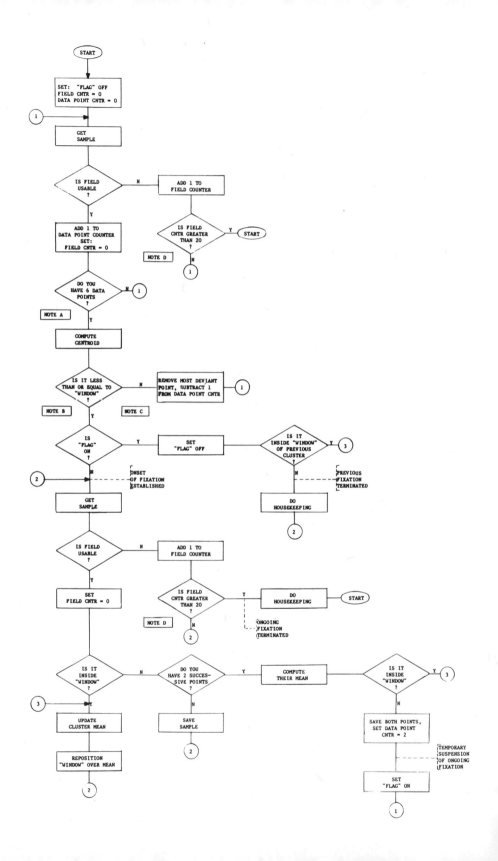

order of fixations, while the circles around each fixation represent its duration.

In this task the subject searched the matrix of numbers to find the number "54." Although *identical raw data* were used to generate each scan path, the paths appear to be quite different. Since the total viewing time remains unchanged, it may be seen that the number of fixations outputted as well as the amount of data lost varies as a direct result of how the algorithm differentially partitions the stream of data based on a simple change of the minimum allowable fixation duration.

Another critical aspect of the fixation algorithm, the spatial boundaries of the "window" (Note B in Fig. 1), significantly affects the same measures. Figure 3 shows the results of taking the *identical raw data* used in Fig. 2 (for the 6–point fixation criterion) and changing only the window size parameter. These scan paths also appear to differ from each other although perhaps not as strikingly as those shown in Fig. 2. As the window size decreases, there are fewer fixations when all other variables are held constant. Conversely, increasing the window size increases the number of fixations. This effect will continue up to some maximal window size and then reverse its course. Theoretically, as the window size approaches the limit of the viewing screen area, the number of measured fixations should approach unity. The proper window size chosen for use is primarily a function of the system resolution. However, empirical considerations related to task parameters and subject behavior also influence the decision. Once the decision is made it is not changed thus enabling such diverse eye-movement tasks as picture recognition (cf. Fisher, Karsh, Breitenbach, & Barnette, this volume) and reading (cf. Shebilske & Fisher, this volume) to be meaningfully compared.

The preceding examples illustrate the effect of separately varying only two criteria. It should be recognized that a wide variety of scan paths can be obtained by simultaneously varying any of the critical criteria used in the algorithm.

A critical step in determining the *onset* of a fixation is the method used to choose the first six data points (Note C in Fig. 1). There might be no problem if the eye behaved in an orderly manner, never wandering off its intended target or suddenly jumping away from the screen and then returning. In reality however, because of just such behavior, there is a likelihood that the first six data points collected will not fall inside the "window" boundaries. More samples must then be selected to find a cluster that meets the criterion. One procedure is to discard the earliest points in a sequence, systematically moving along the sequence until six successive points meet the criterion (an approach similar to that used by Flagg, 1977). Another approach is to continually discard the point most deviant from the mean,

FIG. 1. (*opposite page*) General flowchart of a fixation algorithm.

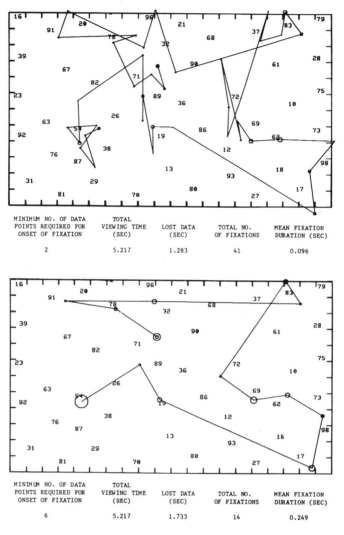

FIG. 2.   Four possible fixation scan paths obtained from *identical raw data*.
Paths are shown to vary as a function of the number of raw data points that
determine the *onset* of a fixation. All other fixation criteria are held constant.
Each inset represents the subject's viewing screen area upon which a matrix
of numbers (as shown) was projected. Inflection points on the scan path
represent points of fixation, the lines connecting them indicate their order of
occurrence and, the circle around each fixation represents its duration. This
data was generated by a subject-paced task of searching the number matrix as
quickly as possible until the number 54 was detected. Detection time was
5.217 sec. The amount of lost data, the total number of fixations measured,
the mean fixation duration and the data point condition used are listed under
each inset.

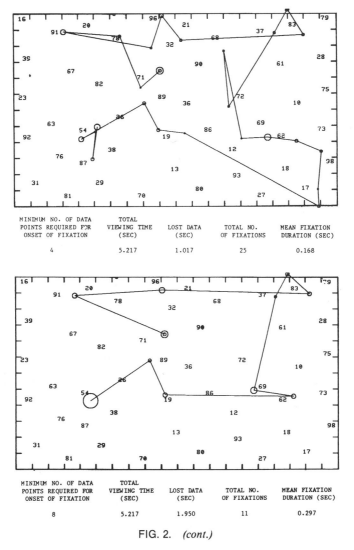

MINIMUM NO. OF DATA POINTS REQUIRED FOR ONSET OF FIXATION	TOTAL VIEWING TIME (SEC)	LOST DATA (SEC)	TOTAL NO. OF FIXATIONS	MEAN FIXATION DURATION (SEC)
4	5.217	1.017	25	0.168
8	5.217	1.950	11	0.297

FIG. 2. *(cont.)*

replacing it with the next occurring point until the criterion is satisfied (the method presently in use at this laboratory). The first approach places more importance on the serial order of data points, while the second approach stresses the amount of dispersion of the cluster, where the most deviant point represents a lower probability of being meaningfully associated with the rest of the cluster. Both approaches have their advantages and disadvantages in terms of their relative data loss (from a data partitioning point-of-view) or more seriously, in terms of their cognitive implications for eye-movement behavior (from a psychological point-of-view).

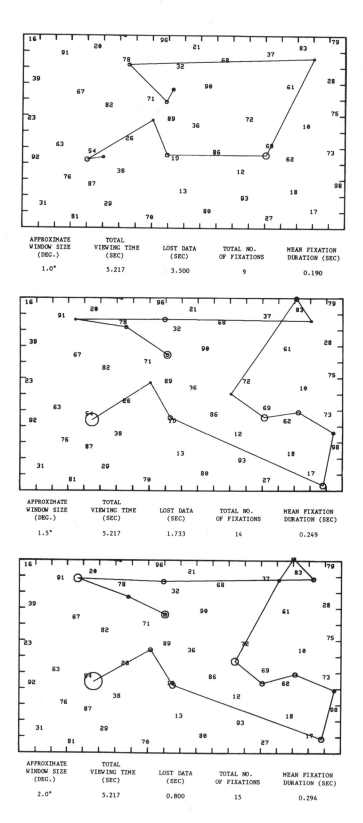

APPROXIMATE WINDOW SIZE (DEG.)	TOTAL VIEWING TIME (SEC)	LOST DATA (SEC)	TOTAL NO. OF FIXATIONS	MEAN FIXATION DURATION (SEC)
1.0°	5.217	3.500	9	0.190

APPROXIMATE WINDOW SIZE (DEG.)	TOTAL VIEWING TIME (SEC)	LOST DATA (SEC)	TOTAL NO. OF FIXATIONS	MEAN FIXATION DURATION (SEC)
1.5°	5.217	1.733	14	0.249

APPROXIMATE WINDOW SIZE (DEG.)	TOTAL VIEWING TIME (SEC)	LOST DATA (SEC)	TOTAL NO. OF FIXATIONS	MEAN FIXATION DURATION (SEC)
2.0°	5.217	0.800	15	0.294

Note D in Fig. 1 relates to a procedure designed to take care of some of the problems associated with data loss caused by specific equipment and task parameters, and also gross head movements which may occur either while the onset of a fixation is being established or during an ongoing fixation. The use of specifically 20 consecutive fields is based on the examination of raw data collected over many years and represents an ongoing experimentation with specific data handling problems in a continuing effort to improve the algorithm.

Decisions concerning a minimum allowable fixation duration (e.g., 100 msec) are not specific to a particular eye-movement recording device or system, although system sampling rates may be a partial factor. The minimum allowable variance (window size or spatial boundary) of a cluster of data points that constitute an ongoing fixation is also not necessarily system-specific. The specific measure of central tendency used, if any, depends upon such things as how a researcher wishes to tie together concepts of system resolution with observable subject behavior. Some considerations concerning different approaches to choosing which data points to include in a fixation and which not to are partially system-specific while other considerations such as procedures used to handle gross head movements may be totally specific to a particular eye-movement system or test contingency. In general, all researchers must arrive at a data partitioning scheme custom tailored to their own specific needs. However, the summary measures of fixation frequency, duration, and location generated by any particular algorithm are quite common and likely to be taken for granted, as though they were produced by some standardized measuring device. The purpose of discussing how these measures are derived using as an example one specific algorithm and, how easily they are affected by subtle criteria considerations, was to illustrate how ambiguous such measures may be if the various criteria used to construct them are left unreported.

SUMMARY

The problem of defining a fixation is one that perhaps deserves more recognition than it has had in the past. Generally speaking, the more complex the system the more complex the task of definition will be. One method of defining a fixation in a complex system was described here merely as an

---

FIG. 3. *(Opposite page)* Three possible fixation scan paths obtained from *identical raw data*. Paths are shown to vary as a function of the size of the "window of resolution." All other fixation criteria are held constant. Further information on these scan paths may be found in the caption for Fig. 2.

example to illustrate the need for more open discussion of the concepts of fixations used by many different investigators and highlight the importance of reporting exactly what approaches to data reduction were employed in any given study. Once these needs are recognized and implemented, comparisons between studies should take on considerably more meaning.

ACKNOWLEDGMENTS

The authors gratefully acknowledge the contributions and comments of the following individuals on various drafts of this manuscript: Joshua Borah, Dennis F. Fisher, Barbara N. Flagg, Robert H. Lambert, Joseph Mazurczak, Richard A. Monty, and David Sheena. A special word of thanks goes to B. Diane Barnette for rendering helpful technical assistance throughout the preparation of this paper. Portions of the research leading up to this paper were accomplished in part under US Army Research Office Contract No. DAAG29-76-C-0022 to Gulf + Western Applied Sciences Laboratory. This paper may be reproduced in full or in part for any purpose of the United States Government.

II CENTRAL AND PERIPHERAL PROCESSING

What might be considered as the fundamental characteristic of the human visual system is its centrally symmetric organization: The visual sensory system is centered around foveal reception. That part of the environmental stimulation which impinges on the foveal parts of the two retinas will be subject to highly detailed analysis, with a progressive degradation towards the periphery. This is a consequence of the fact that the visual resolution power decreases along any radius toward the periphery of the retina. This is due not only to the privileged anatomical structure of the central retina (higher cell density) but also to the further physiological elaboration that the visual message receives on its way to the visual cortex (magnification factor). The second main characteristic of the visual system is its *mobility*: By means of eye movements (combined with head and body movements), the privileged central area processing can be directed to any part of the environment. In addition, the visual receptive system operates as a distance sensor (meaning that it doesn't require physical contact like the tactile sensors, but only directional contact). Thus, this mobility gives the visual system its preeminent position among the battery of senses that connect us to our surrounding world. It is a spatially focused receptor system actively organized in sequential processing. Only a part of the available information is selected at any time for intensive processing: This might have the functional value of protecting the central processors from overload. Following this, at the next instant, a new part of the available information can be chosen and selected for further intake and processing. The way the visual system plays this role of a selective and active interface between the individual and his environment is very impressive.

For the experimental psychologist, this natural device is also remarkable. Since oculomotor activity is an overt behavior that is accessible to recording and measurement, it opens a door to the scientist interested in the organization of perceptual and cognitive processing. To the extent that eye movements are reliable correlates of the sequential centering of attention, we can observe and analyze them in order to understand how thinking goes on. The problem is that this correspondence cannot be completely assessed. More seriously: The hypothetical constructs that are supposed to correspond to the orienting movements of the eyes (mental focus, attention shift, and so on) are not well defined, but themselves result from analogies. There is a danger that this kind of approach becomes tautological, describing only observable motor events without testing their signficance in relation to any separate level of functioning.

However, we can be sure that eye movements testify to changes in successive orienting of the receptive system. *Successive fixations control successive visual inputs* that will be processed, and that are at least characterized by the spatial displacement of high resolution in central viewing and poorer resolution in peripheral viewing. On the other hand, *successive fixations depend on decisions taken on the basis of peripheral vision.* At each pause, a choice of the next position will be made, perhaps as a result of peripheral stimulation by targets that trigger an eye movement in a quasi-reflex mode, or perhaps a move will be made toward an area that has been evaluated as likely to provide further useful information. The reciprocal feedback of visual field input to motor output and of motor output to visual input is a remarkable feature of our visual apparatus. This interplay of temporal sequences involving a spatial focus is an ultimate consequence of the simple fact of receptor inhomogeneity.

Many questions can be raised concerning the functional role played by the differentiation between central and peripheral vision. Among these, a major problem is to understand how the control of eye movements is affected by information coming from peripheral vision. This problem is addressed by the studies grouped in this second part of the present volume. The two first papers concern what useful sensory information comes in from peripheral vision. The following two are more interested in the way peripheral processing governs eye movements. And the last paper in this section investigates the adaptability of the oculomotor system to unusual contingencies. In this introduction, I briefly comment upon the main ideas and new data that these pieces of research have contributed to our understanding of the general problem of the dynamic interplay between vision and eye movements.

FIRST QUESTION: WHAT CAN BE SEEN AND USED IN PERIPHERAL VISION?

Classical data exist to show how acuity decreases across the visual field from fovea to periphery. Most of the studies have measured the decrement either of detection or of discrimination capacity in static situations in which the observer maintains his sight upon a central fixation point and a stimulus is presented in the peripheral field of vision. In contrast, the interest of the present studies lies in their assessment of visual input collected during a fixation while the eyes are scanning the displayed material. H. Widdel records the spontaneous pattern of ocular scanning of scattered elements displayed over a wide area, among which one single differentiated element has to be discovered. Of special interest is the final part of the scanning pattern in which a saccade takes the gaze from some position onto the target. The data show that the target is reached from a greater distance when the density of the display is lower. This is interpreted by the author as a correlate or a measure of mental work load. It might also be the effect of lateral interference reducing the discriminability of the target in peripheral view, which might result secondarily in a trade-off between density and area, keeping constant the amount of material successfully analyzed.

This useful field of view within a dynamic scanning task, which H. Widdel calls "visual lobe area," is also investigated by W. Prinz under the name of "control area" when an observer searches for a certain target letter within rows of non-target letters. This situation is closer to reading and evidence is presented, showing a vertical asymmetry in favor of the lower part of the field where targets have a higher probability of detection at a larger distance than in the lines above the line being scanned. Several reasons can be provided for such an asymmetry. A so-called "structural" source of asymmetry could be augmented sensory sensitivity in the lower field. It seems more reasonable to consider the asymmetry of the scanning task as a powerful incentive to emphasize downward rather than upward perceptual efficiency. This is what Prinz calls the "functional source of asymmetry," opposing it to the "structural" one. He postulates that this functional asymmetry depends on attentionally controlled operations only effective in central vision. The point of interest is the possibility of obtaining a change in the capacity for target detection around each fixation point by changing subject's scanning strategy: for example, using a bottom-up sequence rather than the normal top-down sequence. The experiment shows some effects that can be attributed to the way peripheral information is used while scanning rather to its input capacity. We will encounter again later on these aspects of flexibility of intake and processing, which is a very interesting aspect of this type of research.

SECOND QUESTION: HOW DOES PERIPHERAL ANALYSIS AFFECT EYE MOVEMENTS?

What rules govern saccadic behavior in relation to the demands for visual input in order to accomplish a task efficiently?

In a scanning task which in a way is similar to that used by Prinz, Z. Kapoula examines with great precision how the eyes jump and pause across lines of scattered symbols. One of the main observations is that the mode of scanning shows an important difference dependent on whether or not peripheral information can be used to predict the identity of the next object from the previous fixation position.

If a precise aim is required over the targets, then the organization seems to be different in saccadic timing and efficiency, and fixation durations are longer. This is also in accordance with the result of J. Findlay and T. Crawford in the next paper. When aiming for a target that requires accurate fixation in order to be efficiently processed, the subject's eyes must overcome a seemingly automatic tendency to be attracted by a neighboring target. Repeated practice reduces the overshoot, although the plasticity of the system appears to be limited.

In both Kapoula's and Findlay's situations, a peripheral analysis of the available information is performed in a way that seems to depend not simply on sensory capacities but also according to a particular mode of functioning that may be adapted to the task to be performed.

THIRD QUESTION:
HOW CAN THE OCULOMOTOR
SYSTEM ADAPT TO UNUSUAL
CONTINGENCIES BETWEEN
PERIPHERAL AND CENTRAL INPUT?

In normal conditions, an ocular saccade brings into foveal vision a part of the field that has previously been seen in peripheral vision. Normally, integration occurs between foveally processed information and previous peripheral pre-processing of the information coming from the same source. If this principle is artificially suspended, the adaptability of the system may be tested by its capacity for developing new functioning rules. This is what Kaufman and Coles demand from their subjects, children or adults. They observe that such a trick as having a part of the field disappear when looked at is quite disturbing to their subjects, although they are not consciously aware of the manipulation. Some changes occur in ocular behavior, reflecting the sensitivity of the oculomotor system to the difference from its usual control mode. The kind and speed of adaptation is interesting to analyze. It appears that even such basic mechanisms as orienting response to visual stimulation can be modulated by particular contingencies.

As a conclusion to these general remarks, let us emphasize how current research concerning peripheral and central vision has changed compared with traditional tachistoscopic studies. It is not sufficient to make a direct transposition from static processing capacities in the visual field to those operative while the eyes remain on a fixation during scanning, search or reading. First, because during a fixation, foveal processing of local information occurs within the same period of time as the preparation for the next saccade (probably these processing times overlap, at least partially). Secondly because during this same fixation time, not only is foveal information processed but also peripheral. Thus there can be preprocessing of the next target and probably post-processing of previous ones. This is most evident in reading, since text understanding requires constant reconsideration of the whole set of words that make up a sentence.

This is why current studies such as those presented here are particularly interesting. They don't approach central and peripheral visual processing capacities as rigid sensory properties of separate parts of the receptor system. Instead they investigate how the whole receptor and motor systems behave in normal *dynamic* situations.

This brings us to a second basic problem addressed by these studies, which probably is the most important: What is the *plasticity* of the visual receptor device and of its relationship with the oculomotor plant? Can the limits of peripheral detection or discrimination capacities change as an effect either of training or of attentional attitudes? Experimental demonstrations of such flexible properties of the receptive system are the best demonstrations for an elaborate interplay between passive sensory mechanisms and "higher" active control sources. This interesting approach lies behind most of the current studies presented here. The role of training in peripheral viewing or in accomplishing certain unusual tasks is shown to modify the limits of peripheral detection of targets or the efficiency of latency of ocular responses. Another aspect of flexibility of the system involving a particular combination of peripheral and central processing is the role of intentionality which also seems to modulate the relationship between sensory intake and motor output.

We are only on our way towards understanding how such a complex and elaborate coordination between perceptual visual messages and motor adjustments of the eyes can work. The theories and experiments reported in this volume are a contribution to an active research effort into the models, still incomplete, of our amazingly versatile visual system.

ACKNOWLEDGMENTS

I want to thank John Findlay and Kevin O'Regan for their participation in the discussion of some of the ideas expressed in these comments and in their formulation.

Ariane Levy-Schoen

II.1 A Method of Measuring the Visual Lobe Area

Heino Widdel
Forschungsinstitut für Anthropotechnik
Wachtberg, Federal Republic of Germany

INTRODUCTION

Peripheral vision is used to guide subsequent eye movements to informative regions while looking at a picture (Pollack and Spence, 1968; Gould and Dill, 1969; Antes, 1974). Generally, information is picked up during a fixation, which is the relatively immobile phase of the eye movement behavior, when the control of length and direction of the next saccade is also determined. When the saccade, which represents the rapid part of eye movement behavior, is executed, perception of new information is unlikely to occur. The analysis of the process of visual perception in this immobile period has given rise to intensive research interest.

VISUAL LOBE AREA CONCEPT

The peripheral area around the central fixation point from which specific information can be extracted and processed is the visual lobe area or useful field of view. The size of this area depends, among other things, on characteristics of the visual target and the surrounding context. It is narrow when the target is embedded in a complex background or surrounded by irregularly positioned non-target items (Brown & Monk, 1975), when the density of non-target items and the visual load increase (Mackworth, 1976), or when the similarity of target and non-target items is high (Bartz, 1976).

Usually, the visual lobe area is measured with tachistoscopical techniques. Recent research work using this technique has been attempted by

Mackworth (1976), who measured the visual acuity limit in a peripheral discriminaton task; and by Engel (1976), who analyzed what he called the conspicuity area. This method is quite simple and provides a favorable setting for the analysis of the shape of the visual lobe area because it is not influenced by eye movement strategies and dynamic processes dependent on stimulus material. As Enoch (1959) pointed out, the shape has a longer horizontal than vertical extension, however, Bellamy and Courtney (1981) found that the shape also depends on target characteristics. One disadvantage of this technique may be that measurement is not based on eye movement activities, but rather on static fixation behavior. A similar problem exists with a modified technique used by Mackworth (1976), where he presented the stimulus material moving through two windows. The distance between the windows was altered and subjects had to fixate on one window to detect targets which could appear in either window.

The second technique of measuring the visual lobe area involves the analysis of the interfixational distances. It takes into account the dynamic behavior of eye movements during a visual search task. This method was used in a variety of investigations, e.g., Snyder, and Taylor (1976) or Megaw and Richardson (1979), and is fruitful for specific research questions. It is not a direct measurement of the visual lobe area but allows a deduction of its average size. One disadvantage is that it is illogical to measure the visual lobe size for specific targets or target characteristics. A special measurement technique of analyzing the visual field, used to estimate mental work load, was evaluated by Voss (1981). He analyzed performance in peripheral vision by presenting peripheral light stimuli for detection. Lights were presented with a spectacle frame fixed on the head eliminating the influence of head movement. The calculation of the detection rate of the light stimuli during car driving shows that the functional visual field is sensitive to external load. This method represents a valid new indicator of mental work load, but visual field sensitivity was a secondary task, and it is not appropriate for analyzing specific aspects of visual performance.

A novel method combining advantages of the techniques described for measuring the visual lobe area is now presented. The philosophy is that during a successful fixation in a search task, the target-item can be detected in the peripheral area. The following saccade is determined by this peripheral stimulus and the next fixation will attain the target. A successful fixation is, in these terms, a fixation which is followed immediately by the fixation of the detected target. During a visual search task a subject is executing n fixations; generally $n > 1$. When the detected target is fixated the fixation n is identical with the target fixation and the fixation $n - 1$ is called a successful fixation because the target was detected peripherally. As an example, the

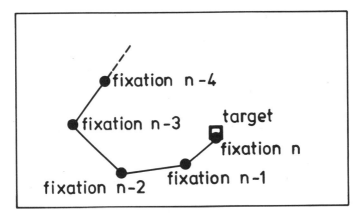

FIG. 1.   Last five fixations of a search pattern. Fixation *n* is the target fixation and fixation *n* − 1 the successful fixation. During fixation *n* − 1 the target is detected peripherally and the saccade to fixation n is determined.

last sequence of a search pattern with the last five fixations is shown in Fig. 1.

In a series of search trials the distances of the fixations $n-1$ to the targets can be measured and the distributions of the distances can be computed. Figure 2 shows an example of such distributions, where the zero-position represents the fixations $n-1$, and the squares represent the relative positions of the peripherally detected target in each trial.

Additionally, those fixations in the vicinity of the target have to be analyzed during the time in which the target is not being detected peripherally. When no target fixation follows, or a target fixation follows without detection of the target, the fixation is considered to be unsuccessful. During an unsuccessful fixation the target is not detected and the length and direction of the following saccade is not determined by the target location. There is a possibility that hitting the target may be a random event. It cannot be prevented that such a fixation would be falsely judged as successful, although it is by definition an unsuccessful one, because of lack of peripheral detection of the target. Such random hits will occur in all experimental situations and measurement procedures, and therefore will be balanced in comparing different visual lobe areas.

One way to quantify the visual lobe area is in terms of (S/S + F)*100, i.e., the number of successful fixations (S) divided by all fixations (S + F), which include the unsuccessful fixations (F), for each unit of distance from target. The operational procedure of the measurement of the visual lobe area has to

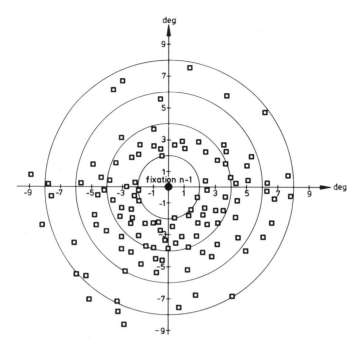

FIG. 2.   Sample distribution of the distances from the fixations $n-1$ to the targets. Zero-point represents the fixation $n-1$ (successful), and the squares represent the relative target positions in each stimulus presentation. Data are from one subject in the first session of experiment I, searching with high density material.

take into consideration the search area near the target. The outer limit of this area has to be established empirically. It is determined by the fact that the frequency of successful fixations approaches zero. This limit is expected to have an approximately circular shape and the area within it is divided into a series of concentric, equidistant rings. The width of these rings, where successful and unsuccessful fixations have to be identified, depends on the visual search problem and may vary from one to two degrees as is shown later.

Experimental investigations are essential for evaluating new methods. Two experiments with visual search tasks have been planned and executed in order to get some indication of the validity of the visual lobe area concept. Both experiments are highly similar and are described in detail below. Apparatus, experimental setup, eye movement measurement technique, presentation mode of stimulus material, and control of experiments are identical in each case.

Apparatus

The eye movement recording system used was the Honeywell Oculometer developed by Merchant (1969). It functions on the principles of the pupil-cornea reflection method, also called the point of regard measurement, as described in detail in Young and Sheena (1975).

The basic operating principle of the oculometer required illumination of the eye of the subject with infrared radiation from a single light source. The radiation reflected from the eye is monitored with an infrared sensitive television camera. The optics of the oculometer include the necessary lens, mirror, and beamsplitters to transmit the infrared radiation from the source to the eye of the subject and to return the optical signal to the electro-optical tracker for conversion to an electrical signal. This electrical signal generated in the circuitry of the electro-optical tracker is processed by a minicomputer and converted to the desired output format as shown in Fig. 3.

The infrared radiation coming from the source irradiates the eye of the subject and is received by the electro-optical tracker. A portion of this radiation passes through the cornea and pupil to the retina and is reflected from the retina, backlighting the pupil. The pupil is then imaged on the face of the television camera as a bright circular disk. The signal processing unit calculates the center and the diameter of this disk. In addition, an image of the infrared source is reflected from the corneal surface of the eye of the subject and is also brought to focus on the face of the television camera.

The rotational movement of one's eye in elevation is accompanied by a corresponding vertical change in the displacement between the center of the pupilar disk and the image of the infrared source. This displacement is scanned and calibrated to provide the elevation look angle of the subject's eye. The azimuth look angle is determined simultaneously in a similar manner from horizontal displacement of the two images. The focus distance of the electro-optical tracker optics provides a measure of the distance of the subject's eye from the sensor. The distance to the instrument panel is de-

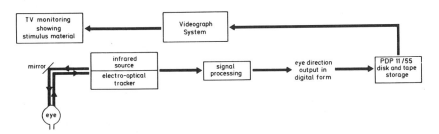

FIG. 3.   Function flow diagram of the apparatus used in the experiments.

rived from the geometry of the setup. The x/y–coordinates of the subject's lookpoint are then computed. The sampling rate of the system is 50 x/y–coordinates of eye movements per second.

The data were stored and processed by a DEC PDP 11/55 computer, which was also used for all task programming and the management of the different experimental sequences. The visual stimulus material was generated by this computer and presented by the Videograph, whch is a color video display controlled by a microprocessor, on a TV screen (see Fig. 3). The subject sat in a darkened room in front of the TV screen at a distance of 52 cm. The head was fixed in a chinrest to avoid rotational head movement.

EXPERIMENT I

The dependence of the visual lobe area size on the difficulty of a visual search task was investigated in the first experiment. It is part of a more complex research question described in Widdel and Kaster (1981). A large number of small, square, meaningless, identical symbols were spread out randomly over the stimulus field with an extent of 27 × 22 cm or 30° in the horizontal and 25° in the vertical dimension. Each square symbol had a size of 0.5°. The symbols were green on a homogeneous background of darker green. The contrast between symbols and background was low, and this provided very difficult conditions for visual perception. A single target-symbol was added to the others differing only in its internal graphical design. Otherwise, it has the same size, color, and luminance as the other symbols. This target-symbol had to be detected by the subjects. A stimulus picture presented in Fig. 4 shows the non-target-symbols ⊞ and the target-symbol ⊡; other target-symbols used were these: ⊟ ⊟ ⊞ ⊟.

The difficulty of the stimulus material was systematically varied by using three levels of non-target-symbol density. The highest density has a stimulus field of 576 symbols; medium and lowest density have stimulus fields of 461 and 352 symbols, respectively. One session was composed of 15 presentations of stimulus fields in a random sequence with each density occurring five times. For each presentation new positions of target- and non-target-symbols were determined by a random counter generator and the stimulus field was regenerated by the Videograph.

Eight subjects took part in nine sessions. One session lasted up to half an hour and the elapsed time between sessions was one day. When subjects detected the target-symbol during a presentation they pushed a button stopping the stampling of eye movement data. Then, the stimulus picture disappeared and subjects had to fixate on three isolated, successively presented points in the vicinity of the former target-symbol with distances between points of 5°. With this procedure, three fixation coordinates of the Honeywell Oculometer associated with the known TV screen-coordinates of

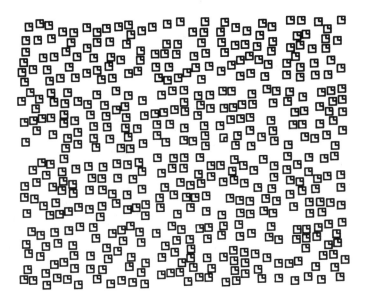

FIG. 4. Stimulus material used in the two experiments.

the three points were sampled as the basis for the required linearization procedure for all oculometer data. Mean search times varied from 9.82 sec to
56.30 sec depending on task difficulty.

Results

The visual lobe area was analyzed for each of the three density levels over all
subjects and sessions. The outer limit of the visual lobe area has a size of 9°
around the target. This critical area was subdivided into nine concentric,
equidistant rings with a width of 1° (as example see Fig. 2). In this area the
successful and unsuccessful fixations were identified. The relations between
them were calculated at the different distance units as described before. The
results are illustrated in Fig. 5.

The illustration shows that the probability of target detection is an approximately linear function of non-target density. The visual lobe area size
is largest with low density stimulus material and is smallest with high density
stimulus material. The size rankings among high, medium, and low density
stimuli is constant across all distance units. This observation is supported
statistically between low to medium and high densities ($p < .01$). In other
words, the fixations on visual search material of low difficulty have a higher
probability of being followed by the target fixation than on visual search
material of medium or high difficulty. Another interpretation of the result
means, e.g., that when a target was detected with a probability of .30, subjects fixated in a distance of 5.5° from the target with low density material
and in a distance of 2.7° from the target with high density material.

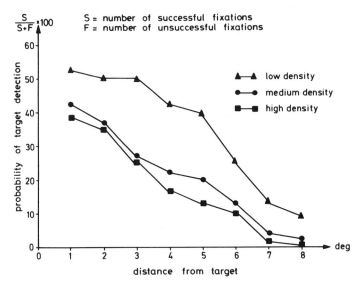

FIG. 5. Probability of peripheral target detection in the visual lobe area depending on density of non-target stimuli. The zero-point of the x coordinate represents the target position in each trial.

EXPERIMENT II

A second experiment was conducted to analyze the conspicuity of five colors. This experiment was aimed towards further validation of the concept of the visual lobe area. It was intended to answer the question, whether the visual lobe area is also useful to measure the conspicuity of the five colors red, blue, violet, green, and yellow.

The experimental arrangement was identical with the first experiment. Only the visual search material was modified and adapted to the object of the research question. The stimulus material had a medium density of 461 identical symbols, each of a known graphical structure. Four colors were randomly assigned to 460 symbols so that each color was represented by 115 symbols. One randomly positioned symbol was assigned a fifth color and represented the target-color to be detected by the subjects. For each presentation, the stimulus material was generated again in the described random strategy, changing the target-color and the assignment of the other four colors to the remaining 460 symbols. One session comprised 30 trials, i.e., each color was presented six times as a target-color. Each of seven subjects had eight sessions for a total of 1680 trials. Thus, for each color, 336 different eye movement patterns had to be evaluated. The mean search time of trials varied from 1.05 sec to 5.61 sec depending on the color.

The five colors presented on a TV screen had to be optimized in order to control the experimental conditions. The only independent variable, which had to be varied systematically, was hue. Other aspects of color had to be kept constant and equalized. The colors were adjusted to a luminance of 65 cd/m² by using a digital color measuring instrument. Furthermore, the saturation of the five colors had to be equalized, using a trichromatic colorimeter. Changing one parameter was followed by a change of the other because luminance and saturation are not independent values. Therefore some small differences between the saturations of the colors resulted. This can be seen in the standard color diagram showing the locations of the colors (Fig. 6).

Results

The visual lobe area was analyzed for each color in the number described previously. The determination of the outer limit of this area turned out to be problematic in comparison with the first experiment. The frequency of fixations for lobe sizes of more than 14° was rather low because of the limited size of the TV screen, and the relatively large visual lobe areas as a

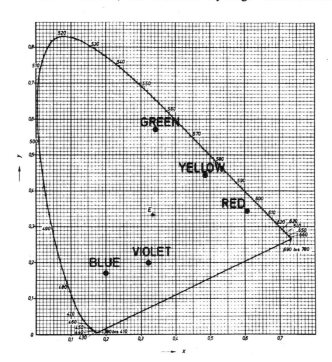

FIG. 6.   Location of the five colors in the standard color diagram.

result of the low task difficulty. The analyzed area around the target was partitioned by concentric, equidistant rings in size steps of two degrees. The probabilities of successful fixations in these areas are illustrated in Fig. 7.

As illustrated in this figure, visual lobe area sizes vary with colors of target. Detection probabilities of colors correspond with their mean search times, not reported here. The differences between green and the four other colors are significant ($p < .01$) as are the differences between yellow and the four other colors. A tendency toward a difference between violet and red or blue was noticeable but insignificant. The visual lobe areas can be interpreted as values of the conspicuities of the specific colors. These results may be useful in applying color to the coding of information to be presented on electronic displays.

CONCLUSIONS

The concept of the visual lobe area as defined and measured by the relation of successful and unsuccessful fixations in the previous work includes the influence of dynamic eye movements. In this sense, a generalization to practical search tasks requiring eye movements and even individual search strategies is possible. Two experiments demonstrated the validity of this method, which obviously has to be supported by further investigations with altering conditions and situations.

The first experiment illustrates the usefulness of the visual lobe area as an indicator of visual load as determined by stimulus density. This finding sup-

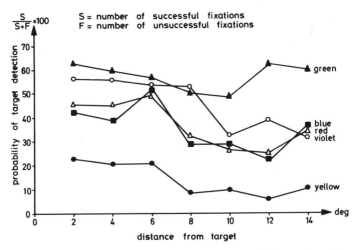

FIG. 7. Probability of peripheral target detection depending on five colors. The zero-point of the x-coordinate represents the target position in each trial.

ports the suggestion that in a more general view the visual lobe area may represent a correlate or a measure of mental work load. It can provide information about attention span as influenced by external or internal conditions.

As indicated in the second experiment, the visual lobe area can be used to analyze the conspicuity of colors. Furthermore, one may suppose that it is appropriate to measure the conspicuity of other kinds of targets and characteristics such as shape, luminance, graphical structure, etc. These problems are relevant mainly in the application areas of information design on displays. Knowledge of the size of the visual lobe area may also help in developing optimization strategies in visual inspection. This could be used to train individuals to use specific search strategies for improving search performance e.g. Lovie and Lovie (1968) reported using the strategy of subdividing the display into smaller areas. The object of these considerations is increasing search performance and reducing faults in perception and decision. In this regard the size of the visual lobe area, as measured during dynamic eye movement behavior, can be an important parameter in modeling visual search activities. Kraiss and Knäuper (1981) simulated visual search tasks with a task network model and predicted differences in search performance depending on random or systematic eye movement strategies.

II.2 Asymmetrical Control Areas in Continuous Visual Search

Wolfgang Prinz
Abteilung für Experimentelle und Angewandte Psychologie
Universität Bielefeld
German Federal Republic

CONTROL AREAS IN VISUAL SEARCH

The experiments reported here explore the size and the shape of functional visual fields or, as we prefer to say, of control areas in a continuous visual search task. Generally the results of these experiments seem to suggest (1) that control areas can be asymmetrical on the vertical dimension and (2) that control area shape is determined by both, functional (attentional) and structural (sensory) factors, which can be complementary.

Basic Method. Our experiments utilize a visual search task of the Neisser type (cf. Neisser, 1963, 1964). A typical search list is shown in Fig. 1. Basically, the list consists of a sequence of letters randomly drawn from a predefined set of non-target letters. At one location in the list the non-target letter is replaced by a target letter. The subject's task is to search for the target. Subjects are instructed to scan the list row by row—just as one reads—and to do so as fast as possible. When they detect the target they have to press a button and name the target letter.

In experiments with this task, subjects frequently report that they detect the target prior to scanning the row that contains it. For example, the subject may detect a target at a certain location in row 8 while scanning through row 5 and fixating some location in that row. In this case, the target would be detected at a (vertical) distance of 3 rows.

For a more systematic study of these detection distances, some device is needed that permits specifying the row that is being scanned at the moment the target is detected. In our experiments, this information was obtained by

```
HHMMXHLLVNNXKMWWVHFLFKTHNXXNFLTTKTFHVHWN
WMKKMNXFLVHFWTNFLMWFNNMNHFKXXWFKXFXFMNMX
VTFMLMHVFTXHFFTHXXTXLLTMMLFVKLNNKWTTHVVF
MXMKWXLXLVHVVLLNHFLHHKNFTTKLMFXFVLMKTLLM
NVTTNTHVNKWKNFWFVWNWKWLNHMLFHNLKKWVFLTXV
VFMKHMKWLVNLWXXMMTLTWVVWMLTLVLWMVLNXXVFK
KTVMVTWVKXHTFMWXKNNNVMWHXWKMTXHTXNVWFWKV
TMHLLMVXHNMKLWXFVLLMWVFNWFTVMKTLTVHTKVTK
VKKHHLXNLMWMVKNXFXVHFFMMHWVHKVLHLFXNXFLL
TFNVKMTMXTVTXLHHMTXKKMXLWVKTVNTWVXTTHLHT
HWWMLDVNWKWHHHNVVHWMVFVTKTMNLHXNHHHHXWWV
FKTWWMFHNVXFLMFLHKTFLVNXHHHNLNTFVLLLFLMVM
NMKXVXWVLLFTNNHWVWKTMHXFLXVXTFKWFXVNMKLW
VKTKTHVFFTWLHFKTLFLFHMWWTHHLLTFHNLTWVNHX
FWHFLKTNKWTMWXMWVWHTXKXVKVXXWKKWTWLFFXFL
VLVTVFWXNMFXVTFMKHMLNVFNHNLTXXNNFTXHNMVM
NWNVXKMFHNLNLXTTMFWHKFMFWFMXNWWKXLFFLNTN
TNXHKTWNVKWFWNMWTLNNMLFMFNFNMFFFTTHNNFKL
XXVLVXNTLHHTXXTXKTKWTKMLXVWFTNWLWKXHLNVT
TNTHNMMXHWWLTWFWWNFTHWTXKLKNNFMVXNKNKLHM
KKKNTFLLVXVNKFTVMKXWVMFVMWVTKTKNKHNKTFLF
TFVLKLMFTWLKMTVWKMVMWLMLWVLKWLXKXWHFKVHN
FKTXNVVLKNVVXKTXLFLXKWXTKFMWHHNXLFVVHXKK
WWLLKFMVNWMHTFHTFMXTXLNWFNXHXNVTXHMXMFWL
XXHVMTLWTMXFNWMMTTNLWVTTWMTWWWTHHMKLTWMV
MLXMXMMHVLHTVMLWLWWVFLXMXTWHTNHXVNWTWFHN
HHMLNWHXKXVWTKXLNXLNWTVWNLNFMHFMMLH TMWV
LKFWVTWNVNFNMFKFWLHVLWTFVFXHTVVKFXWNFNKN
XFKXMHTLTTVHXNLMTTFWWMHTTNTNKWWVWKHMTLNX
FVXNXLHNVVLMHTNXMVKKNLTNXTLLHKFMTFFTNNKN
NHVKLKNVFKNFLLMKNXMWTVFKHNNFLVVHVWNLLTWK
VWKVMVKTMMVXVVTHLLVFMMKTMFXVWTWMLHWNTWTW
```

FIG. 1. Typical search list as used in Experiment 1. Non-target set: *H M X L V N K W F T*. Target: *D*.

recording the horizontal component of the EOG and by counting the number of return sweeps by which the subject returns to the beginning of the next row. So, in the above example, after four return sweeps, the subject would be considered to scan through row 5, and if she detected the target before the occurrence of the next return sweep, the detection distance for that trial would be recorded with size 3.

Previous Results. Though this method may not be perfect, we now have substantial evidence supporting both, its reliability and its validity (see Prinz & Kehrer, in press). Some of the data that were observed in several previous experiments can be summarized as follows:

1. Vertical detection distances range between 0 and about 6 degrees of angular distance. A detection distance of 0 implies that the target is not detected prior to scanning the target-containing row itself. A distance of 6 degrees implies that the target is detected about 6-10 rows prior to scanning the target-containing row (the exact value depending on list size and viewing conditions, of course).

2. Detection distances are clearly related to target-non-target discriminability. For example, an angular letter (such as *A*) has a larger detection distance if it is embedded in a "round" non-target context (composed of such letters as *O, C, B, G*) as compared to an angular context (composed of, e.g., *Z, N, T, X*).

3. When several targets are to be searched for simultaneously, the targets clearly differ in their mean detection distances. For example, when the subject has to search for A and Q simultaneously in an angular non-target context, Q will be detected at a much larger vertical distance than A.

4. There are substantial individual differences in variation of detection distances. In a given simultaneous search task, there are always some subjects who virtually show a random fluctuation about the zero distance (even for "easy" targets), and some others who show clear indication of parafoveal detection (even for difficult targets).

These results indicate that the subject is able to exert some control over the detection of a target not only in the row just fixated, but also over some larger area around the fixation point, depending on the type of non-target context. If this view is adopted, the mean detection distance for a given target is an estimate of the vertical extent of the subject's control area for that target. However, because this method does not permit recording detection distances above the fixation point, this estimate is restricted to the area below the row just fixated, and we have no indication of the extent of the control areas above the fixation point.

With respect to this problem, one of two views may be adopted. The *first view* assumes that control areas are basically concentric in shape, i.e., approximately symmetrical in their vertical extent. According to this view, the upper halves of the control areas virtually possess the same target detecting capabilities as the lower halves. These capabilities are not needed, however, in the present task because the target is always detected in a position below or beside the fixation point. In contrast, the *second view* assumes that the control areas are asymmetrical under the conditions of this task. As subjects are never required to watch for a target above the fixation point it is reasonable to assume that they either learn to concentrate their attention—and thereby their target detecting capabilities—on the zone below the fixation point (leading to an attentional neglect of the upper zone) or that they learn to adapt the sensitivity of various sections of the visual field according to the demands imposed on them by the actual task (leading to a decrease of sensitivity in the upper zone).

VERTICAL ASYMMETRY OF CONTROL AREAS— EXPERIMENTS 1 AND 2

A decision between the first and the second view can be reached under conditions where targets are offered as locations above the fixation point without the subjects' knowledge, i.e., while they are watching for the target only within and below the row just being scanned. There are now two lines of evidence supporting the conclusion that the subjects are virtually unable to detect those targets.

The first line of evidence comes from a closer look at the error data from our previous experiments. The two views differ in their predictions about the chance of detecting a target after first overlooking it. When subjects scan the target-containing row without detecting the target, they continue the search while scanning the next row, further expecting the target only within or below that row. If the control areas were asymmetrical, the upper target would then have the same chance of being detected as a lower target at the same distance. If the control areas were perfectly asymmetrical, upper targets could not be detected at all.

The results of all experiments conducted so far are clearly in favor of this latter alternative. The probability of detecting an upper target that has been overlooked is virtually zero. This may be illustrated by the error data from an experiment where 24 subjects were practiced in a simultaneous search task over 4 experimental sessions, with about 90 trials per session. Though the experiment was conducted for a different purpose it is relevant to the present illustration because the total number of observations (and, correspondingly, the total number of omission errors) is large enough to draw sound conclusions. The total number of trials that were recorded was 8904. In 714 of these trials the target was overlooked until the end of the scan of the target-containing row, corresponding to an overall error rate of 8.02%. The critical observation is that the target was detected during the scan of the next row only in 10 out of these 714 cases. Detection of upper targets was observed in only 6 of 24 subjects, though a considerable number of omission errors—i.e. chances for upper target detection—was observed for each particular subject.

A more detailed analysis was performed on the results of the last two practice sessions where the subjects were well familiar with the task and, correspondingly, the data were less noisy than in the initial sessions. In these two sessions the overall error rate was 4.19% (185 omission errors out of 4402 trials). The details of the results are summarized in Table 1.

The subjects searched for two targets simultaneously, D and Z. As the non-targets in the search lists were drawn from a set of angular letters the two targets differed in discriminability. The "easy" target, D, was overlooked until the end of the scan of the target-containing row in 28 out of 2121 cases, corresponding to an error rate of 1.3%. As can be seen in Table 1, the target was detected during the scan of the next row in none of these 28 trials. The "difficult" target, Z, was overlooked until the end of the target-containing row in 157 out of 2282 trials, corresponding to an error rate of 6.9%. For this target, detection during the scan of the next row was only observed in 2 out of these 157 trials. Part (b) of Table 1 summarizes these results in terms of probability of upper target detection and

TABLE 1
Results of Experiment 1. (a): Absolute Values of Detection and
Error Frequencies. (b): Probability of Target Detection at
Distances + 1, 0 and − 1. See Text for Further Explanation

	Target	Total number of trials	Number of trials where target was detected at distance				was not detected
			$d > 1$	$d = +1$	$d = 0$	$d = -1$	
(a)	D	2121	1267	524	302	0	28
	Z	2281	442	631	1051	2	155

			Probability of target detection at distance		
			$d = +1$	$d = 0$	$d = -1$
(b)	D		.61	.91	.00
	Z		.34	.87	.01

compares them with the corresponding values for lower target detection. These probabilities were obtained by dividing the number of detections observed at a certain distance by the number of trials in which that target had not been detected before. For example, the probability of detecting Z at $d = 0$ is $[1051/(2281 − 442 − 631)] = [1051/(1051 + 2 + 155)] = [1051/1208] = .87$.

It is obvious from these results that upper targets can by no means be detected in the same way and at the same distance as lower targets. The error data rather suggest that the capability for detecting a target is basically restricted to the area below the fixation point and that, in the present task, the subjects are virtually blind in the upper halves of their visual fields.

The second line of evidence comes from Experiment 2, where upper targets were inserted in addition to lower targets without the subjects' knowledge. In this experiment, subjects were required to start their search at the beginning of the middle row of the search list and to scan its lower section in the usual way (left-right/top-bottom). The upper section was completely irrelevant. Each of 4 subjects was engaged in a simultaneous search for D and Z in an angular non-target context again. There were 7 experimental sessions. In the first two sessions, subjects were practiced on the task. They were instructed to concentrate their search on the lower section of the lists (where they would always detect a target if they searched carefully) and to neglect the upper section (where, when occasionally glancing at that section, they would find non-targets only). In the remaining five sessions, an additional target was inserted in the upper section of each list without the subjects' knowledge. In these sessions, there were 80 trials each, divided into 5 blocks of 16 trials. In the first block, the upper targets had a distance of 5 rows from the starting row. In the remaining 4 blocks the upper target distance gradually decreased to 4, 3, 2, and 1 row, respectively.

If the conclusions drawn from the omission errors are valid, it must be expected that additional upper targets cannot be detected immediately. This was actually observed in session 3 where the search lists first contained upper targets. None of the 4 subjects detected them, though each of them had 16 independent chances at distance 1 (and many more chances at larger distances). On the other hand, it cannot be expected that the upper targets remain undetected over several practice sessions. This is the case because the experimental procedure does not preclude an occasional glance at the upper section, which may lead to an occasional detection of a target to be found there. Correspondingly, 3 of the 4 subjects detected their first upper target in sessions 4, 5, and 6, respectively.

Table 2 shows the results for these 3 subjects in terms of detection probabilities for upper and lower targets. As the first detection of an upper target was always related to the easy target, D, the results are only given for this target. The entries for upper target detection are estimated by taking the reciprocal value of the number of independent chances of detection that were needed until the first detection actually occurred. When an upper target at distance $d = 1$ is detected on its 25th presentation at that distance, a detection probability of 1/25 is scored. The entries for lower target detection are calculated from 2 or more sessions, where upper targets were first detected. The results clearly indicate a substantial difference in the order of magnitude in the probability for upper versus lower target detection.

One of the subjects did not report any upper target detection during the experimental sessions. In an interview after the end of the experiment she reported, however, that she had occasionally seen an upper target in the last two sessions and that she had not felt obliged to report it because it occurred in the irrelevant section of the list. Thus, failing to report a detection does not necessarily imply a failure to detect. This observation suggests some caution in the interpretation of non-detections. For the other 3 subjects, interviews at the end of the experiment revealed, however, that they had reported upper targets as soon as they had detected them.

STRUCTURAL AND FUNCTIONAL DETERMINANTS OF ASYMMETRY—EXPERIMENTS 3 AND 4

From the results of the first two experiments it can be concluded that the control areas that are effective in the continuous search task are highly asymmetrical in their vertical extent (or that they are even restricted to the area below the fixation point).

TABLE 2
Results of Experiment 2. Probability of
Target Detection at Distances +1 and
−1 for 3 Subjects ('Easy' Target,
D, Only). (The First Detection of
Upper Targets was Observed in
Sessions 6, 5 and 4 for Subjects
NE, EL and ZW, respectively.)

	Subject		
	NE	EL	ZW
d = +1	.95	.76	.92
d = −1	.04	.05	.08

What is the basis of this asymmetry? As we indicated above, two different explanations may be offered. The failure to detect upper targets may be due to functional or to structural reasons. According to the *functional interpretation,* subjects usually *do not* watch for upper targets because they have learned, in the course of the task, to concentrate their attention on the lower zone exclusively, resulting in an attentional neglect of the upper zone. This view implies that an immediate shift to the upper zone should be possible if and when it turns out to be necessary. According to the *structural interpretation,* the subject *cannot* watch for upper targets because, in the course of the task, the mechanisms underlying target detection have undergone structural changes that result in a decrease of sensitivity in the upper zone. These structural changes cannot immediately be reversed when the task is changed.

Some preliminary evidence bearing on this question may be obtained from the results of the later sessions of Experiment 2. It is interesting to speculate what will occur after the first detection of an upper target. The functional view would predict that subjects will immediately shift their attention to the area above the fixation point (at least during the scan of the starting row) once they have noticed that upper targets do occur. The structural view would predict that the first detection of an upper target will not lead to an immediate improvement of upper target detection because the structural basis of the previous asymmetry cannot be changed instantaneously.

At the first glance, the results from the last sessions of Experiment 2 clearly support the functional interpretation. Once the first upper target has been detected the probability of upper target detection is raised immediately to a level that remains stable until the end of the experiment (by the way, without impairing the detection probability for lower targets at all). This effect was observed in each of the 3 subjects who showed upper target detection during the experiment. However, at the second glance, there is also some evidence in favor of the structural interpretation. Though the detection probabilities are immediately raised, upper targets are usually not detected at the same distances as lower targets. Even two or three practice sessions after the first detection of upper targets, when subjects are clearly aware of their possible occurrence, the detection distances tend to remain asymmetrical. This is illustrated in Fig. 2 in terms of (cumulated) detection

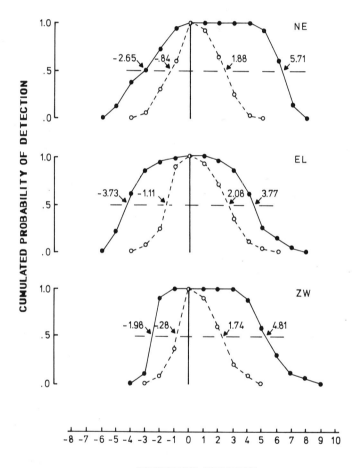

FIG. 2.   Cumulated probabilities of target detection (ordinate) over detection distances (abscissa) in sessions 6/7 of Experiment 2. Solid line: target D, broken line: Z. Same Subjects as in Table 2. Note that the medians cannot be directly read from the direction distance scale. As the scale values are means of class intervals a correction for continuity must be applied when the medians of the cumulated distributions are calculated.

probabilities over detection distances. The curves on the righthand side show the threshold functions for lower target detection; the curves on the lefthand side present the same information for upper target detection. The entries are medians that give an indication of the average detection distances. Except for subject EL, target D, upper target detection is always poorer than lower target detection.

These results seem to support the functional interpretation with a slight indication favoring the structural interpretation. Experiment 3 attempted to further test the structural interpretation. In this experiment there were basically two task conditions: top-down—scan (left-right within and top-down between the rows) and bottom-up—scan (right-left within and bottom-up between the rows). In the top-down condition the subjects had to watch for lower targets as usual. In the bottom-up condition they had to watch for upper targets. Eight subjects searched in 5 experimental sessions each. The first two sessions were considered as practice sessions where only the standard top-down task was applied. Each of the remaining three sessions began with a warm-up phase (16 trials top-down scan) and was then continued by a critical phase where the direction of the scan was reversed on every trial (76 trials in both directions), thus forcing the subject to alternate between lower and upper search on each trial.

The results from the critical trials in sessions 3–5 are summarized in the upper part of Fig. 3. The righthand curves show the threshold functions for top-down search; threshold functions for bottom-up search are given on the left. Each of the four curves is based on a frequency distribution that was obtained from summing up the individual frequency distributions over all subjects. (The alternative procedure of first obtaining individual threshold functions and then combining them into an average function yielded completely equivalent results: The medians of the present functions are virtually equivalent to the medians of the individual functions.)

As is shown in Fig. 3, a pronounced difference between detection distances for upper and lower targets was observed for the easy target, D (absolute size of medians: 4.37 versus .196). This difference was highly reliable with 7 of 8 subjects. For the difficult target, Z, a small but unreliable difference in the same direction was observed (.72 versus .43). As the detection distances for this target came quite close to the floor value at 0, the small size and the low degree of reliability of this effect should not necessarily lead one to neglect it completely.

Again, two factors are needed for a satisfying account of these results. On the one hand, the subjects are clearly able to switch from trial to trial between watching for lower and for upper targets. This again supports the functional interpretation of the factors that govern the extent of control areas. On the other hand, upper target detection is clearly less efficient than lower target detection even if explicit instructions and some practice on the

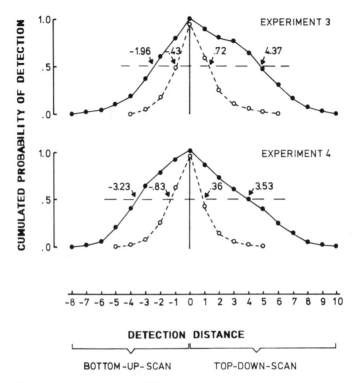

FIG. 3. Cumulated probabilities of target detection over detection distances in Experiments 3 and 4. For further details see Figure 2.

task are provided. This supports the structural interpretation of the underlying factors. It seems that a combined model is needed to account for the asymmetry of control areas in terms of both functional *and* structural determinants.

Experiment 3 originated from the assumption that the structural component of the observed asymmetry is due to a specific adaptation of the sensitivity of various portions of the visual field to the actual task demands and that this adaptation is established in the course of the practice period provided within the experiment. Though the results clearly support the assumption of a structural basis of the asymmetry, they lead one to doubt whether an explanation of this effect in terms of experimental practice tells the whole story. One might argue that it is not very likely that the relatively small lead in practice of the top-down—scan as compared to the bottom-up—scan can really account for the pronounced asymmetry observed (at least for the easy target, *D*). Are there any possible advantages of lower over upper target detection existing prior to and independent of the present task? Experiment 4 was run in order to explore whether the effects observed in

Experiment 3 were either due to the training period provided within the experiment or to some other pre-experimental sources. These two classes of factors can only be separated when Experiment 3 is supplemented by an equivalent experiment where the subject is required to scan in the bottom-up mode during the experimental training sessions and during the warm-up phase at the beginning of the later sessions. This task was performed by 8 additional subjects in Experiment 4. All other aspects of the task were equivalent to Experiment 3.

The results are shown in the lower section of Fig. 3. For the easy target *D*, a slight and unreliable difference in favor of lower target detection is observed (3.53 versus 3.23). A closer look at the individual results shows that for some subjects upper target detection was reliably less efficient than lower target detection, whereas for others the reverse was true. For the difficult target *Z*, upper target detection distances were (unreliably) larger than lower target detection distances.

The combined results of Experiments 3 and 4 suggest the conclusion that structural asymmetry must be decomposed into a pre-experimental and an experimental component. If this principle is adopted, the results can be summarized as follows: for the easy target, there is a pre-experimental asymmetry that favors lower over upper target detection. Under practice with top-down scan (Experiment 3) this asymmetry is reinforced by the experimental task. Under practice with bottom-up scan it is counteracted and—on the average—balanced. However, for the difficult target there is no indication of pre-experimental asymmetry. The results for this target are completely compatible with the view that a slight asymmetry in one or the other direction is established on the basis of the specific practice provided within the experiment.

Interaction Between Structural and Functional Factors

Though the results of the last two experiments look quite confusing at the descriptive level they can easily be accounted for by a simple model. The model postulates that target detection is mediated by two independent mechanisms that operate at different locations in the visual field. With respect to the assumed differences between central versus eccentric vision, the model is loosely related to Trevarthen's distinction between ambient and focal vision (Trevarthen, 1968). With respect to the functional nature of the operations involved it draws back to the distinction between automatic detection and controlled search suggested by Shiffrin and Schneider (Schneider & Shiffrin, 1977; Shiffrin & Schneider, 1977). Though the model was originally developed for a different purpose (explanation of the effects of mental load on search performance in yet unpublished experiments), its application to the present task is straightforward. It rests on three basic assumptions.

1. *Mechanisms:* There are two mechanisms for the accumulation of target evidence in continuous search: automatic detection (AD) and controlled search (CS). Target detection in eccentric vision is mediated by the AD mechanism. Its efficiency at various locations in the visual field depends on the permanent distribution of sensitivity. Asymmetries of this distribution are therefore reflected in corresponding asymmetries of the efficiency of AD. Target detection in central vision is mediated by the CS mechanism. Its efficiency depends on the transient distribution of attention over the visual field. Asymmetries of this distribution are therefore reflected in corresponding asymmetries of efficiency of CS.

2. *Interaction:* The two mechanisms watch for the target independent from each other. On each trial, the target first enters the eccentric region covered by the AD mechanism. If it is detected, the search stops. If the AD mechanism fails to detect the target it gradually enters into the zone covered by the CS mechanism where it has some more chances of being detected.

3. *Pratice:* In principle, practice enhances the efficiency of both AD and CS. However, there is a negative correlation between the efficiency of AD and the amount of practice available for CS. This is because, according to the interaction principle, there will be less opportunity for practicing controlled search to the degree that efficiency of automatic detection is improved.

With these principles in mind the results of Experiment 3 and 4 can be explained as follows. The *easy target, D,* can nearly perfectly be detected by AD under the condition of top-down scan. Under this condition, CS is only very infrequently needed to detect this target. Under the condition of bottom-up scan, AD is less effective (due to some asymmetry of the permanent sensitivity distribution) and CS comes into play more frequently. This explanation is supported by a closer look at the (uncumulated) detection probabilities at various distances shown in Table 3. In both experiments the same general pattern is observed in the *D* data: The detection probabilities at larger distances are clearly smaller for upper as compared to lower targets. This reflects the structural difference in efficiency between the two halves of the visual field. The difference is reversed, however, for the smaller detection distances. In both experiments, the probabilities of upper target detection at distances 1 and 2 are clearly superior to the corresponding values for lower target detection. This reflects the difference in the efficiency of CS, which—according to the interaction principle—is an indirect result of the difference in the efficiency of AD: The poorer the efficiency of AD the larger is the number of opportunities for practicing CS. Whereas

TABLE 3

Probability of Target Detection at Various Vertical Distances in Experiments 3 and 4. (In These Experiments the Angular Distance Between the Rows was About .75 degrees.)

Target	Condition				Probability of target detection at distance						
		0	1	2	3	4	5	6	7	8	9
Exp. 3											
D	top-down scan	1.00	.33	.17	.35	.28	.27	.15	.08	.05	.03
	bottom-up scan	1.00	.51	.38	.23	.10	.07	.01	.01	.01	
Z	top-down scan	.84	.41	.18	.06	.04	.01				
	bottom-up scan	.87	.36	.14	.03						
Exp. 4											
D	top-down scan	1.00	.50	.31	.18	.21	.16	.13	.09	.04	.02
	bottom-up scan	1.00	.67	.38	.35	.26	.16	.02	.01	.01	
Z	top-down scan	.93	.34	.09	.03	.02					
	bottom-up scan	.88	.48	.19	.06	.02	.01				

this general pattern is observed in both experiments, there is also a critical difference that reflects the effects of experimental practice. With practice in top-down scan (Experiment 3), the pre-experimental difference in AD efficiency is even enlarged. In contrast, with practice in bottom-up scan (Experiment 4), the experimental practice counteracts the pre-experimental asymmetry in the efficiency of both mechanisms, AD and CS. Therefore, the differences between the two probability distributions are less pronounced in Experiment 4 than in Experiment 3.

The *difficult target, Z,* can only be detected by CS under both scanning conditions. As there is no interaction with different degrees of efficiency of AD, and as CS is completely independent from the permanent distribution of sensitivity in the visual field, the efficiency of CS is only affected by the practice provided within the experiment. In principle, CS is equally efficient for upper and lower targets, and specific practice on one of the two scanning patterns will lead to an equal increment of efficiency of that mechanism.

Further support for this model comes from the differences between the subjects in Experiment 4. As has been pointed out by Prinz and Kehrer (in press), subjects differ substantially in the amount of target evidence needed for triggering the detection response. According to the present model, subjects who are willing to accept a low amount of target evidence frequently tend to base their detection response on the low amount of evidence made available by AD at peripheral locations, instead of waiting for the higher amounts of evidence made available by CS in central vision. The reverse is true for subjects with a high evidence criterion: They tend to rely on CS rather than on AD. Under the condition of Experiment 4, this difference between low- and high-criterion subjects should be reflected in a difference in their proneness to the assumed pre-experimental source of asymmetry: Low-criterion subjects (with large detection distances) should be clearly affected by that source (mediated via AD) whereas high-criterion subjects (with small detection distances) should be less affected (to the degree they rely on CS instead of AD). This was actually observed in the experiment for the easy target, *D:* When the subjects are ranked according to their mean detection distances for that target, clear indication of (pre-experimental) superiority of lower over upper target detection was observed for the subjects on the first three ranks. In contrast, for the subjects on the last three ranks, there was an equally clear indication of (experimentally induced) superiority of upper over lower target detection. For these three subjects, the results for *D* were virtually equivalent to the overall results for *Z.*

Nature of Structural Factors

Which is the source of asymmetry that is reflected in the difference in the efficiency for upper versus lower target detection? It has long been known that the lower half of the visual field is superior to its upper half in several respects. As was observed a hundred years ago by Johannes von Kries, left eye reaction times to visual stimuli are considerably shorter for stimuli appearing below rather than above the fixation point (von Kries & Auerbach, 1877; von Kries & Hall, 1879). About twenty years later, similar results were obtained in Wilhelm Wirth's left eye experiments in a more difficult visual detection task. Reaction times were shorter and differential thresholds were lower in the lower as compared to the upper half of the visual field (Kästner & Wirth, 1908/09; Wirth, 1907, 1908, 1927).

More recent evidence is also available. In various studies of the visual evoked response it has been shown that the lower and the upper half of the visual field have different electrophysiological properties that are not yet fully understood (Michel & Halliday, 1971; Lehmann & Skrandis, 1979). In the lower half of the visual field, the VER is usually larger in amplitude and shorter in latency as compared to the upper half of the visual field (see also Wildberger, 1981). Most recent evidence at the behavioral level comes from Widdel's search experiments, where it was also observed that targets are more frequently detected below than above the fixation point (Widdel, this volume).

The evidence seems to suggest that some degree of vertical asymmetry is inherent in the human visual system. An ecological explanation of the phenomenon offers itself: For an animal that lives on a solid surface in a terrestrial environment most relevant objects appear in the lower half of the visual field, and, under normal viewing conditions, objects in the lower half tend to be closer to the body than objects in the upper half. Accordingly, it might be wise to furnish the organism with a higher efficiency of detection in the lower than in the upper visual field (cf. Lehmann, Meles, & Mir, 1977).

In conclusion, the results of our experiments suggest that the size and the shape of control areas in continuous search are governed by both functional (attentional) and structural (sensory) factors. The operation of attentional factors reflected in the CS mechanism seems to be restricted to central vision whereas structural factors reflected in the AD mechanism operate in eccentric vision.

In the standard search task these two factors act in the same direction, resulting in highly asymmetrical control areas. When they are separated from each other it is revealed that they act independent of each other. Functional asymmetry arises from an asymmetrical distribution of attention that can be changed immediately if necessary. Structural asymmetry arises from an asymmetrical distribution of sensitivity that cannot be changed in itself because it is related to anatomical and physiological differences between the upper and the lower half of the visual field. Both of these asymmetries can either be strengthened or weakened by specific experimental practice.

These conclusions are well in line with the evidence available from numerous studies on the perceptual span in reading. McConkie (1979) has recently proposed a distinction between (1) the region around the fixation point within which sufficient visual information for a given task is available, and (2) the subregion within that region from which visual information is actually taken during a given fixation. As far as reading is concerned, it seems that both the region from which information can be utilized and the subregion from which it is actually utilized can be asymmetrical in their horizontal extent (Bouma, 1973; Rayner, Well, & Pollatsek, 1980; Pollatsek, Bolozky, Well, & Rayner, 1981). In a similar way we argue that the perceptual span (control area) in our search task is asymmetrical on the vertical dimension and that the asymmetry pertains to both the area where sufficient information is available (structural asymmetry) and the subarea from which the information is actually taken (functional asymmetry).

ACKNOWLEDGMENT

The Experiments reported herein were supported from Grants 2757 and 2735 by the University of Bielefeld. The experiments were conducted by Eva Böcker and Hans-Joachim Bönigk. The author is indebted to the audience at the Bern meeting for many valuable suggestions.

II.3 The Influence of Peripheral Preprocessing on Oculomotor Programming in a Scanning Task

Zoi Kapoula
Laboratoire de Psychologie Experimentale
Paris, France

INTRODUCTION

Our work concerns the control of eye movement activity. Particularly, do time constraints in the visual system allow moment-to-moment control of eye movements by ongoing information processing?

Lévy-Schoen and Rigaut-Renard (1980) and Lévy-Schoen (1981), among others, showed that fixation durations can be determined directly by the combination of the processing done at the current fixation plus processing done on the basis of partial information available in peripheral vision when the eye was at the preceding fixation. This latter kind of processing we call peripheral preprocessing.

The task used by Lévy-Schoen was a simple comparison task of two objects. This situation is very constrained in the sense that the eye must always make the same sequence of two saccades. It might be argued that the simplicity of this task favors peripheral preprocessing, but in less constrained situations fixation durations might also be affected by other factors like general scanning strategies. The preparation of a less constrained routine of eye adjustment could induce a global program for the length of time the eye will remain at every element and there would be no need for moment-to-moment adjustment on the basis of local processing.

To study the relative roles played by global programs and moment-to-moment adjustments, we created a situation that provokes an eye movement scanning routine similar to that found in reading. To avoid the problems of interpretation that arise when the material to be read has a linguistic structure, we used simple symbols as material.

Method

In our experiment, we present lines containing a series of 0's and 8's. The 0 and 8 were chosen as stimuli because used they were of the same luminosity on the CRT and had similar density, contours, and curvature. We hoped they would therefore be about equally easy to see both from central and from peripheral vision. Figure 1 shows examples of some lines presented individually on the computer screen.

In order to vary the amount of peripheral preprocessing that can be done on a given stimulus element, we varied the spacings between successive elements in the line. Preliminary experiments determined the visibility of the two stimuli at different distances into peripheral vision. In these experiments each stimulus was presented at an unpredictable eccentricity while the eye was fixated at the center of the screen. Figure 2 shows the results. We found that the visibility declines in non-central vision but it remains above chance level up to 12 letter spaces from the fixation point.

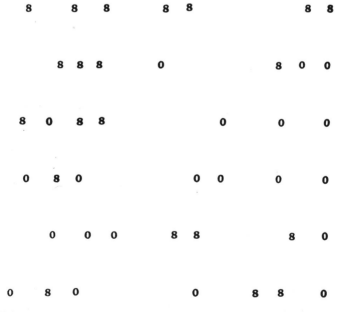

FIG. 1. Examples of lines presented one by one on the screen. From Kapoula, O'Regan, and Lévy-Schoen (1980). Each line shows a different order of the spacings between the third, fourth, fifth, and sixth stimulus elements. There were 6 orders and 8 lines for each order. The number of target stimuli for each of these 8 lines range from 0 to 7.

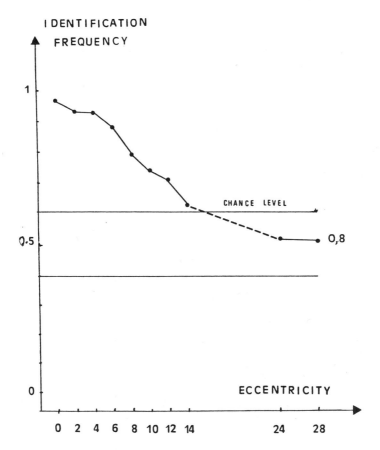

FIG. 2.   Identification frequency as a function of the eccentricity. The 0 or 8 were presented at an unpredictable eccentricity while the eye was fixated at the center of the screen. Chance level was determined by the binomial test.

Based on these preliminary results we selected the spacings of 4, 12, and 24 letter spaces to provide three levels of peripheral visibility.

In the scanning experiment the stimulus elements were spaced in an unpredictable fashion on each line, using these three spacings. This prevented subjects from preprogramming their scanning as a function of a known spacing pattern.

Assuming that the eye will jump from one stimulus to the next, the hypothesis followed that: When a stimulus on the line is preceded by a large space, less preprocessing of it should be possible, so fixation duration on it should be longer. If this is the case, a positive correlation between fixation durations and preceding saccade size is expected.

Procedure

The experiment began with a calibration of the photoelectric eye movement measuring apparatus. Stimulus lines appeared on the screen one at a time while calibration accuracy was maintained. Otherwise the experiment was interrupted and calibration repeated. By use of a computer controlled "smooth pursuit" calibration method (O'Regan, 1978), and by automatic calibration checking, we obtained an accuracy of ½°.

The subject was required to scan each line. The task was to count the number of occurrences of the stimulus indicated as target. After each line was scanned the subject had to indicate whether the number of targets was even or odd.

Results

The results of the analysis were pooled for 5 subjects. Figure 3 illustrates the relation between fixation durations and preceding saccade size. A tendency can be seen for fixation durations to increase when the preceding saccade size increases. The values of the correlation coefficient range from +.2 to +.5 for different subjects, and they are all significant at the .05 level.

This result can be explained by the hypothesis of peripheral preprocessing. The increase of fixation durations following large saccades could be due to the fact that less use is made of peripheral information when the eye makes a large saccade. In other words, the factors shown to determine fixation durations by Lévy-Schoen in a highly constrained situation seem also to be at work in the simplified digit reading situation studied here.

EXPERIMENTS 2 AND 3

To further confirm these results we performed two other experiments where peripheral information was not available. Figure 4 shows examples of lines presented in these experiments.

In Experiment 2, each of the two stimuli 0, 8 were placed between two figural masks. In this way identification of 0, 8 in non-central vision became difficult because of the lateral interference of the mask.

For Experiment 3 we designed two rectangular symbols having the same luminosity and the same density on the CRT screen. The only different feature was the orientation of a bar situated inside the rectangle. Because the distinguishing bar was inside the rectangle, it was very difficult to see it in peripheral vision.

To determine the visibility of these kinds of symbols we also performed preliminary experiments in which we presented the symbols at various ec-

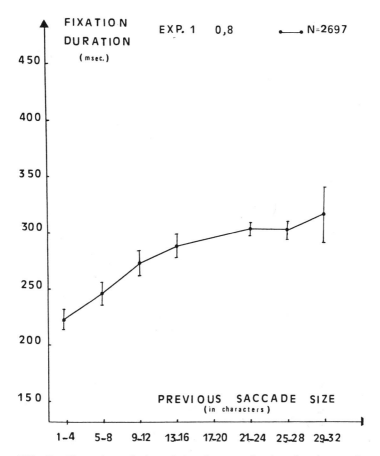

FIG. 3. Illustration of the relation between fixation durations and preceding saccade size. The abscissa shows saccade sizes in character spaces. On the ordinate is shown the mean duration of the fixations following saccades whose length fall in a given saccade class. The vertical bars indicate the standard deviation of individual means ($\sigma/\sqrt{N}$). The curve is based on 2697 fixation–saccade pairs.

centricities while the eye was fixated at the center of the screen. Figure 5 shows the results for each pair of symbols. The visibility of these symbols declines very fast and it attains chance level around two character spaces from the fixation point.

Therefore peripheral information was much more limited than found in Experiment 1. The hypothesis in these scanning experiments was the following: That because of the limited peripheral vision, except when preceded by saccades smaller than 2 letters, fixation durations should be uniformly long

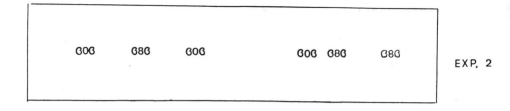

EXP. 2

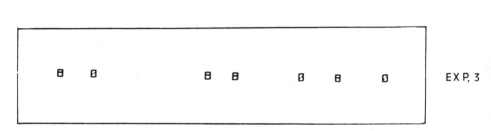

EXP. 3

FIG. 4.   Examples of lines used in Experiment 2 and in Experiment 3. In Experiment 2, the spacings between the target 0, 8 elements were also of 4, 12, 24 letter spaces.

In Experiment 3 the critical spacings were again of 4, 12, 24 letter spaces. The order of these spacings was also counterbalanced.

for all preceding saccade sizes. For this reason we don't expect a correlation between fixation durations and preceding saccade size.

Results

The results of the analysis were pooled for the same 5 subjects. Figure 6 illustrates the relation between fixation durations and preceding saccade size. Contrary to our prediction, we didn't obtain flat curves. Curves are not flat but their shape is not monotonous, for which correlation coefficients are not relevant. For homogeneity with the previous analysis in Experiment 1, we calculated the correlation coefficient. In Experiment 2, the values of this coefficient range from $+.1$ to $+.3$ for different subjects, and in Experiment 3 from $-.2$ to $+.2$. These values are lower and more scattered across subjects than in Experiment 1.

To understand more detailed aspects of these data, in the following study we examine the factors determining the length of fixation durations in each experiment, leaving for the moment the topic of the correlation.

STUDY OF THE LENGTH OF FIXATION DURATIONS
IN EACH EXPERIMENT

First of all, as can be seen in Figs. 3 and 6, fixation durations are longer for Experiments 2 and 3, where peripheral information is not available, than for the first 0, 8 experiment. These longer fixations could be interpreted to be due to the greater amount of foveal processing that must be done on each symbol when peripheral preprocessing is unlikely.

But the fact that fixation durations on the rectangular symbols (Experiment 3) are longer than those on the masked symbols (Experiment 2), sug-

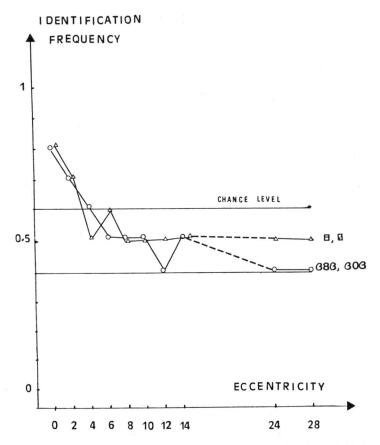

FIG. 5.   Identification frequency as a function of eccentricity for each kind of symbols. We performed the visibility experiment for each pair of symbols separately.

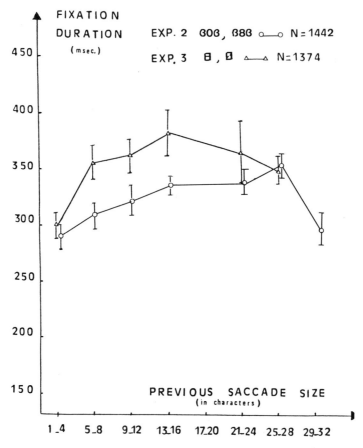

FIG. 6. Illustration of the relation between fixation durations and preceding saccade size for the "Mask" and "Rectangle" experiments. *N* indicates the number of saccade fixation pairs for each curve.

gests that this factor does not fully explain the effect. Fixation durations could also depend on the perceptual difficulty of each kind of symbol.

We performed a test experiment where each kind of symbol was presented foveally and measured the manual response time. As can be seen in Fig. 7, identification time is longer for rectangle symbols than for masked symbols. Identification time for masked symbols is longer than for 0, 8 symbols.

The fact that fixation durations in the corresponding scanning experiments present the same hierarchy suggests that fixation durations depend on the difficulty with which each kind of symbols can be processed. In other words, the length of time the eye remains on symbols depends on the processing done at the current fixation. This result favors the hypothesis according to which fixation duration can be controlled by ongoing information processing.

However, fixation durations could depend not only on the amount of processing but also on oculomotor factors related to the scanning strategies used by the subject.

Some recent data suggest that the duration of fixations is related to the accuracy with which the eye adjusts on the stimulus. Findlay's (1981a) data suggest that saccadic latencies are related to the fixation accuracy.

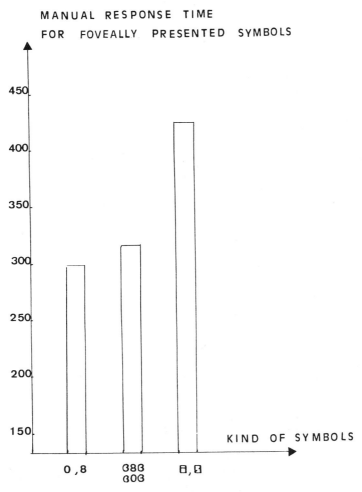

FIG. 7. Manual response time for each kind of symbols. In each experiment we presented only two symbols with an unpredictable order at the fovea for 50 msec.

These results show that the routine of eye adjustments used depends on the information available in peripheral vision: In the first experiment, where peripheral information is available, the subjects do not systematically fixate every stimulus element; elements are frequently skipped. However in the second and third experiments, where peripheral information is not available, the eye almost always lands on every stimulus element of the line. We counted the number of skipped stimulus elements and found that in the first 0, 8 experiment 15% of elements are not fixated, whereas in the experiment with masked symbols as well as in the experiment with rectangle symbols only 3% to 5% of elements are skipped over. This means that in these latter experiments, the oculomotor system calibrates its saccades *more precisely* so that the eye can land on each element of the display.

Bouma (1978), in a pilot experiment in which subjects had to fixate a series of dots spaced at a few degrees, found fixation durations 100 msec longer than that found in reading. He explains these longer fixations by the fact that a more precise *aiming* is required in such situations.

To check for the role of the aiming precision on fixation durations, we performed an experiment where the visual processing on each symbol was simple and had low variability. In this experiment we presented lines containing a series of crosses spaced the same as the symbols in the other three experiments. The subjects were instructed to fixate each cross *accurately,* moving from left to right while counting them.

We were surprised at the fixation durations observed. Mean fixation durations on crosses were 65 msec longer than on the masked symbols, 39 msec longer than on the rectangle symbols, and 100 msec longer than on the 0, 8 symbols.

These findings led us to question whether effects of aiming precision could be working in the other three experiments. In order to evaluate the component of the length of fixations that can be due to this factor, we performed the following analysis.

STUDY OF THE DURATION OF FIXATIONS IN ACCURATE AND INACCURATE FIXATION SEQUENCES

We started with only those fixations that were accurately placed on elements, and divided them into two classes according to the accuracy of the preceding and following fixations. The amount of visual processing was the same for the two classes of fixations. The only difference was the accuracy with which the eye fixated the preceding and the following stimuli. Figure 8a, shows the results of this analysis in Experiment 2. This figure illustrates the relation between fixation durations and preceding saccade size for each class of fixations. The solid line shows data for *accurate fixation sequences.*

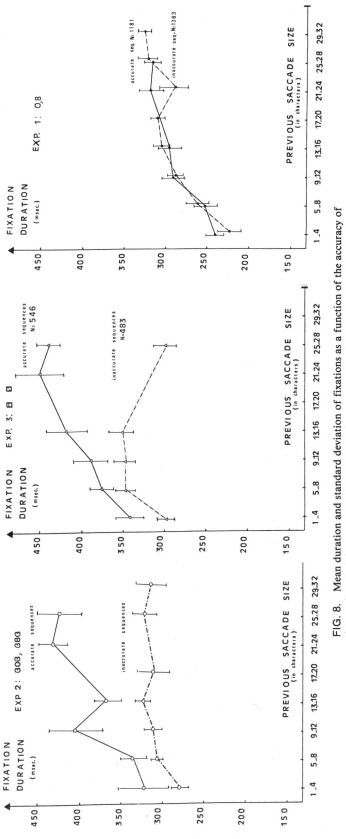

FIG. 8.   Mean duration and standard deviation of fixations as a function of the accuracy of the previous and the next eye adjustment. Both curves (solid and dotted lines) contain fixations placed on elements with an accuracy of ≤ ± 2 characters.

The solid line contains only those accurate fixations for which the preceding and the following fixations were also placed on the preceding and following stimulus with an accuracy of ≤ ± 2. The dotted line contains the fixations for which the preceding and/or the following fixations were not placed with this accuracy of ≤ ± 2 on the respective elements.

111

In other words, this curve contains only fixations on elements for which both preceding and following fixations were accurately placed on the preceding and following stimulus elements respectively. The dotted line shows data for *inaccurate fixation sequences*. That is, fixations accurately placed on an element but preceded and followed by fixations not accurately placed on the preceding and/or following stimulus elements respectively.

It can be seen that fixation durations are generally longer for accurate sequences, and increase as the preceding saccade size increases. On the contrary, fixation durations for inaccurate sequences are uniformly short for all preceding saccade sizes.

Figure 8b shows the same pattern in results of this analysis on the data obtained in Experiment 3: that is, fixation durations are generally longer for accurate sequences; and positive correlation is found between fixation durations and preceding saccade size for accurate sequences.

The general increase of fixation durations for accurate sequences, suggests that the length of fixation durations in these experiments, depends not only on the perceptual difficulty but also on oculomotor factors related to the accuracy with which the eye aims for the stimulus elements.

The correlation found for accurate sequences between fixation duration and preceding saccade size, cannot be explained by a preprocessing factor, because these symbols are indistinguishable in noncentral vision. The fact that we found this only for accurate sequences, suggests that the correlation might be caused by specific oculomotor factors involved in this type of sequence. The following considerations relate to this oculomotor factor: First, it might be that the eye's "settling time" is generally longer for accurate sequences and perhaps even longer after large saccades. Second, it might be that the time needed by the oculomotor system to prepare the next precise adjustment depends on the size of the saccade to be programmed. Perhaps the smaller this saccade is, the longer the oculomotor system needs, which is consistent with data presented by Vidal-Madjar and Lévy-Schoen (1980), suggesting that saccade latencies are longer for stimuli presented at 2.5° eccentricity, than for stimuli presented at larger eccentricities: 5° or 7.5°.

CAN WE EXPLAIN THE CORRELATION OBSERVED IN THE 0, 8 EXPERIMENT, WHERE PERIPHERAL INFORMATION IS AVAILABLE, IN TERMS OF PREPROCESSING?

The fact that a correlation between fixation durations and preceding saccade size was found in Experiments 2 and 3, where peripheral information is not available, throws some doubt on the explanation of the correlation observed in the 0, 8 experiment, in terms of preprocessing. Perhaps the first hypothesis of preprocessing is not the only one. The same oculomotor factor supposed to be involved in the other experiments could also have caused the correlation observed in the 0, 8 experiment. If this is true the same pattern would emerge for accurate and inaccurate types of sequences in this situation, as in Experiments 2 and 3. But if the pattern is not the same this would mean that preprocessing could be at work. To examine this hypothesis we applied the same analysis based on the separation of sequences of higher and lower accuracy. Figure 8c shows the results. Fixation durations for accurate and inaccurate sequences do not differ, but the correlation between fixation durations and preceding saccade size, for both, accurate and inaccurate sequences is verified.

These results suggest that the oculomotor factor supposed to be involved in Experiments 2 and 3 is not involved the same way in Experiment 1. So our first explanation of the correlation observed in Experiment 1 in terms of preprocessing, remains plausible.

Another argument in favor of preprocessing is the effect of peripheral preprocessing on fixation locations. In Experiment 1, the eye adjusts selectively on the target elements skipping over the non-target elements —19% of the skipped elements are non-target and only 10% are target elements. This means the stimuli 0, 8 used in Experiment 1, must have been processed from a distance. So we can deduce that the elements not skipped over could also be preprocessed but with less certainty.

CONCLUSION

It seems that the way the eye functions in Experiments 2 and 3, where peripheral information is not available, is different from the way it functions in Experiment 1, where peripheral information is available.

Particularly in Experiments 2 and 3, oculomotor factors are involved for the following reasons: The masked and rectangle symbols used in these experiments are processed with more difficulty than the symbols 0, 8 used in Experiment 1. The more the perceptual processing of a symbol is difficult, the longer the eye remains on it. This may be partly for maintaining the visual axis on the symbol and partly for programming a precise saccade allowing for fixation of the next element. These two factors may be active simultaneously.

On the contrary, in Experiment 1, the eye doesn't need to control at every instant the accuracy of the present adjustment nor the accuracy of the next adjustment. It seems that in this experiment, the eye moves without great constraints, guided at every instant by useful peripheral information. So both the correlation found and the tendency to more frequently skip over non-target elements suggest that in this case, fixation duration and saccade size can be immediately controlled by peripheral and foveal information processing.

Globally, our results suggest that: (a) The presence or absence of useful peripheral information determines two characteristics of ocular behavior: the time required for foveal processing, and the mode of scanning used by the subject. (b) Fixation durations depend on the amount of local processing, but also on the scanning strategies dictating the precision with which the eye adjusts on the successive stimulus elements.

ACKNOWLEDGMENTS

This work constitutes part of a PhD thesis done under the direction of Ariane Lévy-Schoen & Kevin O'Regan.

II.4 The Visual Control of Saccadic Eye Movements: Evidence for Limited Plasticity

John M. Findlay and Trevor I. Crawford
University of Durham, England

Saccadic eye movements are among the most common and most stereotyped behavioral responses made by human subjects. The eyeball presents a constant load to the oculomotor muscles and thus control may be made by means of a preprogrammed ballistic pattern of activation. The activation pattern is now well understood (Carpenter, 1977) and it is possible to model the flow of information occurring when the eye makes a saccadic response to a target appearing in the periphery (Becker & Jurgens, 1979; Findlay, 1981b). The presence of such a stereotyped system provides psychologists with a valuable "preparation" upon which to base investigations of behavioral plasticity like those found in attentional and expectation effects (Michard, Tetard, & Lévy-Schoen, 1974). This paper explores the extent to which practice can modify a particular aspect of the flow of information from visual stimulus to saccadic response.

A characteristic feature of human saccadic eye movements to targets that appear in peripheral vision is that saccadic response is generally directed by "global" aspects of the visual information (Findlay, 1981a; 1982, in press). Evidence for the assertion has come from examination of the amplitude of saccades generated when subjects are presented with two targets that appear simultaneously in the periphery. For targets appearing in this way either to the right or to the left, the first response of the saccadic system is to produce a saccade that directs the gaze to some intermediate point between the two targets. This may be followed by further corrective saccades but the first response is of considerable interest because of the implications for the way in which early visual information is processed. The size of the saccade can be systematically influenced by the properties of the target in a way that may be described as being directed to the "center of gravity" of the target configuration. This dependence of the "global effect" upon the visual characteristics of the targets suggests strongly that the site of the effect is within the stages of visual processing leading up to the effect response. Thus examination of the plasticity of this effect should throw light onto these processing stages.

A notable feature of the results on the global effect was that it appeared only slightly affected by the context in which the saccadic eye movement was made. Saccadic eye movements are best understood in a wider behavioral context as in an experiment reported earlier (cf. Findlay, 1981a). These first saccades, in a task that was designed to direct attention to target detail, were compared with those in which the same visual stimuli were presented but only the global aspects of the configuration were designated important. A small but significant difference in the first saccade amplitudes was found. Paradoxically, the direction of this effect was opposite to that which might have been expected. In the task involving target detail, the saccades to double targets showed a greater dependence on the global configuration, that is they landed further from the individual targets, than in the other task. This demonstrates that the global effect is not completely determined by the stimulus information and thus some plasticity can be expected.

The immediate consequence of the global effect is that the gaze is directed at some location *away* from the actual target. If two targets are presented, one at 5° and the other at 10°, the mean first saccade amplitude is about 6.4°. Thus, immediately following this saccade, the 5° target is seen at an eccentricity of 1.4° in peripheral vision. It is well known that visual acuity declines steadily with eccentricity in peripheral vision. However, the rate of this decline is relatively slow and many visual discriminations can be made when the stimuli are presented in the near periphery (cf. Bouma, 1970, 1978, and Widdel, this volume).

The situations in which the global effect was found in saccadic eye movements were made without any precise determination of the useful field of view for the discriminations concerned. Thus, it was not possible directly to state whether or not the saccades that land away from the individual targets were or were not *maladaptive*, that is, whether they took the eye to a location in which the targets were in a region of peripheral vision in which the discrimination was more difficult. However, an informal psychophysical study suggested that the gap detection task described in Findlay (1981a) could indeed be carried out if the targets were presented at 1.4° in the periphery. It was also found that some subjects performing this task showed a pattern in their response times that supported this possibility. Thus when a trial involved responding to a gap in a square at 5° eccentricity, responses were as fast as they were when there was also a square at 10° as when the 5° square was present alone, although in the former case the first saccades were landing away from the target. This suggests that with double square targets subjects are able to make an "attentional scan" of each target in turn, starting with the near one, which is unaffected by the eye misalignment. It is further possible that the globally directed saccades represented an attempt on the subject's part to produce an optimal strategy such as directing the gaze to a location in which both targets were discriminable in the visual periphery.

Consideration of these questions prompted the present investigation in which a task was devised insuring the global effect to be maladaptive. Preliminary studies demonstrated that a numerosity judgment task fulfilled the requirement for a discrimination where the useful field of view was confined to a narrow region around the fovea. The main hypothesis under investigation was whether the global effect could occur in conditions where it could be predicted that it would be maladaptive.

Additional questions related to the effect of practice on the saccadic behavior. If the subjects did produce globally directed, maladaptive saccades, would these eye movements change with experience on the task? Several possibilities were envisaged in which subjects might be able to voluntarily reduce or eliminate the global effect. For example, a reduction might occur in conjunction with an increase in saccade latency, since it has been demonstrated (Findlay, 1981a) that longer latency saccades show less global effect. Thus a form of speed–accuracy trade-off might occur (cf. the paper by Kapoula in this volume).

McLaughlin (1967) has shown evidence for plasticity in the system generating target directed saccades. He presented subjects with a target at 10° eccentricity and during the ensuing saccade, the target was moved to a new position 1° closer. With practice a subject changed the saccadic amplitude to 9.1°. Later work (Cavicchio, 1975) confirmed that this represented a parametric adjustment of the saccade "gain control."

THE FUNCTIONAL FIELD OF VIEW FOR THE DISCRIMINATION TASK

A number of preliminary studies were carried out in order to find a visual discrimination that could only be made close to the fixation point, and could also be generated on the computer controlled $X-Y$ display available. Eventually, the most satisfactory solution proved to be the task of numerosity judgment illustrated in Fig. 1. Brief presentations were made of dot micropatterns presented at a fixed location on a Tektronix 602 oscilloscope (spot size 0.5 min arc; spot luminance 400cd/m² against a background of 10cd/m² measured with a UDT photometer). Each stimulus consisted of a micropattern containing either four or five dots, always surrounded by a square frame. The dots in each micropattern occupied positions chosen at random from a 3 × 3 array of possible locations (certain combinations such as 2 × 2 clusters making 4 dots were eliminated). Examples of the stimuli are shown in Fig. 1. The separation of the dots in the array was 2.8 min arc and the length of the side of the square was 9.1 min arc.

The functional field of view for this discrimination was determined by a tachistoscopic procedure similar to that used by Bouma (1970). In order to allow an appropriate comparison with the eventual experimental situation, a procedure was used that gave the subjects minimum uncertainty about where the stimulus on a particular trial would be located. This was achieved by running blocks of 50 trials with the stimulus at the same position (i.e., the same side and same eccentricity) on each occasion. A fixation point was presented for 800 msec and following this the stimulus was presented for 100 msec. The subject was required to indicate with a forced choice response whether 4 or 5 dots had been present. A check was made for an-

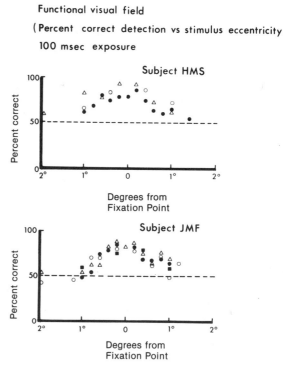

FIG. 1.   Plots of the functional visual field for the numerosity tasks for two subjects. Different symbols correspond to different sessions (in the order: filled circles; triangles; squares; open circles).

ticipatory eye movements by recording eye position during some of the blocks; no eye movements were found to occur. Thus the records give a true measure of peripheral discrimination capacities in the situation.

Figure 1 shows the curves representing the functional visual fields for two subjects (one being the author), both of whom possessed 6/4 vision. The curves are quite similar and show that the functional visual field is very restricted. Discrimination is substantially poorer at 0.5° from the fixation point and is almost at chance level at 1° from the fixation point. The curves appear quite reproducible and show little effect of practice. Those pratice effects occurring probably relate to the subjects' experiences of being able to "learn" the patterns of certain dot configurations. This was a possibility because of the constraints on the generation of the micropatterns. It may be noted that the narrowness of the functional visual field is largely attributable to the masking effect of the square surround; when tests were carried out without the mask the discrimination didn't change out to two or three degrees into the periphery.

The results demonstrate that the dot discrimination task is suitable for attacking the problem described above, namely whether the global effect with saccadic eye movements will remain under conditions where it will be maladaptive. If saccades direct the eye to a location that is one degree removed from such targets, it is clear that a large performance decrement would be anticipated, if the discrimination is carried out at the point where the first saccade lands. The possibility of second corrective saccades introduces a complication that might result in a response time rather than response accuracy effect, so regretfully the predictions are somewhat less clear.

EXPERIMENT TO INVESTIGATE THE GLOBAL EFFECT WITH THE NUMEROSITY DISCRIMINATION TASK

It has been shown in the previous section that the numerosity discrimination task is significantly impaired when the stimuli are presented as little as 0.5° away from the fixation point. Accordingly, the prediction may be made that if a situation is set up in which a subject's saccades take the gaze to a point at this distance, or further, from a target, efficiency will be impaired. The following experiment investigates this prediction.

The design was similar to that described in Findlay (1981a). On each trial the subject was presented with either a single or double target of the type investigated in the preliminary experiment. The subject used two response buttons and was asked to respond with one if a five dot configuration appeared, in either square in the case of double targets. The other button was used if a single target had four dots or if both squares in the double targets had four dots. All targets had the sizes used in the preliminary experiment (square side 9.1 min arc, dot spacing 2.8 min arc). The eccentricities used were 2° and 4°. Greater eccentricities were precluded by the range of the eye movement recorder being used. From the data reported in Findlay (in press) it can be deduced that, if the global effect is unaltered in the current task, the saccades in the two square configuration will direct the gaze to an eccentricity of about 2.8°. This region is where discriminability is low (see Fig. 1) for the 2° target and nearly impossible for the 4° target.

The stimuli were again presented on a Tektronix 602 display screen. Each trial commenced with the appearance of a fixation cross that remained visible until the subject lifted her finger from a hand key, when it disappeared and was replaced by the target stimulus. Trials were run in blocks of 64; the eight first trials were not analyzed and the remaining 56 contained 16 single 2° targets, 16 single 4° targets (in each case 8 having 4 dots and 8 having 5 dots), and 24 double targets (8 with 5 dots at 2° and 4 dots at 4°; 8 with the reverse, and 8 with dots in both positions).

The horizontal eye movements of the subject were measured using a development of the method described by Findlay (1974). Before and after each block a calibration record was taken. This showed that, with the exception of one block, the subject's eye position could be estimated with an accuracy of about 0.2°. However, the phenomenon noted in Findlay (in press) that intra-block variability in saccade amplitudes was less than inter-block variability again appeared suggesting that static calibration procedures may be subject to systematic errors. For this reason it was decided to use the amplitude of saccades to the single target squares as a baseline measure and the extent of the global effect has been assessed by comparison with this baseline.

Two subjects were tested, SC and AH, both female postgraduate students who volunteered to perform in a number of sessions. The subjects were introduced to the discrimination task by participating in a block of 50 trials of the preliminary experiment with the target eccentricity set at 0.2°. The procedure of the main experiment was then explained and the subjects were told that the experiment was concerned with their ability to improve the discrimination with practice. They were aware that their eye movements were being recorded but were naive about any details of the hypotheses under investigation. Two experimental blocks were then run and this was repeated each day for one week (the blocks on successive days are labeled 1A, 1B, 2A, 2B . . . etc.). This pattern was completed fully for subject AH (sessions 1A to 5B). In the case of subject SC, sessions 5A and 5B had to be postponed until the following week (5 days after session 4) and a further two sessions 6A and 6B were also run on the following week.

Results

Saccade Amplitudes. Saccade amplitudes have been plotted for the double square targets in terms of the percentage overshoot in comparison with the saccades to single 2° squares in the same direction. In effect this may be regarded as forming a calibration procedure in which the saccades to single square targets are used as the standard. Figure 2 shows the mean percentage overshoot for each subject as the experiment progresses.

Figure 3 demonstrates that the effect is systematic. It shows each individual trial in one of the blocks of the first session (Subject AH, Block 1B). It can be seen that with the double square targets, the variability in sac-

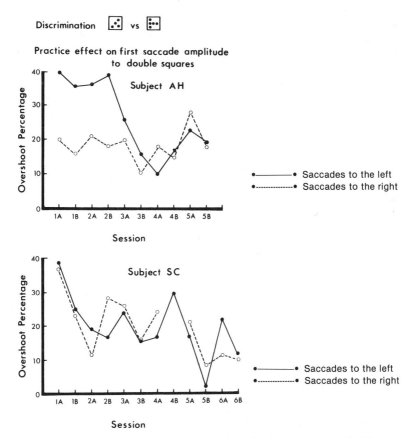

FIG. 2. Session by session variation in the amplitude of saccades to double square trials (one square at 2° and the second at 4°). The amplitude is expressed relative to the amplitude of saccades to single 2° squares.

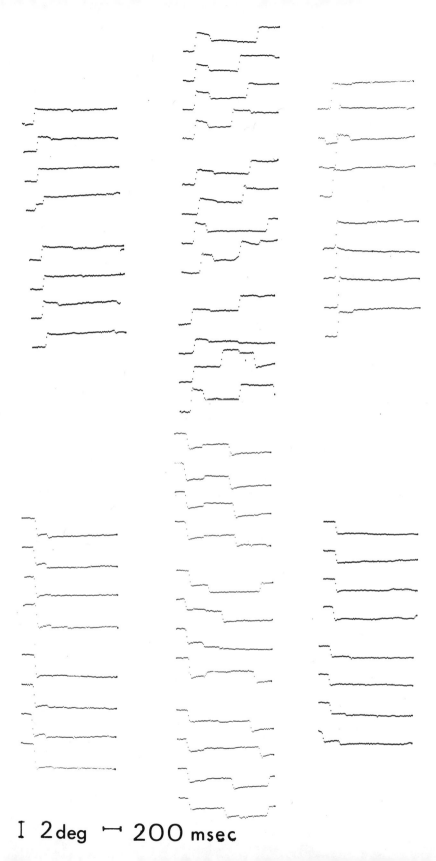

I 2 deg ⊢ 200 msec

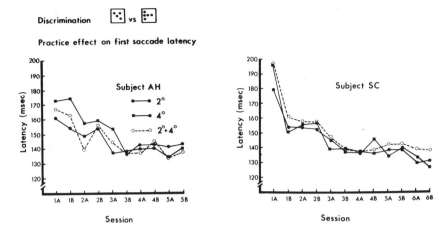

FIG. 4. Session by session variation in the latency to initiate saccades to the various target configurations.

cade amplitudes is slightly greater than for the single square targets. In the majority of cases with the double square targets, the first saccade is followed by a second corrective saccade back to the actual target position. An interesting feature that also may be noted in this set of records is that following the first saccade in the double square conditions the eye shows a systematic drift in the opposite direction. Since the first saccade is overshooting the near target, this drift may be similar to the effect reported by Kowler and Steinman (1979), that attending to a target in a particular direction will cause the eye to drift in that direction.

Saccade Latencies. Figure 4 shows the changes in mean latency that occurred over the course of the trials. Both subjects show a systematic decrease as the sessions progress. There are some suggestions of systematic effects of the stimulus configuration upon saccade latencies at various

FIG. 3. Complete records for one block (subject AH, Block 1B). The first column shows saccades to single 2° squares; the second column to the double squares and the final column saccades to the single 4° squares. Note the consistent pattern of overshoot and return saccades to the double square targets.

points (for AH latencies to the single 4° target is longer in the early sessions etc). However these effects are idiosyncratic and the data appear to be in accord with the position developed by Findlay (1981b), where a review of available literature suggested that no systematic effect of eccentricity existed on saccade latencies in the range of eccentricities from 1° to 20°.

Errors. Figure 5 shows the percentage of errors made on each type of stimulus as a function of practice. Both subjects made substantially more errors on the double targets than on the single targets. Only a small fraction of the differences can be accounted for probabilistically as a result of the fact that the a priori probability of an error is higher on double targets. If it is assumed that there is a constant probability, p, of making an erroneous discrimination with a single target, then the probability of making an error on double targets will be given by $2 \cdot p \cdot (1 \bar{p})$. (This expression ignores the possibility of simultaneously making an erroneous discrimination on both targets, the effect of which depends upon the target configuration; with the observed error proportions, this may be neglected). However, the differences in error proportions between single and double square targets are much greater than those predicted on this basis.

The initial hypothesis of the experiment was that with the double square targets, the globally directed initial saccades would be maladaptive and thus result in errors. If it is assumed that the subject processes the double squares at a perceptual level by treating firstly the near target and secondly the distant target, the initial maladaptive saccade should effect the processing of the near targets. This is supported by a breakdown of the errors made in the

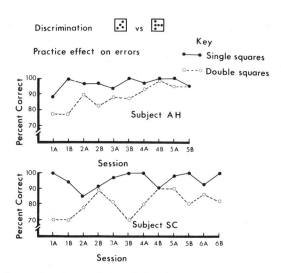

FIG. 5. Session by session variation in accuracy in the numerosity discrimination task.

double square configurations. In cases where the error consisted of a failure to detect a 5 dot configuration, it was usually the 2° target position. (Subject AH missed 10% of such targets in the 2° position compared with 5% of targets in the 4° position. Subject SC missed 30% of targets in the 2° position and 9% of targets at 4°.)

Response Times.   Figure 6 shows the response times (times for manual reaction) as a function of practice session. No clear pattern emerges from this analysis, other than the increased reaction times for double square targets, irrespective of target position. It is possible that the instructions emphasizing accuracy resulted in the subjects processing both targets even though a response could in some instances be made on the basis of the first target.

Subjective Reports.   Both subjects were aware of making errors in the early sessions. Subject SC, after four days practice, reported the following. "I have been trying in the last sessions to scan the targets more systematically starting with the near one. In the earlier sessions I found myself scanning in the other direction—I don't know why." Both subjects were surprised when eventually they were shown the pattern of their eye movements. It has been found generally that subjects are not aware of making the large overshoot and the corrective saccades when presented with double targets.

DISCUSSION

The experiment was designed to investigate whether the global effect in saccadic eye movements would appear in situations where precise fixations are necessary. It has been demonstrated that it indeed does. In the early sessions, when presented with a double square configuration, both subjects produced saccades that took the gaze to an intermediate target position (2.6°–2.8°). The magnitude of the overshoot in these sessions was close to that reported in other tasks by Findlay (in press). Furthermore, the results show reduced accuracy to be a direct result of the magnitude of the misdirected saccade.

Additionally, however, there is convincing evidence that the global effect is to some degree modifiable. Three of the measures taken show gradual and systematic changes with practice. Firstly, the overshoot shown in saccades to double targets decreases; secondly, the latency of initial saccades to both single and double targets decreases; thirdly, the subjects' discrimination accuracy improves. No consistent changes appear in the fourth measure taken, the discrimination time (manual response). However, this measure also shows high variability and since the instructions emphasized accuracy it seems advisable to disregard this result. Although it is tempting

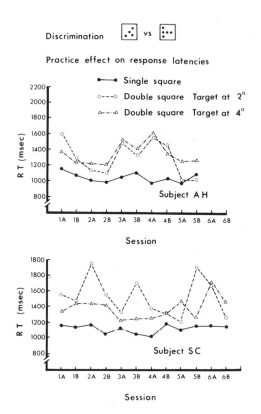

FIG. 6.   Session by session variation in response time for the numerosity discrimination task.

to attribute the improvement in accuracy to the more precise direction of the saccades to the double targets, this conclusion cannot be justified on the available data. The improvement in accuracy could simply be a result of increased practice with the discriminations necessary.

One of the suggestions made above was that subjects might reduce the global effect by delaying their saccades. It has been shown that the global effect is reduced for saccades with longer latencies and this has been confirmed in unpublished studies that show some voluntary control over saccade latencies. However, the present results show a systematic decrease in saccade latency occurring in parallel with the decreased overshoot. The steady decrease in latency is itself interesting. It has been suggested (Findlay, 1981b) that saccade latency is influenced more by non-visual factors, like the internal preparatory state of the subject, than by visual variables. The targets in this experiment were subject initiated, so it is possible that the effect resulted from improved familiarity with the properties of the control buttons. This might allow finer tuning of some general preparatory system.

In both subjects, continued practice resulted in a reduction in the over-shoot although neither subject eliminated the global effect. One possibility is that subjects learned to "recalibrate" their saccades in a similar, but more complex, way than that shown by the subject of McLaughlin (1967). Thus it is possible that all saccades that would have taken the eye to 2.8° might be redirected to (say) 2.4° without saccades to 2° and 4° being affected. The possibility seems unlikely, although regrettably no control of presenting single targets at intermediate positions between 2° and 4° was made. A more plausible alternative is offered below that relates to concepts of attention and accessibility.

The consistent finding is that when first encountering a task involving double targets, all subjects will produce saccades that appear to be responses to the overall target configuration rather than the individual targets. This result seems to be independent of the visual task. An interpretation may be offered in terms of current modeling of the visual system. A large body of work, following the early studies of Campbell and Robson (1968), has suggested that visual information is analyzed in a number of separate "channels," which are responsive to different spatial frequency ranges. The demonstration of the global effect suggests that under normal circumstances, the visual information used by the saccadic system is coming from channels tuned to low or very low spatial frequencies, which "see" the target pair as a single, unresolved pattern of activity. It is possible, however, for information of other channels to be accessible to the saccadic system and, possibly, for the low frequency global information to be disconnected. It appears that this occurs when the subject makes a conscious attentional effort to direct the eyes (cf. the report of one subject concerning scanning). This may correspond to a visual analogue of the well-known phenomenon in audition that a particular frequency channel may be assigned attention, resulting in improved detection for that frequency (Swets, 1970). This is somewhat different from the suggestions made earlier (Findlay, 1981a; in press) that the fine-grained information is simply not available until sufficient time has elapsed from the commencement of the stimulus. The weaker argument now appears stronger.

A final comment may be made on the relationship between eye position and visual processing. Although very fine control is possible in the positioning mechanism of the eye (Ditchburn, 1973), the demonstrations of this have generally required that subjects are explicitly instructed to fixate. In more dynamic situations, the positioning of the eye seems much less precise (see also records presented by A. Gale in this volume). Normally, subjects are unaware of the lack of precision because the difference between the gaze position and point of visual attention is much smaller than the functional field of view.

Effects on Eye Movement Functioning of an Oculomotor-Contingent Spatial Stimulus

II.5

Jean-Louis Kaufmann and Peter R. Coles
University of Geneva
Geneva, Switzerland

When recording eye movements the researcher is usually interested in one of two principal objectives:

1. as an end in itself, that is, in studying the biomechanical properties of eye movements
2. as an index of a presumed cognitive activity and/or the ways in which such activity may develop with age, practice, etc.

Although both areas of interest are seductive and have given rise to a large number of research projects and papers, the results of the second are frequently less clear and may even be contradictory (Sigman & Coles, 1980). One criticism of this approach is that intrinsic properties of the oculomotor system are usually treated as "noise," relative to the task requirements, which has to be eliminated from analysis (Pailhous, 1970). An example of this "noise" might be resting positions of the eye not directly related to information intake. Alternatively, the imperfect correspondence between "looking" and "seeing" complicates analysis of visual search tasks.

A compromise providing a mixture of the two areas concerns the "plasticity" of the oculomotor system and the extent to which its automatized functioning may be disrupted or modified. This theoretical position allows eye movements to reflect not only information intake, but also properties of the oculomotor system itself. A pathological example of plasticity might be seen in adaptations to oculomotor activity shown by patients with visual field deficits. Another example in normal life might be the deliberate "looking" with parafoveal or peripheral areas when fine discrimination is required in poor light conditions. The compromise approach allows us to consider the possibility that eye movements may themselves be the *object* of a cognitive activity and not simply the external sign of such activity (Pailhous & Bullinger, 1978; Mayer, Bullinger, & Kaufmann, 1979). This might be especially true during the initial phases of adaptation to a disruption in ordinary oculomotor functioniong. (Such an approach maybe applied to any sensorimotor system, not only vision.)

The experiment presented adopts this compromise position. We attempted to disrupt highly automatized oculomotor functioning by making stimulus presentations contingent upon eye position. This was achieved by dividing the stimulus field into two approximately equal parts with a virtual boundary between them. The stimulus stayed "OFF" if the gaze remained in the left half of the field and remained "ON" if the gaze stayed in the right half. Crossing the boundary caused the stimulus to appear or disappear depending on the direction of eye movement: toward the left turned the stimulus "OFF," toward the right turned it "ON."

In general it was expected that the eye movements recorded under these conditions would show disruptions compared to those under free or habitual conditions. Secondly, it was felt that a kind of exploration of the contingent rule might appear initially, for instance by frequently crossing the virtual boundary, as suggested by a previous pilot study (Kaufmann & Bullinger, 1980).

METHOD AND EXPECTATIONS

Eye movements were recorded using a version of the "bright pupil" technique. The X coordinates of eye position were used to control the stimulus presentations. This was achieved by on-line analysis of a video image of one eye at a rate of 10 Hz. A computer program analyzed the previously digitized video signal to determine the locus of gaze, control the stimulus presentations, and store the parameters of oculomotor activity—time, center of pupil, center of corneal reflection—for further off-line analyses. Given the precision of the eye movements apparatus and the inter-element distance of the grid of $4° \times 5°$ "squares", all fixations falling in a square were treated as approximately equal (i.e. biased by the exact locus). Ten children aged 5.6–7 years, ten aged 7.6–9 years and ten adults were examined. Because of technical problems and relatively uncomfortable conditions, particularly for the youngest subjects, valid analyses were possible for 5 of the youngest children (Gp. 1), 7 of the older children (Gp. 2), and 6 adults (Gp. 3). The subjects were seated on a chair with their head resting on a chin-rest in front of a stimulus subtending $+20°$ horizontally and $+15°$ vertically at a distance of 90 cm.

They were required to look at a configuration of identical elements (dots) in order subsequently to reproduce them, or for the youngest subjects, to recognize the pattern. This choice of pattern minimized the importance of individual elements but emphasized their relative spatial positions.

Subjects were told that they would see the configurations of dots in a peculiar way but they did not know that we had established a rule linking their oculomotor behavior to the appearance or disappearance of the stimulus. When the stimulus had been seen for a total of 15 seconds (20 for the youngest subjects), subjects were required to make a drawing of it from memory, or to recognize it among similar patterns. These were the *explicit* task instructions and it would have been possible to execute these without necessarily attending to the intermittant stimulus presentation.

However, it was expected that such an unfamiliar setting would lead the subject—or a least his oculomotor system—to explore the surroundings, either to understand the source of perturbation, or to accomplish the task efficiently. Such an exploration of the perturbation itself would constitute an *implicit* task requirement. In order to evaluate the extent to which this implicit requirement had consciously influenced subjects' behavior, interviews were taken after completing the drawings. The subjects were asked to tell us what they had done with their eyes and to comment if they could on the nature of the intermittance of stimulus presentation. The most important expectations were that for the implicit requirement:

1. Fixations in the "OFF" part would reflect a reaction of surprise or waiting, for example longer durations, less diffuse distribution.

2. There might be more or less systematic alternation between left and right parts of the field in order to explore the rule, or a concentration of fixations around the central border for the same reasons.

3. Towards the end of the exploration there might be more fixations on the right ("ON") part than on the left in order to execute the explicit task requirements.

4. Age effects might be expected on: (a) the explicit task because of incomplete elaboration of instruments for understanding spatial tasks and, (b) the implicit task because the child's body schema is less differentiated and so oculomotor activity will be less amenable to adaptation under cognitive control. In other words, the child does not know he moves his eyes in order to look and see and will be less inclined to change fixation.

In phase two, contingent displays were eliminated and subjects had to analyze other configuration of elements or dots and subsequently recognize or draw it. The stimulus was presented continuously for 5 seconds for the youngest subjects and, for those of Gp. 2 and Gp. 3, for as long as they required with a maximum of 60 seconds. Subjects were asked to close their eyes when they felt they could reproduce the stimulus adequately.

RESULTS

Free Versus Contingent. We will first examine some examples of exploration patterns during the free and contingent conditions. It should be pointed out that these patterns show high inter-individual variability. This is most obvious in the free condition (Fig. 1a, b) where exploration patterns are more or less diffuse, more or less close to the elements, as if guided by the structure of the stimulus field, and more or less redundant as previously identified by Sigman and Coles (1980).

Although the instructions given to the subject were sufficient to point out the object of the stimulus examination, that is, to reproduce it in a drawing, they were of no use in guiding the visual examination itself. Further, as pointed out by Pailhous (1970) the relevant information for the examination of spatial relations concerns the relationships between elements as much if not more than their exact positions. In other words, oculomotor activity could be oriented in different ways by the structured field.

As we can see in Fig. 2a and 2b there is a greater homogeneity in eye movement patterns during contingent conditions than during free conditions.

There seems to be a certain polarization close to the virtual boundary, but more "erratic" eye movements (relative to free exploration patterns) appear in the left or "OFF" part than in the right or "ON" one.

There are several explanations for the apparent polarization around the boundary. Subjects could use this location as a resting position when they have looked at the left-hand parts of the field and when the stimulus had disappeared. Alternatively, it could be a strategic position either to foveate the left "inaccessible" part when the stimulus appears by "chance" (due to oscillations of the regard around the boundary). Looking at the boundary area could also serve to keep the stimulus in privileged peripheral retinal regions.

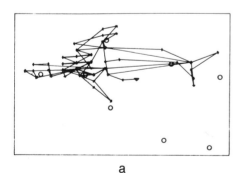 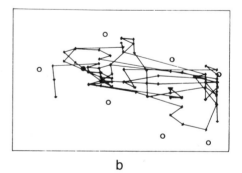

a   b

FIG. 1.   (A) Examples of free exploration by a child of 8 yrs and (B) an adult (○ = stimulus elements).

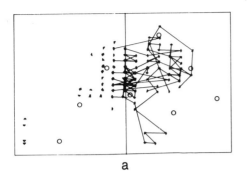
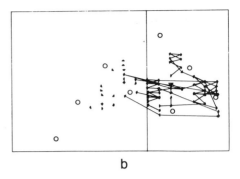

a   b

FIG. 2.   Examples of exploration with the contingent rule (boundary shown with vertical line) by a child of 7 yrs (A) and an adult (B). (Solid line = stimulus ON, loci only = stim. OFF).

With the exception of some of the youngest children, all subjects could reproduce something of what they had seen. Naturally their drawings reflected their cognitive level for analyzing such a spatial stimulus. The youngest subjects said they had seen a set of dots and their particular arrangement did not seem important (Fig. 3a). For those of Gp. 2 the arrangement became more relevant and even the need to use all of the space on the paper seemed important. Adults retained arrangement of dots and the overall shape of the configuration (Fig. 3b).

All subjects tended to begin their drawings to the left and reproductions were usually more diffuse on the left than on the right. We are unable to say whether this is due to writing habits or whether it reflects a salience acquired by the left half of the stimulus as a result of the contingent rule.

Since the youngest subjects Gp. 1 and 2 mentioned the number of elements as an aid to memorize the configuration, two independent judges coded the drawings. By qualitative examination, scores of fidelity were at-

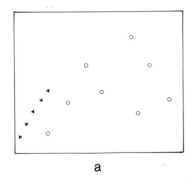
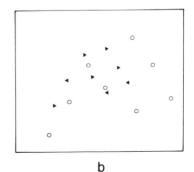

a   b

FIG. 3.   Examples of reproduction (▲) of the figure (○) by a child of 6 yrs (A) and an adult (B).

tributed regarding number of dots, relative position, whole shape of the configuration (cf. Table 1).

These general measurements seem to indicate that the youngest subjects did best on the contingent displays, adults did equally well on the contingent and free viewing and the older children did best on free viewing.

The scores in this table are group means and tempered by large intragroup variability and the fact that only four of the younger children reproduced the stimuli in both contingent and free conditions.

Interview

We have illustrated some general effects of the contingent rule. At which level of cognitive or sensorimotor behavior may the rule be operating? From the brief interview that followed each subject's visual exploration and reproduction there is no evidence that a conscious cognitive control of eye movements is working in this situation. None of the subjects was able to specify the contingent rule although one 8-year-old did say "I have to move my eyes and the stimulus appears." Two adults felt that there was a rule and that the appearance of the stimulus was not regular. One of them also said "It depends on the velocity of the analysis of my gaze." For the remaining subjects it was "the computer" or "chance" that controlled the appearance and disappearance of the stimulus.

PERTURBATIONS OF OCULOMOTOR BEHAVIOR

We found no evidence of conscious representation of either the rule or of the control of eye movements. Nevertheless the contingent rule did not prevent subjects from carrying out the task and did seem to modify the exploration patterns. The effects of the rule on oculomotor behavior may be seen in a number of parameters. First, we take the mean percentage of fixation in the left, center, and right parts of the field (cf. Table 2).

TABLE 1
Ratings of Fidelity Between Drawing and Model
(1: Good, 2: Partial, 3: Bad Fidelity)

| Age | Contingent | | | Free | | |
	number	position	form	number	position	form
Gr 1	1.5	2.3	1.7	2.4	2.8	2.6
Gr 2	1.4	2.7	2.4	1.5	2.3	2.0
Gr 3	1.0	1.7	1.4	1.1	1.6	1.3

TABLE 2
Mean Percentages of Fixations in 'Off,' Boundary, and 'On' Parts

Age	off	Contingent bound.	on	off	Free bound.	on
Gr 1	38	34	28	23	29	48
Gr 2	31	30	39	30	21	49
Gr 3	22	40	38	27	12	61

The comparison of the contingent conditions to the free one (analyzed as if it were explored with the same virtual boundary) reveals that there is a polarization in the "boundary zone" for all groups. The youngest children, whose fixations are less concentrated in the "boundary zone," attempted to look frequently at the "OFF" zone. Older children, on the other hand, tended to concentrate fixations in that zone equally in contingent and free condition. The adult's fixations seemed even to avoid the "OFF" zone of the field in the contingent condition.

These results suggest that under the constraint of the contingent rule the center of the field is a "privileged" place for the eyes, as here they may acquire a new function. It is possible that the nature of this function operates in different ways for each age group.

A second parameter revealing the effects of the contingent rule concerns the horizontal component of eye movements during exploration. The presentation of the stimulus in fact depends directly on this parameter. Figures 4a and 4b show examples of the horizontal components of exploration for one child of Gp. 1 and one adult respectively.

We may observe different kinds of interactions between the horizontal component of the eye movements and the contingent rule. The children oscillate between the "ON" and "OFF" parts and then stop at the boundary—especially when the gaze returns from the "OFF" or left part. This alternation seems more regular and appears after an initial period spent in the "OFF" part for children (Fig. 4a). For adults (Fig. 4b) there are more attempts to keep the stimulus "ON" especially towards the end.

When the eye movement records are collapsed to the X-dimension alone, an interesting result emerges for all subjects that is rather reminiscent of oculomotor patterns recorded with hemianopics. Movements from the right to the left part are more direct than those from left to right. Left to right (i.e., "OFF" to "ON") movements seem to be carried out as a series of small "steps." We measured the proportion of subjects showing stepwise movements in both directions (cf. Table 3).

The difference in the number of "steps" versus "direct" movements is quite large for all groups and strengthens the impression that oculomotor

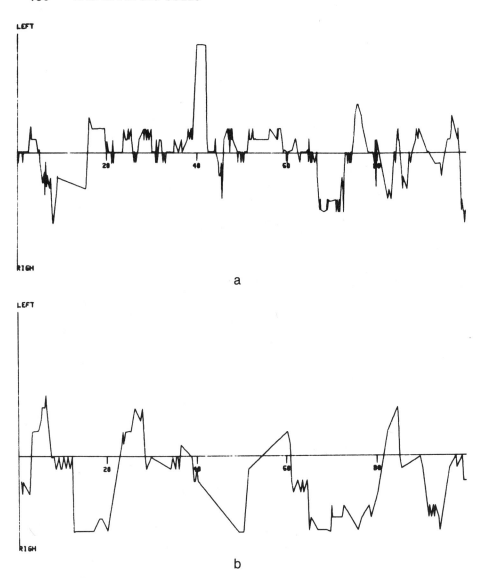

FIG. 4.   Horizontal component of eye movements over exploration time under the contingent condition by a child of 7 yrs (A) and an adult (B). (Numbers indicate percentages of exploration time.)

functioning is disrupted by the contingent rule. These two kinds of movement (direct or stepwise) are possibly due to the fact that from right to left (''ON'' to ''OFF'') saccades crossing the boundary are guided by visible elements of the stimulus. In the other direction (''OFF'' to ''ON'') this is no longer the case and the eye seems to wander or creep towards the center, without the support of visible stimulus elements.

TABLE 3
Proportion of Subjects Showing "Step" Movements According to Direction of Crossing the Boundary

Age	Right – Left	Left – Right
Gr 1	.25	.75
Gr 2	.28	.71
Gr 3	.28	.71

Saccade Amplitude and Fixation Duration. As discussed above, there are general effects of the contingent rule on the dispersion of fixation loci. It's of interest to speculate whether these effects are reflected by the saccade amplitudes and the fixation durations—both classical parameters of eye movement analysis. If so, would there be a difference between free and contingent conditions for example in "ON" and "OFF" parts? If there are modifications, do they differ between age groups?

Despite the small subject numbers and relatively weak differences on both parameters, it may be seen that the small amplitudes and higher fixation durations go together—in the contingent condition for the "OFF" part of the field. These findings agree with our hypotheses in as much as they suggest surprise or waiting states following the sudden disappearance of the stimulus.

Other data indicate a form of processing that analyses the left side of the field in a dynamic way starting from the right side and crossing the boundary, whereas exploration of the right side may proceed without such adaptations.

CONCLUSIONS

This experiment has shown that a disrupted environment has different effects according to age on oculomotor functioning. There is, however, no evidence for cognitive control of the observed modifications. The supposedly automatized functioning of this sensorimotor system is not drastically but rather only slightly modified. This may have been due to some kind of confusion between explicit and implicit task requirements. We believed that the visual effects of the contingent rule would orient the cognitive activity towards the rule itself and hence to the interaction of stimulus appearance and eye movements. Further experiments where the implicit task becomes the explicit one (i.e., "find the rule governing the appearance of the stimulus") are necessary in order to test this belief, and are now planned.

ACKNOWLEDGMENTS

This research was carried out with the support of the Swiss National Science Foundation (F.N.S.) Grant No. 1-828-0.78.

III PICTURE VIEWING AND VISUAL TRACKING

Know thou thyself: Presume not God to scan
The proper study of mankind is—man.

Alexander Pope (1688–1744)

One tends at first to divide scientific experiments into two types. In one type, (principally the experiments of physics and chemistry), the experimenter sets up precisely defined conditions which he chooses and then makes his measurements. He usually chooses conditions such that the interpretation of the results will be unambiguous and lead directly to new and precise information about the physical world. On the other hand the geologist and the astronomer have to accept the conditions which nature provides. In their main studies they can only observe; they cannot experiment.

The biological sciences form an intermediate type. The anatomist can cut 1000 slices from a brain and examine each one minutely in an electron microscope, but interpretation is seldom simple and unambiguous, and in any case he is experimenting on a dead brain and wishes to deduce something about the function of a living brain. The psychologist can do certain experiments (such as the determination of the absorption of light in the photo-receptors by Rushton, 1962) that are essentially physical or chemical experiments. These lead to fairly precise numerical results and the deductions to be drawn from them are fairly simple. In electrophysiological experiments on animals such as the experiments of Hartline (cf. Hartline, 1934) and numerous others on electric signals produced by vision, the experimenter wishes to interfere as little as possible with the normal life processes of the animal. Yet, in the higher animals at least, he must use anaesthetics and has great difficulty in establishing conditions for reproducible experiments—which are still representative of the normal nerve function of the living animal.

The psychologist is in a rather special position. He studies man, the human mind. He can choose at one extreme merely to observe behavior, being careful to conceal from his subjects the fact that they are being observed, or at the other extreme he can do laboratory experiments in which he endeavors to set up precise experimental conditions and to study the response of his subjects to accurately predetermined stimuli. This kind of experiment demands the cooperation of the subject who knows that he is under test. However willing the subject and however good his intentions, this cooperation is never complete. It is never like the cooperations that the chemist receives from his chemical balance.

Within the laboratory experiments, the psychologist has a further choice—whether to set up conditions of normal life using more complicated stimuli—with an inevitable difficulty in interpreting the more complicated results. Each of these conditions carries its own advantages and disadvantages, and it is probably essential that both types of experiment be done. My own prejudices are in favor of setting up conditions that are as precise and simple as possible. This is probably due to the fact that I spent nearly twenty years in pure physics before I entered the, to me, more treacherous ground of psychophysical experiments. Moreover, though I no longer experiment in physics, I retain a strong interest in certain branches of it, so the contrast between physical and psychological experiments is continually before me.

The authors of the first three papers in this section are concerned with different aspects of the survey of a picture. The first paper deals with the effect of eye movements on the alternations of an ambiguous figure. If I had wished to experiment on this subject I should have chosen the simplest ambiguous figure I could find—probably the Necker cube. The authors have chosen to study the much more complicated old woman/young woman picture. The second paper seeks to apply knowledge of scanning strategies to more uniform stimuli (i.e., X-ray chest plates) in an attempt to further examine the utility of teaching strategies that might optimize target detection. In fact, the results were mixed. First, with short learning times no differences were found between training and non-training groups in detection. Second, with longer training better detection occurred, but then the criterion was found to become lax, off-setting any benefits in performance. Certainly, better training and experimental controls are needed to verify these findings.

The third paper deals with the ability of subjects to survey pictures quickly and to recognize differences between somewhat similar pictures. Here again I would have chosen targets consisting of dots or patterns of arrays of simple geometrical shapes. The authors have chosen real life scenes and have created the differences by moving or removing some parts of the pictures. The results in each case are in a certain sense more interesting than those which would be obtained with the simpler figures, but in each case the conclusions require a certain measure of interpretation. There is some room for differences of opinion between experts on some points in the interpretation. The amount of work required to produce any meaningful results is very great and one may congratulate the authors on what they have achieved in experiments which are inherently very difficult.

May I suggest, in connection with visual survey experiments, the use of what may be called "imperfect stabilization" experiments. If, unknown to the subject, the position of the eyes can be monitored to about $10'$, the signal can be used to control a television display in which the subject is forced to direct his fovea to different portions of a picutre, the choice being made by the experimenter. None of the fade-out effects will be obtained (except in the peripheral field). Also, the subject may be placed under various handicaps, e.g., it can be arranged by manipulation of the electronics that either the central field is blacked out or that only the central field is seen. The picture may be made to drift across the subject's retina at any chosen speed. This has been done by Kelly and Burbeck for simple sinusoidal grating papers. The study of vision under the wide variety of experimental conditions which can be produced in this way should yield interesting results.

The authors of these papers recognize that when a subject fixates a certain point there is an area within which he can shift the center of his attention. In the early experiments on stabilization, we set up a target consisting of a line of print, and viewed it under imperfect stabilization conditions. It was found that, starting from the center, each letter could be read in turn by deciding to pay attention to it. Then, at a certain distance from the center, it suddenly became impossible to read the next letter. Similarly, with the Necker cube, it was found that if the corner was placed fairly near the center of the fovea, the alternations could be induced by deciding to direct the attention to the corner (even though the picture remained fixed on the same part of the retina). When the corner was too far from the foveal center, the attention could not reach it and no alternations were observed. May I suggest that there is a considerable opportunity for detailed study of areas of attention using what I have called the imperfect stabilization method.

The last three papers in this section are concerned with eye movements made when tracking a moving target. The paper by Bouis and Vossius proposes a new theory of the response of the eye when the target is gradually accelerated so that the subject has difficulty in tracking it with smooth movements. They propose that there is a high level decision whether to continue to use smooth movements as long as possible or to make a saccade. This decision is made so as to reduce the mean square error to a minimum. This is an interesting idea and I hope the present paper is only a preliminary to one in which the mathematical calculation will be completed and the idea developed more fully. I myself believe that when a target is accelerated the first reaction is to follow a little behind it and move the center of attention to the target position; as the target speed is increased the eye speed is at first increased, but when at some fairly high level it is realized that this tactic is going to fail, then a saccade is ordered. The size of saccade has to be calculated (which takes another 60 msec) and the calculation/organization process must take account of the increase of error in the interval between the decision for a saccade and the making of a saccade. It may be that the kind of mechanisms proposed by the authors enters into the decision about the time of the saccade, but I am not convinced about this.

The last two papers are concerned with the eye movements of schizophrenics and other mental patients when tracking a moving target. These experiments are beset with severe difficulties. The available number of subjects in each group is not large enough, the patients are all under treatment with drugs (it is not clear whether the dosage per unit body weight is the same for all patients), and whether normal cooperation is available must be doubted. The E.O.G. method of observing eye movements was used. It may be the only one possible for the patients but it is not suitable for eye-tracking experiments owing to its zero drift. It may indeed be that the patients are too anxious to cooperate, and come under a psychological strain as a result. There do appear to be differences between the results given by the patients and the results of some normal subjects. It is, however, impossible to say whether these differences are due to the illness, to the drugs, or to an overreaction caused by anxiety to do well in the tests. These difficulties are not the fault of the experimenters who have been unfortunate in that the differences found are fairly small and their interpretation is therefore extremely difficult. Perhaps the most important result is that the patients do track moderately well.

Robert W. Ditchburn

III.1 Eye Movement Patterns in Viewing Ambiguous Figures

A. G. Gale
Division of Radiology, University Hospital
Nottingham, England

J. M. Findlay
University of Durham, Durham, England

Interest in the role of eye movements in the perception of ambiguous and reversible perspective figures has existed for over 150 years (cf. Brewster, 1826). One major concern has been whether a causal relationship between an eye movement and the alternation of the figure could be established such that an eye movement necessarily precedes an alternation of the stimulus percept or whether an eye movement is simply the result of such alternation.

One of the first studies investigating eye movements was carried out by Flugel (1913) who used several reversible perspective figures and different viewing conditions. He concluded that eye movements were not responsible for the alternation as, for instance, when a subject was fixating on a point midway between two reversible perspective figures, it was found that they could reverse together and in opposite phase. According to Flugel, this should require two simultaneous eye movements in opposite directions. No direct recording of eye movements was made in this work, instead their occurrence was assessed by relying on the observer's introspective reports of the movement of an afterimage.

Eye movements were recorded by Zimmer (1913) who found that a movement occurred after a reversal was reported. His measurement technique has been criticized by Glen (1940) who, using an elegant recording method, found a low correlation between frequency of eye movements and reversal rate. Eye movements appeared to be distributed on either side of the reversal response. Glen concluded that a multitude of factors affected the relationship between eye movements and reversals. A similar conclusion was also reached by Wallin (1910).

Using the Schroder staircase figure, Sisson (1935) found that eye movements occurred both before and after a reversal took place and concluded, in a similar manner to Zimmer, that factors more central than eye movements are important. In a later study again with the Schroder staircase Pheiffer, Eure, and Hamilton (1956) found that reversals preceded an eye movement. More recently Flamm and Bergum (1977) using Rubin's vase and the Necker cube found that eye movements both preceded and followed reversals. Such previous studies where eye movements have been recorded have therefore produced inconclusive evidence about the necessity of executing an eye movement before an alteration of the stimulus occurs.

A second point of interest is in the fixation location of the observer as he views such figures. Sakano (1963), using a corneal reflection technique, examined both Rubin's vase and Boring's ambiguous figure. Different conditions of instructions were used, which elicited different scanning patterns (cf. Yarbus, 1967). Instructions to attend to one aspect of the ambiguous figure produced fixations in a restricted area of the stimulus, demonstrating that eye movements at least help to maintain the appearance of an aspect.

Evidence that individual differences in eye movement patterns exist was presented by Holcomb, Holcomb, and De La Pena (1977). They used Mach's book figure and the Necker cube, and on the basis of their results were able to divide their subjects into two groups of high and low scanners. This was based on their extensiveness of scanning, which was related to individual differences in motivational styles. Kawabata, Yamagami, and Noaki (1978) examined fixation locations of observers on the Necker cube and the Schroder staircase. These workers found that fixation position affected which aspect was reported as figure, explaining this in terms of the processing of local depth structures within the fixation region. A somewhat similar relationship between fixation position and aspect reported was found by Ellis and Stark (1978). A series of Kopfermann-like cubes were used and both the loci and fixation durations occurring during reversals were examined. Longer fixations were associated with reversals.

The finding that fixation position is related to the reported aspect is consonant with the view that perception is related to eye scanning (Hochberg, 1968). Most of these studies use techniques where the observer is aware that his eye movements are being recorded either by the rather obvious nature of the recording technique or by the use of calibration trials before the experimental trials take place. It may be that these procedures in fact contaminate the data by making the subjects aware of the experimenter's interest in his eye movements.

A difficulty for any theoretical approach arguing the importance of eye movements in the perception of such figures is the observation that reversals also occur when the eye muscles are paralyzed (Loeb, 1887; George, 1936; Zinchenko & Vergiles, 1972). This would appear to be strong evidence against the involvement of eye movements. However, Matin (1976) reports that in such conditions when the subject attempts to move his eye the visual field appears to move in the direction attempted, which may be related to the subject's intention to move his eye.

A second argument against the involvement of eye movements is that figure reversals still occur when a retinal image of a reversible perspective or ambiguous figure is stabilized. In one study Pritchard (1958) presented stabilized images of a Mach book figure and a Beaunis pile of cubes using a contact lens systems. Reversals were still possible although affected by where the subject was attending on the stimulus. This finding was later extended by Pritchard, Heron, and Hebb (1960) with a variety of different targets including the Necker cube with a target size of 2°.

Such results have been taken as evidence that eye movements cannot be related to reversals as any movements while viewing in such conditions will not produce a change in retinal stimulation. However the fact that reversals still occur in such conditions may be related to the slippage of the contact lens producing inaccurate stabilization, which is a problem with this technique (Pritchard, 1961; Barlow, 1963).

An alternative method for producing stabilized images that overcomes these possible problems has been to produce an after-image of the stimulus by using an electronic flashgun. Evans and Marsden (1966) and also Magnussen (1970) have used this approach and found that reversals still occur.

It seems reasonable to conclude that alternations can occur in conditions of such stabilization. In these studies the size of stimulus typically used is small, generally less than 5°, and it may be that with such small stimuli subjects can attend to different parts of the stimulus without the necessity of executing an eye movement. Few studies record eye movements in such conditions the main problem being that the resolution of many eye movement recording devices with such a small stimulus would result in an extremely crude data matrix. In recording eye movements there is trade-off between recording resolution and stimulus size. The small size of stimulus in stabilized conditions is generally in marked contrast to the larger size used in most eye movement studies.

In one study large stabilized images of several reversible perspective figures, 15°–25° square, were used and eye movements recorded (Zinchenko & Vergiles, 1972). Eye movements were found to occur in association with the reversals of the percept even though as these workers point out such movements were to no avail. This result suggests that the tendency to make an eye movement (which may be consequent on an attentional shift) in such conditions is the important factor (Hochberg, 1970a).

The ability to alternate the perception of stabilized images is hypothesized here to be a function of the generally small size of these stimuli, such that attention can be moved about the stimulus without the need for eye movements. When large stabilized images have been employed and eye movements recorded then movements have been found despite their futility. Thus it is proposed that the important factor in the perception of ambiguous figures in selective visual attention and the importance of eye movements lies in them being part of this attention process. Thus in afterimages or where the image is created post-retinally, as with stereograms, the observer is able to shift attention about the stimulus and so alternation occurs.

In an earlier study (Gale & Findlay, unpublished manuscript) Boring's ambiguous figure was presented to subjects as a large (36° × 28°) stabilized image so that subjects could focally attend only to parts of it. To facilitate good afterimage appearance, the ambiguous figure was first simplified to a line drawing containing 4 elements representing the facial features in the display. The line drawing and these elements are shown in Fig. 1. Prior to painting the afterimage of this stimulus, subjects sat in a darkened room and fixated a luminous point in one of several locations on the line drawing (Fig. 2). An electronic flashgun was discharged creating the afterimage of the stimulus. The results demonstrated that the response of old or young women to the stimulus was determined by the fixation position on the stimulus (Fig. 3). A fixation position near the YE element elicited more response of the young woman aspect (YW aspect), whereas a fixation near the M element gave rise to more old woman (OW aspect) responses.

When one or more of these elements were then omitted prior to painting the afterimage and the fixation position was also altered it was found that not only did the response depend on the fixation position but also on what elements were present near this position. This was taken as demonstrating that the response was dependent on what elements the subject could attend to in the afterimage. Fixation towards the YE element produced more reports of the young woman (YW) aspect, whereas fixation towards the M element produced more old woman (OW) reports. It was argued that the ambiguous figure could be considered as comprising elements that are differentially biased in their likelihood of evoking one or other aspect. The response of figure is thus largely dependent on which areas of the stimulus the subject is attending to. The use of a large stimulus in a stabilized condition enabled investigation of this selective process.

The term element is used here to refer to a line or collection of lines that together represent an identifiable attribute of the object represented by that stimulus. Thus, in a line drawing of a face, an eye will essentially be com-

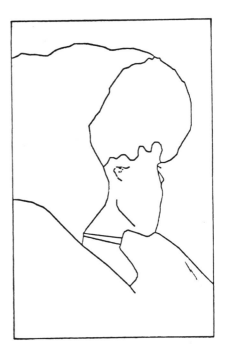

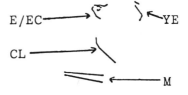

FIG. 1.   The line drawing of the
ambiguous figure with the 4 facial
elements detailed beneath.

posed of several lines, angles, etc., but these separate features together constitute an element, namely an eye, which is recognized. This definition comes close to that used by Kennedy (1974) in describing pictures and is similar to the "distinctive features" of real objects (Hagan, 1974). We have earlier presented a somewhat similar definition (Walker-Smith, Gale, & Findlay, 1977).

It is hypothesized here that the purpose of eye movements in a nonstabilized condition is largely to shift selective visual attention between such weighted parts. The problem underlying previous eye movement work with such figures is that the existence of any such parts had not been first established before eye movement recordings were made. Thus the need for a

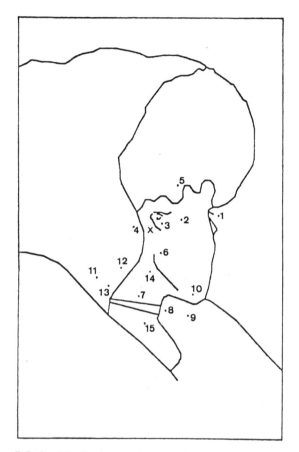

FIG. 2.   The fixation positions used in the afterimage study.

particular eye movement associated with alternation had not been adequately established. It is suggested here that the alternation of ambiguous figures occurs due to attention lapses, some of which involve re-interpreting an already fixated point in the display and some of which involve an eye movement and consequent new fixation location with no expectation of interpreting the stimulus elements at this distal location as one particular aspect. Thus eye movements will sometimes precede alternations and on other occasions there will be no such relationship.

EXPERIMENTAL INVESTIGATION OF EYE MOVEMENTS

The following experiment was designed to investigate the role of eye movements in the perception of Boring's ambiguous figure. To record eye movements without the subjects' awareness, an inconspicuous technique was developed. The ambiguous figure was viewed in various conditions and with different instructions. Subjects were first naively shown in the figure. They were then familiarized with both aspects to overcome any bias to perceive only the one aspect. They were then instructed to concentrate on one and then the alternate aspect. Finally after familiarization with the response procedure they were presented with different versions of the figure and asked to record their percepts.

The following hypotheses were investigated:

1. Controlled Viewing. The results from the previous afterimage experiment showed that a fixation near the YE element elicited more YW responses and a fixation near the M element elicited more OW responses. It was hypothesized that if a subject who could perceive both aspects in the stimulus was instructed to concentrate on the YW aspect then his eye movements would be localized around the area of the YE element. If instead he was instructed to concentrate on the OW aspect then he would fixate more toward the M element. Two relatively distinct patterns of fixations were therefore hypothesized to occur in these two conditions of concentrating on each aspect.

2. Fixation Locations. In normal viewing of the ambiguous figure for a period of time alternations occur. It was hypothesized that as the subject's perception of the stimulus altered so too would the subject's fixation loca-

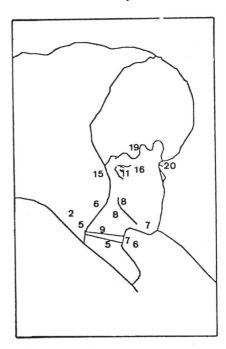

FIG. 3. The number of Young Woman responses (N = 20) elicited by each fixation position.

tions. The subject would fixate more towards the YE element as he responded YW and more towards the M element as he responded OW. The subject's response of figure would coincide with him fixating in similar regions as in the conditions of controlled viewing when he was concentrating on the same aspect.

3. Initial Percept. It is argued earlier that the response of figure depends upon the subject attending to certain stimulus elements. If the elements were then removed from the stimulus and the subject fluctuated between the two aspects then it was hypothesized that the effect of omitting the elements should be to affect the first response. If the response of OW is highly dependent on the presence of the M element then the absence of this element should elicit a first response of YW. Similarly if the response of YW is largely dependent on the presence of the YE element then the absence of the YE element should elicit a first response of OW. These two conditions come close to the biased versions of the ambiguous figure that have been designed to only elicit one aspect (Leeper, 1935; Neisser, 1967).

It is more difficult to predict a specific effect on the initial percept for the absence of the other two elements.

4. Alternation Fixation Locations.   Removing the elements from the stimulus raised the question of where do the subjects fixate when they perceive each aspect on such altered stimuli. If they generally fixate towards some element on the normal ambiguous figure as they are perceiving each aspect, then in the absence of that element do they fixate elsewhere or in the same region when making the same response? If a schematic map explanation for the perception of such stimuli is appropriate, then the subjects' fixation locations will not solely be determined by the stimulus attributes and so it is hypothesized that they will still fixate in generally the same stimulus regions whether elements are present or not.

In these conditions of one or all elements missing two explanations can be given as to why the subjects should still fixate in such regions. Firstly, the line drawing is simple and so a missing element area may be fixated as part of a search for this missing element. Alternatively the subject may actually need to fixate that part of the stimulus in order to respond to that particular aspect. Predictions can be made about the length of time spent fixating in such areas when an element is absent. If the former interpretation is correct and fixation time is dependent upon the surprise fact that the element is absent then longer time is predicted to be spent in this area. If the presence or absence of the element is of little importance (i.e., the observer's internal schema is driving his fixation position) then no difference in fixation time in this area would be expected whether the element is present or absent. If however the current stimulus information also affects the schema than it is predicted that a shorter time should be spent fixating in this region. Both of the latter interpretations are consonant with a schematic map proposal (Hochberg, 1970b) where the subject's map effectively tells him where to fixate so as to maximize the likehood of a response to that aspect.

5. Eye Movements and Alternation.   Examination of the eye movement immediately preceding an alternation response will allow an assessment to be made of whether a movement from one element area to another favoring the alternate aspect is necessary for alternation to occur. It is hypothesized that in some instances this will be the case but on other occasions such a movement will not be necessary. In these latter cases alternation occurs while the subject fixates the same general area of the stimulus. This follows a schematic map explanation where an already fixated stimulus part can be re-interpreted into the alternate map.

Subjects

Five undergraduate subjects took part. All were run individually and had volunteered to take part in an experiment on visual perception.

Apparatus

The apparatus is shown in Fig. 4 and consisted of a large viewing box with a rear projection screen at one end and a face mask at the other. A three channel tachistoscope was used to project stimulus slides onto this screen. A combination of chin rest and the face mask helped prevent large head movements. Eye movements were discreetly monitored by a multiple-source corneal reflection technique that is insensitive to the effects of small head movements (Cowey, 1963).

Four small infra-red light emitting diodes (LEDs) were positioned at the corner of the projected stimulus on the rear projection screen and served as marker lights for the eye movement recording technique. Two other infra-red l.e.d.s were positioned in the right eye piece of the mask and were used to increase the contrast of the pupil-iris boundary. A large half-silvered mirror immediately in front of the subject's position enabled a silicon diode television camera to view the subject's right eye at great magnification. In addition, the field of view of this camera also picked up a stimulus timer and response lights operated by two push buttons that were hand-held by the subject. Eye movements were video recorded for later analysis.

Stimuli

Seven stimuli were presented to subjects as rear projected 35 mm. slides. All stimuli were black line drawings. One of these was the line drawing of the face stimulus used by Noton and Stark (1971c). The others were versions of

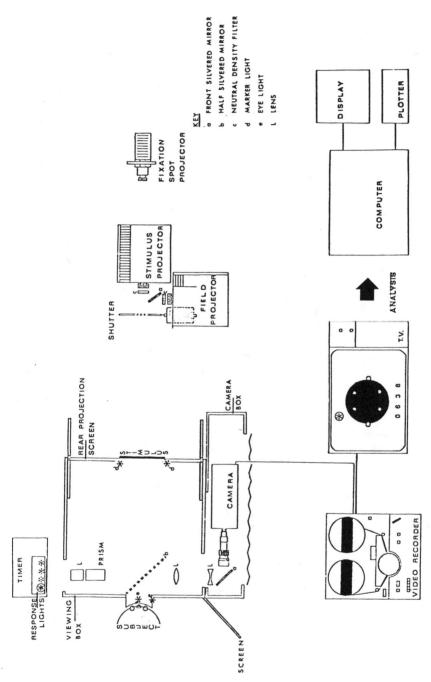

FIG. 4. The apparatus used to record the saccadic eye movements of each observer as they viewed the stimuli. The television monitor shows the pupil of the observer's right eye together with the corneal reflections of the four marker lights and the eye lights. One of the response lights is also shown.

154

the line drawing of the ambiguous figure. The six versions of this figure are shown in Fig. 8. They consisted of the normal line drawing, four versions each with one of the elements omitted and a version with all of the elements missing. The projected stimuli subtended $24° \times 16°$ at the subject's eye.

Procedure

Subjects were seated at the front of the viewing box where all the rest of the apparatus was hidden from view. Subjects were instructed that there were several parts to the experiment and that they would first be shown a sequence of slides and all that was required was for them to look at them. Each stimulus was then shown for 10 sec with a blank inter stimulus interval (I.S.I.) of 5 sec. During the last 1 sec of the I.S.I. a central fixation cross appeared on the screen which the subjects were asked to fixate prior to the next stimulus.

The first stimulus was the face stimulus followed by the full ambiguous figure line drawing, facing either left or right. After the second stimulus the subject was asked to describe it. Subjects were then shown a photograph of Boring's ambiguous figure and also asked to describe it. Both aspects in the figure were then verbally described to the subject in a manner similar to Leeper (1935) and the line drawing described as being derived from this photograph. The subject was then allowed a few minutes to practice alternating between the two aspects on the photograph.

Using the same procedure as before the full line drawing was shown twice and the subject instructed to first concentrate on one aspect for ten sec and then the other aspect, the order being randomized across subjects.

The subjects were then given the two buttons and instructed to use them to indicate which aspect they saw by pressing and holding down one button for each aspect. When it appeared as neither aspect then they were to press neither button. The subject was allowed to practice this response procedure while viewing the photograph of the ambiguous figure. Once subjects became familiar with this response procedure they were shown a series of line drawings similar to those seen previously and that instructed to indicate which aspect was seen using the response buttons. The six different versions of the line drawing were then shown. The first presentation was of the full line drawing and the rest were of the five missing element versions in random order.

After viewing these stimuli a calibration trial was run for each subject where a series of known points on a calibration slide were fixated, the subject using one of the response buttons to indicate when he was fixating each point.

EYE MOVEMENT ANALYSIS

Saccadic eye movements were analyzed by replaying the recorded videotape and examining the fixation location every .2 sec of recorded time. This analysis rate was modified either when the subject altered his response or blinked. Readings taken at the onset and offset of the response lights on the television monitor were corrected for the system response time delay due to the combination of rise or fall time of these lights and the recording television camera lag.

Two techniques of analysis were used, both of which related the pupil center to the corneal reflection of the four marker lights. The first technique employed fitting a series of concentric circles to the television monitor so as to give the pupil center. These circles were etched into both faces of a sheet of perspex and a no-parallax method used to give the best fit. A second perspex assembly contained a matrix that was then fitted to the corneal reflections of the four marker lights. A spatial coordinate reading of the pupil center was then obtained by ascertaining the pupil center with respect to this matrix.

An on-line analysis technique was also developed where the coordinates of the corneal reflections and points around the pupil edge were semi-automatically determined.

Fixation data from the calibration trial was used to establish individual correction constants that were then applied to the rest of that subject's data. This corrected for errors inherent in the corneal reflection technique of recording eye movements (Slater & Findlay, 1975). The resolution obtained with this technique had previously been estimated as 0.5°. The recording and analysis technique is more fully described in Gale (1980).

To offset a false saccadic rate in the experimental trials due to the data sampling rate, a weighted mean of sequential fixations falling within 0.5° of each other was used. This did not apply to any fixation involving a change in response or a blink.

RESULTS AND DISCUSSION

Naive and Single Aspect Conditions

The eye movement data obtained in the first three conditions of naive presentation and concentration on a single aspect are shown in Figure 5 plotted as arrows joining each sequential fixation position. A dotted line indicates a change in fixation location produced by a blink. The number of fixations falling within 1.5° of any part of the stimulus elements was also calculated by first estimating the fixation density per degree of visual angle.

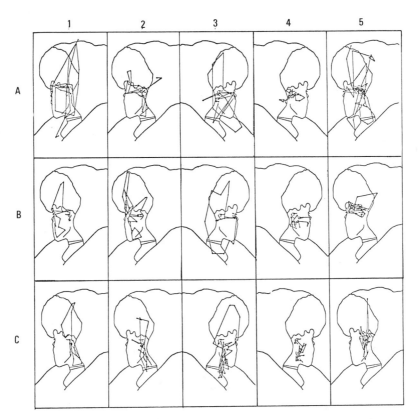

FIG. 5.   The saccadic eye movement patterns of each subject as they naively
viewed the abmiguous line drawing (A) and when instructed to concentrate
on the Young Woman aspect (B) or the Old Woman aspect (C).

An equal area around each element of $3° \times 3°$ was then taken to represent a
fixation falling on or near that particular element, which allowed for
measurement errors (Fig. 7). The number of fixations per element area is
shown for each subject in the graphs of Fig. 6 where it is expressed as a
percentage of the total number of fixation on that stimulus. The overall
percentage of fixations made by the subject in all four element areas is also
shown above each graph.

Naive Presentation

The first stimulus of a face was used to establish a set to perceive the subsequent ambiguous line drawing stimuli as faces. Eye movement patterns for
this initial stimulus are not presented here but demonstrated that subjects
fixated informative facial regions such as the eyes and mouth.

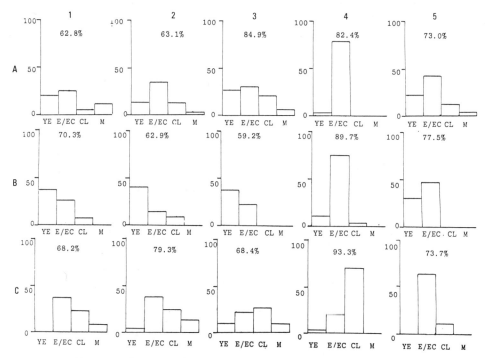

FIG. 6.   The number of occasions when each subject fixated within the four element areas expressed as a percentage of the total number of fications made by that subject in the three conditions of naive viewing (A), concentration on the Young Woman aspect (B) and concentration on the Old Woman aspect (C). The overall percentage figure for the fixations made in all four areas is also shown.

On the intial presentation of the ambiguous figure different patterns of scanning were exhibited by each subject. Fixations tended to concentrate on the eyes of the figure (Fig. 5a), as also demonstrated by the fixation density analysis in Fig. 6a. Such individual differences in eye movement patterns have also been reported elsewhere (Buchsbaum, Pfefferbaum, & Stillman, 1972; Walker-Smith, Gale, & Findlay, 1977).

Controlled Viewing

When instructed to concentrate on the young or old woman aspects, fixations were limited to distinctly different parts of the stimulus. For the YW aspect, fixations were generally made in the upper part of the face region with an absence of fixations near the M element (Fig. 6b). In contrast, when asked to concentrate on the OW apsect fixations were largely made between the E/EC and M elements as shown in Fig. 5c. Fewer fixations were made in the YE area (Fig. 6c) for each subject than in the previous condition. For two subjects no fixations were made in this area.

These results confirmed the first hypothesis in that two distinct fixation patterns were found when subjects were asked to concentrate on each aspect. These results also agree with those of Sakano (1963) who similarly asked subjects to concentrate on each aspect of this ambiguous figure.

Alternation Conditions

In the subsequent alternation conditions the fixation locations are shown plotted according to the subjects' response states (Fig. 8). When the subject alternated on the full line drawing fixations clustered around the four elements as shown in Fig. 8a. As in the previous two conditions the YW aspect was generally reported when the subject was fixating near the YE and E/EC areas with the OW aspect reported between the E/EC and M elements.

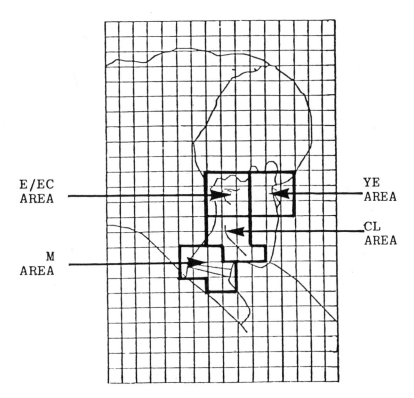

FIG. 7.   The four element areas used for the fixation density analysis. Each grid is 1° visual angle.

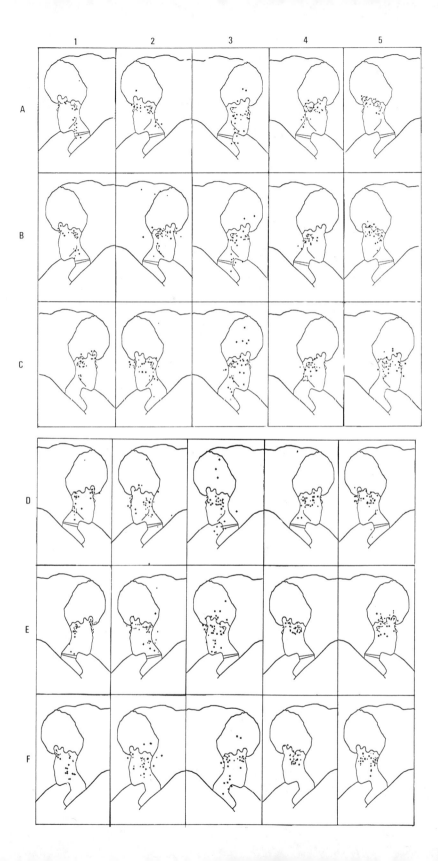

When one or all elements were omitted the majority of fixations were again largely made in the areas encompassing the four elements with YW or OW aspect reported in similar areas as in the previous conditions (Fig. 9). This result confirms the second hypothesis in that subjects still fixated in this regions and similarly reported each aspect as in the controlled viewing condition. Fixation location was meaningfully related to the response of figure.

Initial Percept

On the alternation conditions four subjects initially perceived the YW aspect on the full line drawing. When the YE element was omitted it was hypothesized that the subjects' first response would be as the OW aspect, in contrast three subjects first reported the YW aspect. This finding may be related to the fact that for these subjects the direction of their first eye movement was to the upper part of the facial area of the ambiguous figure. This finding of the YW response is then in agreement with the afterimage work in that the response was determined by the fixation location.

When the M element was omitted a first response of YW aspect was predicted. In contrast an OW aspect response was first made by four subjects. This was again in agreement with the stimulus areas first fixated by these subjects. Four subjects did not fixate in the M element area at all.

No such definite predictions about the effects on the initial percept of omitting the CL and E/EC elements had been made. In the absense of the E/EC element subjects still fixated in this stimulus area and for three subjects this was the area most fixated with two of them first perceiving the OW aspect. Only three subjects fixated in the CL element area when this element was omitted and two subjects perceived the OW aspect.

Complete absense of all of the elements elicited fixations in the regions of the missing elements (Fig. 8f) with four initial percepts of the YW aspect.

One of the characteristics of a schematic map is to tell the subject what to expect at some location and if this information is not subsequently found there then the map must be capable of alteration to accommodate this. The present results suggest that in the case of the different versions of the ambiguous figure the map did not change but rather acted to drive the subject to fixate a particular stimulus region whether or not the expected element was located there.

FIG. 8.   *(opposite page)* The fixations made by each subject in the six alternation conditions of: full figure (A), YE element absent (B), M element absent (C), E/EC element absent (D), CL element absent (E), all elements absent (F). Each fixation is shown plotted according to the subject's response: No response (.), old woman aspect (+), young woman aspect (×). The initial fixation position when each stimulus was presented is also shown (◊).

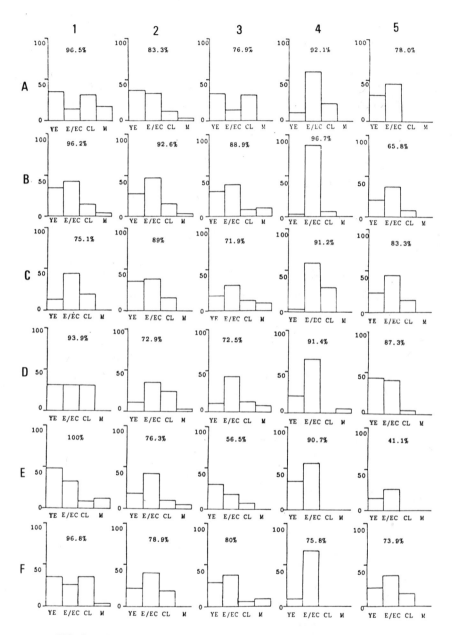

FIG. 9. The fixation density analysis for each of the six alternation conditions of: full figure (A), YE element absent (B), M element absent (C), E/EC element absent (D), CL element absent (E), all elements absent (F).

162

Alternation Fixations

When fluctuations occurred, fixations were subsequently made to an area of the stimulus as determined in the previous afterimage experiments that favored one or other aspect. Previous work in this area has attempted to determine whether a saccade precedes or follows a change in subjects' response of perceived aspect. As pointed out earlier, the "high probability areas" of a stimulus are typically not first established so that the occurrence of an eye movement to such an area cannot meaningfully be determined. In contrast such areas were ascertained here.

Subjects were instructed to report any fluctuations; they were not instructed to either "drive" the fluctuations as fast as possible or to attempt to inhibit them. The response technique allowed for the occurrence of a "neither aspect" response. From examination of the time course of the alternation conditions a NO aspect response was found to occur for every subject between response of YW or OW aspect. This would seem not to be a peculiarity of the response technique itself as several saccades were made during this period and individual differences were evidenced in the duration of such neither aspect responses. Such intervening eye movements where neither aspect is reported may represent "perceptual idling" as proposed by Hochberg (1970a).

The effect of removing each element upon the amount of time spent fixating in that stimulus region was examined. When the YE element was removed a significant decrease in the fixation time in this area was produced (t = 2.94, df = 4, p < .05) compared to the full ambiguous figure. This was accompanied by a similar decrease in the total amount of time spent reporting the YW aspect again compared to the full line drawing (t = 3.04, df = 4, p < .05). This was offset by a slight increase in OW response time. With absence of the M element no significant effect on fixation time in this stimulus area was found (p > .8). Compared to the full ambiguous figure absence of the M element did not produce a significant difference in the amount of time spent reporting the OW aspect but it did result in a significant decrease in time spent reporting the YW aspect (t = 34, df = 4, p < .05).

Absence of the CL element compared to the full figure did not result in a significant difference in fixation time in this area or affect the time spent reporting either aspect. A similar nonsignificant result was found for these variables when the E/EC element was omitted. However for four subjects the omission of this element led to an increase in the time spent fixating in this region. There was no significant difference in the amount of time spent reporting "neither-aspect" in each of the missing element conditions compared to the full ambiguous figure.

These results of no difference in fixation times in the element area when the element was omitted support the proposal that the perception of figure is highly dependent upon the observer's schema. The result for the YE element indicates that current visual information is also important. In the case where all the elements were absent it is difficult to understand how subjects can perceive both aspects in such a stimulus without having earlier seen the full ambiguous figure. Thus again recourse to an explanation invoking the subject's schema is appropriate in this situation. In this situation of all elements absent no significant difference in time spent reporting either aspect was found.

Eye Movements and Alternation

By examining the time course of each trial it was possible to isolate those eye movements which occurred when a change in response took place. This was when the subject indicated by his response the beginning or cessation of one aspect of the figure. These eye movements occurred at various locations on the stimulus and each individual exhibited some consistency in these locations over the different experimental conditions.

On some occasions before a change of response was made an eye movement occurred from one element area to another favoring the other aspect, but in the majority (68%) of cases a change of response was not immediately preceded by an eye movement from one element area to another. Most of these alternation movements occurred within either the YE or E/EC areas. Thus alternation can occur without a major change in fixation location first having taken place, although the finding of the intervening no response state between the two aspect responses complicates this.

One technique of changing fixation location was blinking, which was occasionally found for four subjects. This occurred both during a response of either aspect and during the change from one response to another. Blinking has previously been reported as a technique used by some subjects to alter perception of such stimuli (Wieland & Mefferd, 1967; Ammons, Ulrich, & Ammons, 1959).

A MODEL FOR FIGURE PERCEPTION

For each subject fixations tended to recur in similar locations. This is shown by the superimposition of fixations and by the percentage of fixations occurring in each element area. Such repetitive eye fixations have earlier been reported (Yarbus, 1967; Zusne & Michels, 1964). Noton and Stark (1971 a, b, c) have argued that such repetitive movements were related to the recognition of the stimulus. They proposed that the sequence of eye movements and fixation locations were involved in the representation of that stimulus in memory. This is rather like Hochberg's schematic map proposal, except that Noton and Stark argued that for the later recognition of the stimulus essentially the same sequence of eye movements and fixations (termed a scanpath), as performed by the subject when viewing the stimulus the first time, is executed. To allow for internal shifts of attention, the internal representation of the stimulus, a feature ring, was elaborated into a feature network with the scanpath being a preferred sequence in this network.

This scanpath proposal has not been without its critics (Spitz, 1971; Didday & Arbid, 1975). Eye movements and fixations may be involved in the representation of an object in memory (Loftus, 1972), but such movements are not solely determined by an internal plan as in Noton and Stark's theory. Elsewhere we (cf. Walker-Smith, Gale, & Findlay, 1977) have argued that the finding of regular scanning sequences in a face recognition task did represent some degree of structuring of the eye movements, but that this was not solely a result of an internal strategy determining the next fixation. Rather, it was proposed that current peripheral information executed some control over the next fixation location in interaction with the internal schema.

From the preceding results, the following conceptual model is proposed to account for the role of eye movements in the perception of ambiguous figures.

It is proposed that any two-dimensional representations of a real world object can be considered as a constellation of picture elements. These elements are themselves composed of one or more features as discriminated in the display by the observer. Each element is defined as representing some part of numerous objects in the real world. Thus each individual element can be interpreted by the observer in several different ways. Each of these possible interpretations can be assigned a weighting representing the likelihood that the element will be interpreted in a particular manner. This weighting depends upon several factors, such as the observer's prior experience with real word objects. The possible interpretations of each individual element are neither infinite nor made in isolation but are limited by the same factors that serve to define the possible ways in which the various elements represent parts of real objects.

A two-way process is then proposed to exist between the real-world expectations as they are applied to these elements, which themselves are sequentially attended to and abstracted from the display. The elements are both "fitted" into the expectations and the expectations partly govern the elements sequentially attended to. Norman and Rumelhart (1975) have made a similar proposal calling these two strategies "bottom-up," where the processing starts from the stimulus, and "top-down" where it starts from the schema. This is also essentially what is meant by Hochberg's (1970b) peripheral and cognitive search guidance. The importance of this two-way process is that the ongoing schematic map cannot only be modified by the stimulus information, as in Neisser's (1976) "perceptual cycle," but on occasions the schematic map can effectively over-ride stimulus data that conflicts with the map expectations.

Each interpretation of the stimulus is governed by a schematic map that functions as an expectancy testing program, predicting what will be perceived at various locations in the stimulus. Eye movements about the stimulus function to alter selective attention to different stimulus elements both in accord with expectation from this map and also as a result of current peripheral visual information. Thus eye movements are not solely determined by the schematic map, nor by the stimulus information, but by an interplay between both.

In Hochberg's (1968) theory each schematic map is considered to be a sequence of visuo-motor expectancies such that the intention to make an eye movement with a definite expecation is all important. Littman and Becklen (1976) have similarly proposed that eye movements depend on perceptual anticipation rather than acting to initiate a perceptual act. This meaning of schematic map is adhered to here although with experience or with small stimuli these expectations, and accompanying eye movements, may possibly become largely internalized shifts of attention as suggested by Noton and Stark (1971b). The schematic maps must be flexible to allow for the recognition of mirror-image stimuli or for stimuli of different magnification. The expectations of each map are ultimately governed by ecological contingencies; i.e., they depend upon the structure of the real world. In another context the role of real-world schemata in the recognition of pictures has been considered by Biederman (1972) and also Biederman, Glass, and Stacy (1973). Mandler and Parker (1976) have more recently demonstrated that such schemata affect memory for spatial relations.

The majority of ambiguous and reversible perspective figures are proposed to be represented by two almost equally plausible interpretations, two schematic maps, into which the elements can be fitted. Less plausible interpretations will also exist. For each schematic map, representing the two alternative aspects in these stimuli, the distribution of the element weightings is proposed to be spatially different. This distribution of each set of weightings across the stimulus can be likened to the contour lines on a map joining areas of equal bias towards one interpretation of the stimulus. For some stimuli the difference in this spatial distribution of bias toward each aspect will be small, whereas in other stimuli it will be more extreme.

For any give fixation point on the stimulus the observer will be able to attend to only specific elements. Other elements and features will be more peripherally viewed and will be more "globally" analyzed by the pre-attentive process during that fixation. For example, Biederman, Rabinowitz, Glass, and Stacy (1974) have shown that in a single fixation both particular elements and a more global characterization of the stimulus are extracted by the observer. The immediate response of figure when the observer views the stimulus will depend upon the relative weightings of the elements to which he can attend as they fit into each schematic map. At each fixation position the visual system is considered to apply a secondary weighting process to these elements depending upon how foveally or peripherally they are viewed. This secondary process will depend upon factors such as peripheral visual acuity, so that some elements may not need to be foveally fixated or alternatively elements may be "screened off" as not being important. The observer's response is proposed to be due largely to the sum of these weightings as they affect each alternative schematic map, with the map chosen by the observer as "figure" being the "best-bet" of all this information, which then creates expectations of how subsequently attended elements will be interpreted.

The stimulus area to which the observer can attend in a single fixation is proposed to be not simply that encompassed by the fovea. An essentially dual visual system has been suggested by several researchers with a foveal identifying system and a more diffuse peripheral monitoring and locating system (e.g. Trevarthen, 1968; Didday & Arbib, 1975; Mackworth & Morandi, 1967). While generally accepting this distinction, it is proposed that the observer can attend to an area larger than the fovea. This area is determined both by stimulus and observer parameters which together serve to effectively widen or narrow this attentive field. Mackworth (1976) has used the term "useful field of view" to define the area around the fovea from which information is effectively processed. This area is affected by the density of irrelevant items in the display (Mackworth, 1965; 1976). The amount of information being processed by the fovea also affects this "functional visual field" (Sanders, 1970) such that as the foveal load increases, this field shrinks (Ikeda & Takeuchi, 1975). Experience or training with the stimulus may overcome this shrinkage (Engle, 1971). Edwards and Goolkasian (1974) demonstrated that, with practice, observers could attend to objects peripherally presented and proposed several "fields" extending from the fovea to the periphery such that there was a general falling off in recognition, identification, and detection performance. Elsewhere Gould (1976) has used a zoom lens analogy to describe how observers can selectively attend to different sized areas of a display.

If the observer is free to scan the stimulus, then both peripheral information and the ongoing schematic map instigated by the first fixation (Chastain & Burnham, 1975) serve to determine the next fixation location. An eye movement (saccade) will be made to this location with an expectation, dependent upon the schematic map, of interpreting information foveally viewed there. Due to the ballistic nature of saccades an eye movement is made to informative regions (e.g. Baker & Loeb, 1973; Antes, 1974) as assessed by the peripheral processing during the present fixation (Gould & Dill, 1969). If the information at this fixation confirms or modifies the current map, then subsequent eye movements will be made with an appropriate expectation. In the free viewing of such stimuli the observer may make several eye movements before responding. This may reflect the testing of the schematic map over such fixations.

With ambiguous and reversible perspective figures, alternation occurs so that a different response of figure is given for the same stimulus. This is due to the current map faltering and an alternate one, representing a different stimulus interpretation, is then undertaken. This alternation may occur because the observer fixates an element that has a low weighting in the current map but a relatively high weighting in the alternate map. It may also be because of some form of local satiation that results in an already encoded element being re-interpreted. Thus in some instances eye movements will be made to an alternate element of the stimulus before a change of response of figure is made, and in some cases this change will occur with the observer generally fixating the same element.

A period between responding as either of the two alternate aspects may occur when the current schematic map has been relinquished and the observer is attempting to test the alternate one. This is suggested to be more likely to occur in stimuli in which the high probability areas favoring each aspect are relatively spatially separated.

This model, developed to account for the perception of figure particularly in ambiguous and reversible figures, is largely based on that of Hochberg (1968). It differs from this by proposing that more than two alternative maps can exist for such stimuli and by positing that stimulus parts can be weighted in such maps. In this latter respect it is like Chiang (1976). It further emphasizes the comparison between the ongoing map and the extracted stimulus information in which it is similar to Norman and Rumelhart (1975). The way in which the attended-to information can affect the schema has similarities to Neisser's "perceptual cycle" (1976).

ACKNOWLEDGMENT

AGG was supported by a Science Research Council Studentship.

III.2 The Utility of Scanning Strategies in Radiology

A. G. Gale and B. S. Worthington
Division of Radiology
Queen's Medical Centre
Nottingham, England

Efficient radiological performance requires the ability to readily appreciate what constitutes variations in normal radiological appearance as well as being able to identify the abnormal. Correct interpretation of normal appearances is confounded by the inherent ambiguity present in most radiological images due to their two dimensional representation of internal anatomy which necessarily results in structures overlaying one another. Such ambiguity can be reduced either by additional views of the patient or by alternative radiological techniques such as tomography. Nevertheless radiological diagnosis remains a complex pr' cess and has been shown to be subject to error rates as high as 20–30% (G 'and, 1959; Yerushalmy, 1969; Guiss & Kuenstler, 1960). Errors can occur either due to the inadequate registration of the abnormality by the imaging technique or in the interpretation of the medical image by the radiologist (Gale, Johnson, & Worthington, 1979). Suggestions have elsewhere been made for the improvement of radiological performance (Llewellyn-Thomas, 1969). One such suggestion has been the adoption of some structured approach to examine radiographs (Riebel, 1958) and in particular the chest radiograph.

The chest film is a good example of the complex radiographic image facing the radiologist and is the most frequent radiograph that the radiologist has to examine (Kendall, Darby, Harris, & Rae, 1980). The anatomy of the chest is typically treated in radiological textbooks as divisible into delineated anatomical sections which are each considered separately. These same texts extol the radiologist to use some form of routine systematic search in examining the radiograph (e.g. Sutton, 1980), especially when undergoing training (Armstrong & Wastie, 1981).

It has generally been argued that the adoption of such a set examination routine is necessary as this leads to the better and complete appreciation of the background radiological anatomy. Particular strategies for examination where each anatomical region is sequentially examined have also been proposed as shown summarized in Table 1. As is evident from this Table there is disagreement about the preferred order in which this examination should occur, and Armstrong and Wastie (1981) have recently suggested that the precise order is unimportant as long as some routine is adhered to. The lack of consideration of the technical quality of the film by some authors in the Table probably represents the assumption that this has already been accomplished by radiographers and other technicians rather than the assertion that this is an unimportant factor in radiological diagnosis.

This advice to examine radiographers in a particular fashion is contradictory to the evidence from various studies where the eye movements of radiologists have been reported. In these investigations attempts have not been made to differentiate fixations into the specific anatomical areas of Table 1. In most cases this would be difficult due to the overlaying nature of the internal structures, e.g., a fixation in the lowerleft lung field may represent examination of this area, the diaphragm, or of the heart shadow. Instead the analysis has been concentrated upon consideration of the general areas fixated or of the search patterns of the radiologist. These studies have singularly failed to demonstrate that practicing radiologists adhere to any common predetermined search strategy. Individual differences in scanning (Llewellyn-Thomas & Lansdowne, 1963) and non-uniform coverage of the film (Tuddenham & Calvert, 1961), together with concentration on particular informative areas of the film (Kundel, 1974) have all been reported. These findings demonstrate the similarity between radiological search and other picture viewing situations where parallel results have been found (see Gale & Findlay this volume).

The visual search pattern of a radiologist is affected by the prior clinical information given to him about the patient (Kundel & Wright, 1969) and is somewhat dependent on radiological experience (Kundel & La Follette, 1972). Three types of search pattern have been distinguished by these workers based on the grouping of fixations and extensiveness of scanning. A different type of scanning was exhibited by the same radiologist depending upon the experimental task (Kundel & Wright, 1969). Other work (Kundel & La Follette, 1972) has demonstrated the evolution from one type of scanning to another with increasing radiological experience. While we agree with their conclusion that the improvement of visual search of radiographs develops as a result of increasing radiological knowledge, the classification of the three scanning types remains somewhat arbitrary and worthy of quantification.

In summary, studies of the eye movements of radiologists demonstrate

TABLE 1

Some Suggested Routines for Examining Chest Radiographs. To Facilitate Comparison Purposes Some Condensation in Terminology Has Been Made

Simon (1967)	Fraser & Pare (1970)	Kreel (1971)	Meschan (1976)	Bretland (1978)	Armstrong & Wastie (1981)
1. Diaphragm	1. Soft tissues	1. Technical quality	1. Localize abnormality	1. Technical quality	1. Diaphragm
2. Sub diaphragm area	2. Bony thorax	2. Soft tissues	2. Diaphragm	2. Soft tissues	2. Heart and Heart position
3. Heart	3. Mediastinum	3. Bony thorax	3. Sinuses	3. Diaphragm and sub diaphragm area	3. Mediastinum
4. Trachea	4. Diaphragm	4. Diaphragm	4. Lung fields	4. Bony thorax	4. Hilar regions
5. Hilar shadows	5. Pleura	5. Trachea	5. Apices	5. Central shadow (trachea, mediastinum, heart)	5. Lung fields
6. Lung fields	6. Lung fields	6. Hilar regions	6. Hilar and Mediastinum	6. Hilar regions	6. Bony thorax
7. Bony thorax		7. Lung fields	7. Bony thorax	7. Lung fields	7. Technical quality
			8. Soft tissues		
			9. Sub diaphragm area		

the use of free search rather than the use of any systematic search pattern as proposed in radiological textbooks. Even the three types of patterns classified above do not represent such stylized patterns of examination. One of the problems of free search is that large areas of the radiograph are not foveally viewed even when relatively long viewing times are employed (Llewellyn-Thomas, 1968). This may be a reason why some abnormalities are missed which are readily seen in a second viewing (Gale, Johnson, & Worthington, 1979). The adoption of a scanning technique that ensures more foveal coverage of the whole film may lead to the possibility of detecting abnormalities which would otherwise be missed using free search. An approach like this was considered by Tuddenham (1962) as being of some possible utility particularly during radiological training.

In a different situation Townsend and Fry (1960) have demonstrated the feasibility of an automatic scanning aid in a task employing searching aerial photographs where observers had to detect Landolt C targets on a map. The scanning aid consisted of a 3° window through which the display could be viewed and which moved over the display in a prescribed manner. Observers had to follow the window as it traversed the display thus ensuring a more uniform display coverage than by free search. Such structured search, where the observers had to follow the window, was found not to be as good as free search when the targets were of a high contrast and thus relatively easy to detect. However, for low contrast targets, the scanning aid was found preferable.

One of the problems of a scanning device utilizing a window is that peripheral vision of the rest of the display is omitted and so may prevent the observer from readily developing an appropriate schema for the whole picture. In a task where the observer has to detect a Landolt C target this may not be important, but in a coin lesion detection task, peripheral vision is important in constructing an appropriate schema for the radiograph (Gale, Johnson, & Worthington, 1979). The role of peripheral vision in schema development in other tasks has been described elsewhere (Walker-Smith, Gale, & Findlay, 1977).

The following survey was subsequently carried out to determine whether it was feasible to train observers to use a predetermined scanning strategy which did not preclude peripheral vision and furthermore to examine whether its use led to better observer performance as measured by the detection of coin lesions.

Coin lesions or lung nodules are small and low contrast targets that are frequently used in radiological search tasks employing chest radiographs. These lesions can represent several diseases and their detection in clinical practice has been described as being "fortuitous" (Wright, 1973).

THE SEARCH STRATEGY

The first objective was to determine a suitable search strategy that possessed some radiological validity, and that could then be used in a subsequent experimental study of its utility. This was accomplished by carrying out an initial survey in which 13 radiologists were presented with an outline drawing of a chest radiograph which also had a central cross. The radiologists were asked how they would advocate searching for lung nodules starting at this central point. The results can be characterized as falling into five groups as shown in Fig. 1. From this finding a set of 8 lung field outlines were constructed. Each field was vertically divided into four quarters and the center of each quarter was depicted by a small circle. On seven of the drawings the circles were joined together to represent a particular order of scanning these sections. Five of these scanning patterns were based on the results of the previous survey. Two others were randomly constructed and the final one was left blank (Fig. 1).

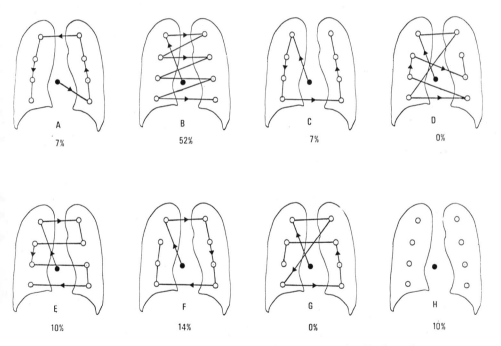

FIG. 1.   The lung field outlines with superimposed strategies. Versions, A, B, C, E, and F were drawn from the results of the first pilot study. Versions D and G were randomly constructed. The percentage of occasions when each version was selected in the second pilot study is also shown.

A second survey was then carried out where these eight drawings were circulated to the radiology departments of five hospitals. In instructions accompanying the form each radiologist was asked to indicate which pattern most typically described how he would search for lung nodules. Each circle was described as representing a general area of each lung field and the indicated search patterns represented idealized patterns of search, they did not represent a definite sequence of fixations and eye movements. Thus the topmost circle included search of the lung apices and the bottom ones included examination of the costophrenic angles. If none of the patterns was suitable, then the radiologists were instructed to draw their own version using the blank outline.

The results are shown in Fig. 1, expressed as percentages of the total number of radiologists taking part (29). The second pattern (1B) advocating a lateral comparative search process from top to bottom was the preferred one and was selected by 52% of the radiologists. Furthermore pattern 1E, which is a variant of this strategy, was selected by an additional 10%. This result is in agreement with the advice proferred on how to examine the lung fields and particularly the rib spaces advocated in radiological textbooks (e.g., Bretland, 1978). The blank outline was only selected 10% of occasions and the 2 randomly drawn patterns were not chosen.

EXPERIMENT 1

Having selected a suitable search strategy for examining chest films, one that could be used to train observers, the following experiment was carried out to investigate whether it was possible to train subjects to adhere to this strategy and furthermore to examine whether its use led to improved performance. The task was to detect coin lesions. This seemed an appropriate target to use as, due to its small size, foveation or near foveation is required. Kundel, Nodine, and Carmody (1978) have shown that 90% of nodules (0.8° in size) are detected by fixating within 2.8° of them. It was hypothesized that a scanning strategy that ensured better coverage of the film should lead to the detection of more of these lesions than in a comparable free search situation.

The detectability of coin lesions is related to their conspicuity (Kundel & Revesz, 1976) and so measures were taken to ensure a similar conspicuity for each nodule. Previous work has also demonstrated that rapid termination of search can occur upon an initial abnormality detection (Llewellyn-Thomas, 1969). To encourage subjects to continue searching past any first detection, which may in any case be a false positive detection, in order that their search patterns could be elucidated, a few radiographs were presented with 2 lesions present.

Subjects

Twenty third year medical students took part.

Apparatus

Normal postero-anterior (P-A) chest radiographs were presented to each subject via a television system that permitted the creation of artificial coin lesions (size 1°) that could be superimposed anywhere over a normal film. A 2 channel projection tachistoscope was used to present either a central fixation across or a normal chest film onto a rear projection screen. This was viewed by a television camera feeding a video mixer. A second camera similarly monitored an oscilloscope which also fed into the mixer. By creating spots of light on the oscilloscope and suitably mixing the two camera outputs, coin lesions of known size and brightness could readily be superimposed in some determined location over a normal chest radiograph. The composite picture was then viewed by the subject on a high definition television monitor. A microprocessor (Intel 8080) was used to control the experiment, create the lesions, and to record the subject's responses. The apparatus is shown in Fig. 2 and is more fully described in Gale, Johnson, and Worthington (1982). The clinical approximation of these artificially created lesions to real nodules had earlier been confirmed by a Consultant Radiologist.

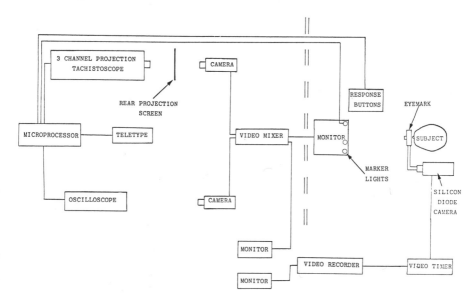

FIG. 2.   Schematic outline of the apparatus. (From Gale, A. G., Johnson, F., & Worthington, B. S., 1982, reprinted with the Editor's permission.

Both the subject's eye and head movements were monitored by a modified NAC Eyemark recorder. This device typically produces an image of the corneal reflection from the subject's right eye, of a small light source superimposed over the scene being viewed. In the present arrangement, the scene lens of the Eyemark was filtered so that only infra-red illumination from the environment was recorded in addition to the corneal reflection.

Small infra red light emitting diodes (l.e.d.s.) positioned above the subject's monitor were systematically flashed during the experiment at a rate controlled by the microprocessor. By means of a silicon diode television camera and associated tape recorder linked to the Eyemark these l.e.d.s. were recorded as additional points of light. The recorded location of these l.e.d.s. altered if the subject moved his head. By this means a record was obtained of both the subject's saccadic eye movements and also his head movements with respect to the display (Gale, Johnson, & Worthington, 1978).

Stimuli

Using direct copy film 35 mm. slides were prepared of 35 P-A male chest radiographs which had previously been adjudged normal by a Consultant Radiologist. Fifteen radiographs were randomly selected to be presented as the "abnormal" films containing one or two artificially created coin lesions. Of these, 5 were presented with 2 lesions present and 10 with 1 lesion. Fifteen others were selected to be presented as "normal" films, and the remaining 5 were used to familiarize subjects with the appearance of the nodules.

To determine the location of each nodule on the selected chest films, the experimenter initially viewed the subject's monitor, which displayed each of the "abnormal" radiographs in turn. Under microprocessor control, a coin lesion was then generated in the center of the radiograph. Using the subject's response buttons as digital positioning controls, the experimenter then moved the lesion to some randomly chosen location, the coordinates of which were then recorded. This was repeated for each of these radiographs in turn.

To obtain a similar conspicuity for each lesion a pilot study was performed where observers were presented with each of the radiographs in turn. A microprocessor program was run whereby these subjects used the response buttons to systematically increase the brightness of each lesion from an initial null value until they detected it. This brightness was then recorded. The brightness was then further increased and then decreased until the subject could just identify it and again the brightness was recorded. This procedure was repeated several times for each observer and a mean brightness figure for each lesion was computed. By this means a similar conspicuity for each lesion was empirically determined.

Procedure

The subjects were randomly divided into 2 groups. Each subject was first familiarized with the appearance of coin lesions. The subject was then seated in front of the television monitor so that the displaced radiograph subtended some 20° square. The Eyemark was then mounted on the subject's head and the subject instructed that he would be shown a series of chest radiographs, some of which would contain 1 or 2 coin lesions that could be present anywhere in the lung fields.

Each radiograph was preceded by a central fixation cross for 5 sec. During the last second of this ISI a warning buzzer sounded when the subject was instructed to fixate this cross. The radiograph was then presented for 10 sec when, if not already terminated by the subject, it was automatically terminated and replaced by the fixation cross. The subject then had to respond before advancing to the next slide.

Subjects had 2 response buttons with which to indicate their decisions about each radiograph. One button terminated the stimulus slide. The other was used to indicate lesion presence and subjects were instructed that they were to press this button when they were looking directly at what they took to be a lesion. If they detected more than one lesion then they were to press this again when they were looking at the further lesion. When satisfied that they had detected all the lesions present on the film, then they were to press the first button to terminate the slide. If they thought the chest radiograph was normal then they were to press the first button only which would terminate the slide.

The subjects were first shown the practice slides until they were familiar with the experimental procedure. After a short break the experimental slides were then shown, the slide order being randomized. For each trial the overall viewing time of each stimulus was recorded as well as the subject's decision about the slide. When the subject indicated the detection of a lesion, this response time was recorded and in addition one of the marker l.e.d.s was flashed to indicate detection of a lesion on the recorded videotape.

After completion of the experiment, a calibration trial was carried out where subjects fixated known points on a calibration slide and a program was run whereby these fixation locations were recorded without any intervening eye movements.

One week later, the subjects were again tested. Prior to this session the experimental group was shown a training videotape to encourage them to adopt the prescribed search pattern. Subjects in the control group received no such training but were given an equivalent amount of time to freely view normal chest radiographs on the monitor in order to equate both groups for viewing chest films prior to this session. Both groups of subjects were then shown the practice slides followed by the randomized experimental slides and finally the calibration trial as in the first session.

The training videotape first showed Fig. 1b on the subject's monitor. Subjects were instructed that they were to consider each lung field as comprising 4 quarters and that they were to follow the set pattern of search, starting from the center of the film and examining each quarter in turn. It was emphasized that the training pattern depicted a stylized pattern and did not indicate a sequence of specific fixations to be followed. The rest of the videotape contained a sequence of chest films alternating with this strategy and subjects were encouraged to practice the strategy on each succeeding film. The training tape lasted 2.5 min.

The experimental subjects were then instructed to adopt this search pattern on the experimental slides. If the subjects had completed the search pattern but wished to further examine the film then they were instructed that they could then search in any manner that they pleased. Conversely, if they were satisfied that the film was normal or that they had detected all the abnormalities present then they could terminate the film prior to completion of the complete search pattern.

EYE MOVEMENT ANALYSIS

The videotaped record of eye movements were input to a variable level video detector interfaced to the microprocessor (Johnson, Gale, & Worthington, 1978). This detected the position of the corneal reflection and the infra-red l.e.d.s and output both their spatial coordinates and the elapsed recorded time to a minicomputer (PDP 11/10). Further interactive analysis on this second computer enabled the recorded saccadic eye movements of the subject to be corrected for head movements by referring the corneal reflection location to the constantly updated position of the l.e.d.s which indicated the display position.

Corneal reflection errors were accounted for by relating the subject's fixation location during the calibration trial to the known position of each point fixated. Correction constants were generated from this trial which were then applied to the rest of the subject's data. Spatial resolution of this automated analysis technique is less than $0.25°$ and the accuracy of the Eyemark after correlation is better than $1°$.

Results

Search Patterns. No common patterns of search strategy were found in the eye movement patterns of both groups of subjects on the first trial. In contrast, the eye movements of the experimental group on the second trial demonstrated that these subjects did adhere to the prescribed strategy throughout the series of radiographs. Figure 3 illustrates this for an experimental and a control subject on both the first and second trial. Individual differences in these scanning patterns were evident even for the same subject on different films. No such overall common search patterns were evident in the eye movement records of the control subjects although 3 subjects on the second trial did tend to use some form of repetitive search strategy on a few of the films.

Subjects from both groups continued to examine the radiograph after detecting a possible lesion and rapidly terminated their examination of that film on detecting two lesions.

Detection Performance. The data was also considered in terms of the detection performance of the subjects. After training the experimental subjects made more false positive and negative responses than the controls although such differences were not statistically significant (Fig. 4). The control subjects on the second trial made more true positive and negative responses than the experimental group although the differences were again not statistically significant (Fig. 4). There were no significant differences within the two groups on either of the two trials.

Discussion

This study demonstrated the ease with which it was possible to train subjects to adhere to a set pattern of visual search. The prescribed pattern had been restricted to 8 generalized movements around 8 areas of the radiograph to aid this process. The experimental subjects after training used this pattern without difficulty throughout the series of radiographs.

Individual differences in such patterns were evident indicating that subjects were not learning the training strategy as a strict set of fixations and eye movements which would be evidenced as a repeatable scanpath (Noton & Stark, 1971c). In contrast, the role of current peripheral vision on scanning behavior was indicated by the variations in these generalized search patterns for each subject on different radiographs. That the experimental subjects did adhere to this strategy is somewhat contrary to the prediction of Llewellyn-Thomas (1969), who has argued that this is only feasible with a mechanical search aid.

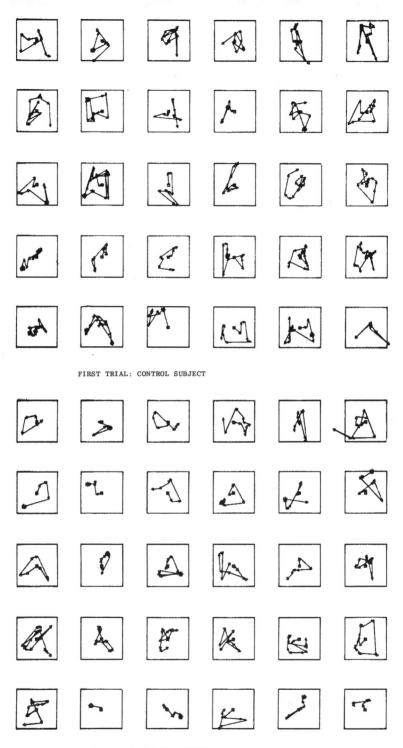

FIRST TRIAL: CONTROL SUBJECT

SECOND TRIAL: CONTROL SUBJECT

FIG. 3. Eye movement patterns for an experimental and a control subject recorded while viewing the 30 radiographs on both trials. For simplicity the radiograph facsimiles are not shown. Each square represents the projected stimulus area of 20° × 20°. An asterisk represents detection of a possible lesion.

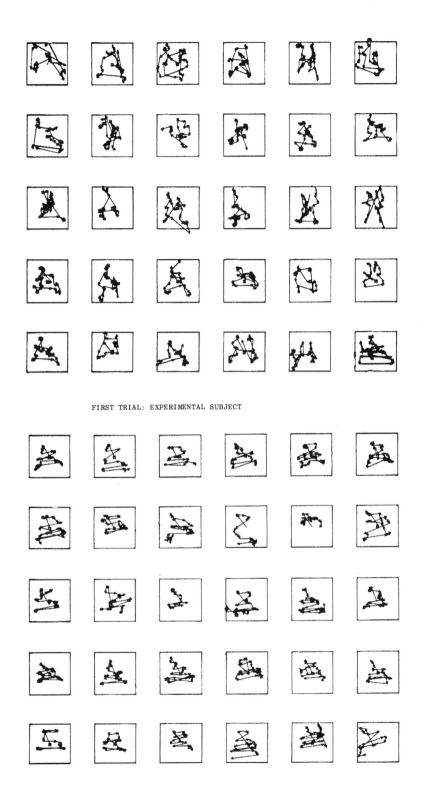

FIRST TRIAL: EXPERIMENTAL SUBJECT

SECOND TRIAL: EXPERIMENTAL SUBJECT

FIG. 3. *(cont.)*

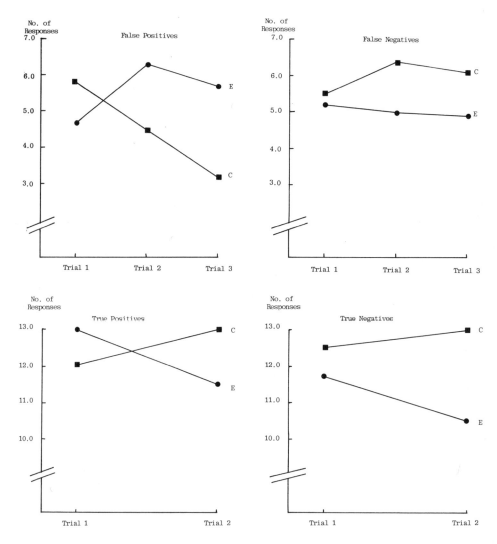

FIG. 4.   Mean number of responses for the experimental (E) and control (C) groups on both trials.

On detection of the first lesion, subjects did not immediately terminate their search, which is evidence of the role of the instructions concerning the possible existence of 2 lesions. On other tasks where a single lesion has served as the target, we have found rapid search termination and detection of the sole target. The purpose of the additional lesions was to encourage such additional scanning. Detection of a lesion did not affect the experimental subject's search pattern.

In performance terms the experimental group fared no better or worse than the control group, and, apart from the fact that the experimental subjects adhered to a set strategy of search on the second trial, there were no measurable differences between the two groups. If anything, the control subjects appeared to be performing better than the experimental subjects in that they made more correct responses (true positives and negatives). However the performance differences were not significantly different. In signal detection theory terms the two groups appeared to be operating with a similar criterion, but for the experimental group there was more overlap between the signal (lesion) and noise distributions than for the controls, i.e., the experimental group had more difficulty in actually discriminating the signal.

This may be for two reasons. First, the use of a search strategy, although feasible for subjects to follow, may not improve performance in terms of leading to a greater likelihood of detecting coin lesions. Thus, although a prescribed scanning pattern may result in ensuring foveal coverage of more of the film than free search, it does not result in better detection performance. The strategy used here was simple so that subjects would have little difficulty in remembering it. Within such bounds it attempted to encourage subjects to foveally view as much of the film as possible, although in this respect it did not go as far as Townsend and Fry's technique in virtually ensuring foveation of the whole film.

Second, the experimental subjects had to adhere to the search strategy and at the same time search for abnormalities. These two tasks may compete for attention allocation particularly given the relatively short amount of training. Thus although the experimental subjects could readily adhere to the general pattern, this was only attained at the cost of inadequately searching for lesions.

EXPERIMENT 2

To examine which of these interpretations was valid, the experiment was repeated with a third test session where the experimental group again trained in the use of the scanning strategy. If the performance of the experimental group on the second trial was affected by the problem of trying to adhere to the prescribed pattern and at the same time search for lesions, then this additional training opportunity should help to overcome this effect. In addition, a more detailed training videotape was used.

It was hypothesized that the experimental subjects would again adopt the scanning strategy. If structured search improves the detection of lesions, then the experimental subjects should make significantly more correct detections than the controls, particularly on the third trial.

If the experimental group in the previous study was affected by the difficulty in searching while using a search strategy, then this should be apparent here, and it was hypothesized that there would be an increase on the second trial in the response times to make correct decisions of normal or abnormal (lesion detection). These times should then decrease on the third trial as the subjects became more accustomed to the strategy. Furthermore, lesions positioned so as to coincide with the initial part of the strategy should be detected faster by the experimental group than lesions located in the lower parts of the lung fields which are examined later.

Subjects

Twenty staff members of the Radiology Department served as subjects. They were all familiar with the general appearance of chest radiographs but were not radiologists.

Apparatus

The experimental arrangement and stimuli were the same as in the previous experiment.

Procedure

The procedure closely followed that of the previous experiment. The subjects were first randomly divided into 2 groups. On the first trial both groups were familiarized with coin lesion appearance as well as the experimental procedure and were then shown the randomized series of radiographs during which their eye movements were recorded. This was then followed by a final calibration trial.

Prior to the second session, the experimental group was trained to use the scanning strategy. The training videotape first described the set pattern. This was followed by a series of chest radiographs alternating with the scanning pattern, as in the previous study, each radiograph being shown for 10 sec. Subjects were encouraged to practice the scanning strategy on each succeeding radiograph. Eye movements of subjects were monitored as they did this and positive feedback given if the general pattern of scanning observed on the experimenter's monitor approximated the set pattern. The final portion of the videotape showed several radiographs with the scanning pattern superimposed for 10 sec and these alternated with the central fixation cross. The subjects were asked to fixate the cross prior to scanning the next slide and were instructed to search the radiograph in the order shown. Again their eye movements were monitored as they did this and feedback of their performance given.

The control subjects spent an equivalent amount of time freely viewing the same number of radiographs for the same amount of time. No instruction to search the film in any prescribed way was given and although their eye movements were monitored as they watched the videotape no feedback of their search process was given. The training and control videotape both lasted 5 min.

Both groups of subjects were then shown the practice slides followed by the randomized experimental slides and finally the calibration trial was run.

The third test session was performed in the same way as the second session. Each session was carried out at weekly intervals.

Results

Eye Movement Patterns.   As in the previous experiment, there were no common search patterns evidenced between subjects in either group on the first trial. However on the second and third trials the experimental subjects did adhere to the general predetermined search pattern. Individual patterns of search were found, although the overall pattern followed the training strategy (Fig. 5). In contrast, no control subjects demonstrated any systematic search pattern on these trials.

Lesion Detection.   The results can be considered in terms of true and false positives/negatives as giving rise to a 3×3 matrix of 0, 1, and 2 lesions present/detected. Ignoring the data for the double lesions (as this gives rise to categories for both correct/incorrect detection), the detection results for the single lesions were examined and are shown in Fig. 6. There was a significant difference in the number of true positives (TP) responses made between the 2 groups on the second ($U = 18.5$, $p < .05$) and third trials ($U = 15$, $p < .05$) with the experimental group making more TP responses on each occasion. The experimental group also showed a significant increase in false positive (FP) responses ($T = 4$, $n = 9$, $p < .05$) and decrease in true negatives (TN) ($T = 4$, $n = 8$, $p < .05$) between the first and second trial.

The control subjects demonstrated a significant decrease in TP responses ($T = 4.5$, $n = 10$, $p < .02$) between the first and second trials and an increase in TN ($T = 6$, $n = 10$, $p < .05$) between the second and third trials. Comparing the overall difference between the first and third sessions, the control subjects showed an overall significant decrease in TP and FP responses ($T = 2$, $n = 10$, $p < .01$) and ($T = 6$, $n = 9$, $p < .05$) respectively with a significant increase in TN responses ($T = 5$, $n = 10$, $p < .02$).

Response Times.   The mean response times for both groups of subjects where they correctly reported the radiograph as normal (TN) are shown in

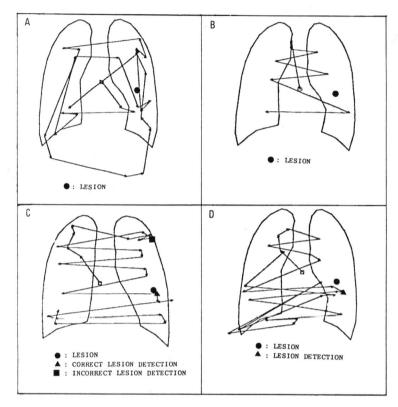

FIG. 5.   An example of the eye movement pattern of an experimental subject when examining the same film before (A) and after training (B) when the scanning strategy was used. In each case the lesion was missed. Further examples of the same subject examining other radiographs after training are shown in C and D. While in each case the subject uses the strategy, large differences in the precise eye movement patterns are apparent.

Fig. 7a. There was no significant difference between the two groups on each of the three trials but the increase in response time for the experimental group between the first and second trial was significant (T = 5, N = 9, $p < .05$) as was the decrease in response time for the control group between the second and third trials (T = 2, N = 8, $p < .02$). The response time data for correct detection of the single lesions was examined in terms of the time for the subjects to correctly identify the lesion and also the time for the subjects to then terminate the radiograph. These are shown in Figs. 7b and 7c respectively. In terms of the "hit" time there was a significant difference between the two groups on the second trial with the experimental group taking longer to correctly identify the lesions (U = 21.5, $p < .05$). The increase in response time for the experimental group between the first and second

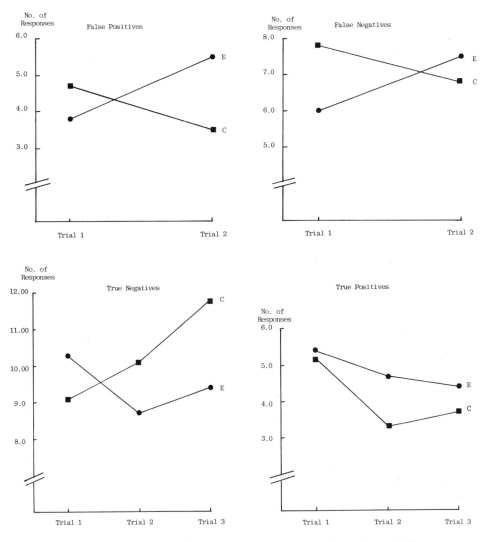

FIG. 6. Mean number of responses for the experimental (E) and control (C) groups on the three trials.

trials was also significant (T = 2, N = 10, $p < .01$). Also between the first and second trials there was a significant increase in the time taken for the experimental subjects to terminate the radiograph after they had correctly identified a lesion (T = 0, N = 10, $p < .01$). There was no demonstrable difference between the two groups of subjects on each trial in the time taken to correctly identify each of the ten single lesions.

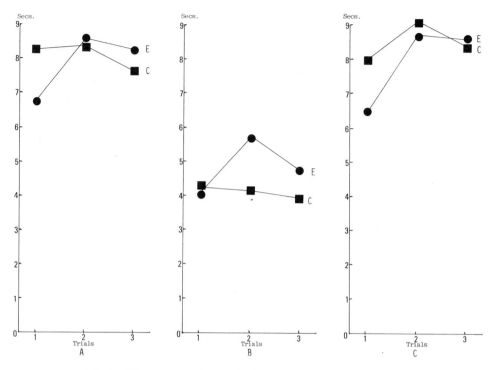

FIG. 7.   Mean response times for both the experimental (E) and control (C)
groups on the three trials. The true negative response times are shown in A.
The time taken to correctly detect a lesion and the overall viewing time of
such true positive detections are shown in B and C respectively.

GENERAL DISCUSSION

Both experiments demonstrated the ease with which subjects were able to
adopt a simple search strategy. The actual pattern of eye movements
evidence were subject to individual differences and demonstrated that the
search pattern was amended by the current visual information. These variations indicate that subjects cannot use a precise search strategy without
some artificial aid, although a simple pattern as employed in these experiments can be used.

The first experiment used a relatively short training session and found no
significant effect of the use of a predetermined search strategy. Indeed from
the pattern of results the implication was that the experimental subjects had
greater difficulty in discriminating the coin lesions than did a comparable
group of control subjects. When the experiment was repeated with a longer
training session involving feedback to the subjects and also the addition of a
third test session then somewhat different results were obtained.

In the first study after training the experimental subjects were making fewer TN and more FP responses than the controls. This was again found in the second study, both of these differences being significant. In contrast the controls made significantly more TN responses across the experiment and fewer FP responses. However, whereas the experimental subjects in the first experiment made more FN and few TP responses this pattern of results was reversed here on both the second and third trials. After training the experimental group detected significantly more lesions than the controls on both of the later test sessions. However, at the end of the third session both groups were detecting fewer lesions than initially, the controls significantly so. This may well reflect an increasing awareness over sessions of the similarity between possible lesion and other areas of normal radiographic mottle.

The overall pattern of detection results at the end of the second experiment imply that both groups of subjects had a somewhat similar ability to discriminate the lesions but that whereas the control subjects were using a rather conservative criterion the experimental subjects used a more risky criterion. Thus the short training resulted in difficulty for the trained subjects to discriminate the lesions whereas longer training largely overcame this but led to a more lax criterion of what constituted an abnormality.

The two experiments used different populations of subjects for reasons beyond our control. Neither of the two groups were radiologists. Nonradiologists were used as subjects because of the advocated use of a set pattern of scanning in radiological training. While this difference in subjects may underlie some of the differences in results between the two experiments, it is unlikely to be the sole explanation. Both groups of subjects were selected as having previous knowledge of radiological anatomy.

The present results seem to bear out that the poor performance of the experimental group in the first experiment was affected by the dual task demands of search and adhering to a strategy. This is supported by the significant increase in response time for the experimental group on the second trial both for true negative and true positive detections of the single lesions. For both these variables these response times then fell on the third session indicating some diminution of effect. Comparable results for the control subjects indicate a general decrease in response times for both variables over this period.

On both the second and third trials, control subjects were faster in correctly identifying normal and abnormal radiographs, although this difference was only significant for the TP results on the second trial. This is of importance in that these search times for the experimental group using a regular search technique were not half that of the free search group as predicted by Howarth and Bloomfield (1968). The systematic search did therefore not benefit the subjects in terms of these search times.

The time taken to abort the slide for a correct detection increased for both groups on the second trial, and, although this decreased on the third trial, it was still higher than initially. As a result of a general practice effect a decrease in this time would be expected. This increase indicates that the subjects became more aware of the need to continue search after detecting an initial possible target. This is not readily explained except for an increased general awareness in both groups of the possible presence of extra target-like areas and as such may reflect the downward trend in correct detections. The extra time taken to terminate the slide after correct detection had been made by the experimental group increased linearly across trials.

It was hypothesized that for different lesion locations a difference in response time would be found between the groups. Thus a lesion located in the top left of the radiograph should be detected quickly by the experimental group as they would arrive at this area first, whereas lesions in the lower regions should have a much longer detection time. In contrast, there should be no such ordered differences in the detection times of the controls. This did not prove to be the case. For all lesions the controls were faster at detection and there was no significant difference between the detection times of the experimental group for different lesion locations. The individual variability overlying the set scanning strategy would seem to have occluded any possible variations in these times.

After training, the experimental group detected significantly more lesions than the controls. This may be taken as indicating the utility of a scanning strategy for clinical use. However, this increase was only made at the expense of making significantly more false/positive and significantly fewer true/negative responses after the first training session than originally. Even after an additional training session there was little difference in these variables. These findings are in marked contrast to the controls who showed an overall significant decrease in false/positive and increase in true/negative responses.

Is radiological diagnosis best served by radiologists using conservative or liberal indices of abnormality present? In clinical practice false/positive reports may result in healthy patients having needless investigative surgery that is both costly to the patient and also in terms of hospital resources. On the other hand, false/negative reports have more effect on the individual patient as the early detection of an abnormality is postponed.

CONCLUSION

The adoption of a structured scanning strategy, although feasible, is not recommended on the basis of these results, as it leads to the rather liberal decision of what constitutes an abnormality. The suggested use of such approaches in radiological textbooks is not based on any evidence save possibly that of introspection.

Why should such an approach be risky if it leads to a more uniform coverage of more of the film? We have proposed elsewhere that visual search in radiology involves the matching of expectations about the medical image to actual stimulus information (Gale, Johnson, & Worthington, 1979). Such an approach has been well elaborated by Hochberg (1970a) and also Neisser (1976). The interaction between the selective sampling of the stimulus information which is directed by an appropriate schema and which is also capable of modification by the sampled information has been termed a perceptual cycle (Neisser, 1976). This would seem to provide an adequate explanation, in cognitive terms, of free visual exploration. However when trying to adhere to a predetermined strategy of search, the stimulus information is either prevented from or at least has a weakened effect upon the ongoing schema, which is itself directing the search. Thus, while individual differences in search patterns are found—evidence that information fed back from the stimulus is affecting the search pattern—the overriding general strategy remains unaffected. This then leads to a breakdown in the ability to adequately search. In particular, the need to compare a region of ambiguity (possible lesion) with surrounding areas and also normal areas elsewhere on the film is prevented, resulting in an increase in false detections.

Carmody, Nodine, and Kundel (1980) have recently used a technique where a chest film could either be examined as a whole or in a piecemeal fashion. The latter approach, when observers selected in what order particular segments of the film could be examined with the rest of the film occluded, led to an increase in false/positives. Viewing a segment prevented the observer from comparing that area of the radiograph with other areas just as in the present study adhering to a strategy prevented such comparisions.

The present strategy was stylized and simple to reduce memory load on the subjects. This does not however answer the question of whether a more complex search strategy would have been useful. It is proposed that the individual variations evident in the scanning records indicate that it would be very difficult for observers to use a more complex strategy. This is supported by other work where it has been reported impossible to teach observers to use a particular search pattern in a military context (Clare, 1979) where in some situations the use of a structured search pattern is considered optimal.

ACKNOWLEDGMENTS

We gratefully acknowledge the help of the following people. Dr. J. Pitfield assisted with the first pilot study. The first experiment was performed with M. Adams in conjunction with Dr. K. Millar. Our research assistant Mrs. E. Pawley performed much of the data analysis.

III.3 Eye Movements and Picture Recognition: Contribution or Embellishment

Dennis F. Fisher, Robert Karsh, Francis Breitenbach, and B. Diane Barnette
Behavioral Research Directorate
U.S. Army Human Engineering Laboratory
Aberdeen Proving Ground, Maryland

If we assume that all saccadic/fixation sequences are more or less encoded and stored for subsequent use, the daily task of eliciting about 230,000 fixations provides a formidable challenge for any system's capacity for recognition. This is not to deny the durability of the recognition process, as Nickerson (1965), Standing, Conezio, and Haber (1970), and Standing (1973) have demonstrated recognition for up to 10,000 pictures to be over 90% accurate. Although these high levels of recognition accuracy are impressive they may be challenged on the range of differences between these pictures. As in the case with similar words in verbal learning, the more similar the pictures, the more interference in recognizing differences between pictures could be expected.

While there has been substantial interest in the topic of eye movements and fixations in picture processing, most of that interest has been aimed at and biased by an a priori assumption that eye movements are essential for perception of pictures and hence, for their subsequent recognition. The bulk of the available empirical evidence seems to be aimed at verifying one of four possible purposes for the eye movement/fixation sequences. First, the maintenance of vision—that is, without eye movements, scenes and pictures fade from view. Second, eye movements and their fixations are directed by perception—that is, fixations fall on locations judged to contain high information like contours, objects, shading, or locations that have some overall semantic value. Third, eye movements and their fixations are responsible for perception—that is, they exhibit a psychomotor program, or schema related to the particular picture or scene being viewed. This program may be scene specific but it is generally considered a reflection of the viewer's cognitive strategy. And fourth, the eye movement/fixation sequence allows for the encoding, storing, and subsequent reconstruction of the retinal images of specific surface details of the scene or picture.

The purpose of the present chapter is to re-evaluate the role of saccades and fixations during recognition, not from the standpoint of challenging their normal occurrence, but as a challenge to assumptions about the essential nature of the fixation/saccadic sequences to the recognition process. To mount this challenge, two variables need to be examined. These are the temporal factors in viewing and the spatial scatter of the fixations.

TEMPORAL FACTORS

Intraub (1980, 1981) used a technique devised by Potter (1975, 1976) in which different pictures were shown on successive movie frames at rates of 113 msec to 245 msec per picture, speeds too fast to allow for eye movements to occur. She found 60% accuracy when subjects were asked to identify/detect a target picture by name or by class, 35% accuracy when they were asked to find a non-category, "target is not a food," but only 11% were remembered. It is her contention that the high degree of identification possible with these rapidly presented pictures is due to each being momentarily "understood" at the time of viewing but then forgotten. For her, the source of interference is not at the identification level but at the encoding level necessary for retention. These data then might indicate that the detection processes seem to be quite durable and selective even at these very rapid rates, but that the memory processes are very volatile, demanding multiple or overlapping subsequent views, hence the necessity of additional eye movements/fixations to enhance that memory.

Loftus and Kallman (1979) exposed pictures from 50 to 1000 msec to a detail-naming group and a non-naming group and found that occasionally some detail could be named but primarily it is the general visual information or *gist* that is recalled. In a subsequent experiment Nelson and Loftus (1980) monitored eye movements while exposing stimuli from 750 to 3000 msec, then subjects examined pairs of stimuli to find the previously seen picture. They found that there was increased probability of encoding detail with each successive unit of time which in effect produced a greater likelihood of finding critical features, essential for recognition, as time progressed. They also concluded that it is quite unlikely that specific detail is encoded in the more rapid presentations. More recent support was provided for this view by Loftus (1981) when attempting to tachistoscopically mimic fixations. Little or no improvement was found for multiple 50 msec flashes equalling 200 or 400 msec, but longer fixations (2 × 200) or 400 msec lead to the best performance. Loftus considered these data as further support of Biederman's (1972) contention that little more than gist is accumulated in that brief time frame.

Friedman and Liebelt (1981), Antes (1974), and Antes and Penland (1981) examined the time course of viewing in a free viewing situation. Although the stimuli between these two research efforts differed somewhat, they both examined the role of expectancy in picture perception, e.g., the subjects' task may have been to find a clock and other modern items in a log cabin setting. In essence, these researchers established a *frame theory* or gist notion of perception. They provide evidence of a hierarchically stereotyped and relatively invariant viewing pattern. Although there were some individual differences, they found that expected objects were initially inspected for shorter durations than when re-inspected later during the viewing period, while unexpected objects were initially fixated longer than they are later in the fixation sequence. Overall however, the novel items demanded more attention than did the expected items.

SPATIAL FACTORS

Mackworth and Morandi (1967) were among the first to characterize fixations and picture viewing. They found that the saccadic sequence tended to follow the few outstanding areas of a picture based on their high information or unpredictable content and that these areas received the greatest ratio of gaze. Yarbus (1967) also illustrated the variability in viewing. In what may seem to be an interminable viewing time of 3 minutes, Yarbus shows that fixation sequences over these sustained viewing periods tended to follow content areas, contour areas, and lightness and darkness patterns. He found that although there were substantial individual differences, substantial within-subject differences between seven viewings of the same picture for the same purpose and for the same subject viewing the picture for seven different purposes, the resultant fixation patterns still seemed to be concentrated on the objects within the picture rather than diffusely scrambled over the entire scene.

Nelson and Loftus (1980) addressed the issue of quality of viewing in that they found that when varying exposures between 700 and 3000 msec, the added fixations increased the likelihood of picking up items to be remembered. Although it is possible that the unusual method of having target and distractor simultaneously exposed during recognition may have tempered the results, they found that there was a 2° critical window region required for "seeing" critical detail. That is, when subjects failed to fixate within 2° of the critical detail they failed to detect the target. It is possible that their highly controlled viewing conditions and selected exposure durations tended to force the specificity of this conclusion. Because, when methodology is pushed to extremes like giving unlimited viewing time, nearly every object in the picture will be found to fall within a 2° critical viewing region of some fixation, and consequently no room would exist for errors in perception or recognition. Such a notion is seen as inordinately delimiting during very brief exposures allowing a single central fixation, but the subject is still able to correctly identify the changed or target object.

Stark and Ellis (1981) provide a very elaborate explanation of the qualitative role of the saccade/fixation sequence. In their view, eye movements are controlled by cognitive models already present in the brain and although each individual provides their own preferred order of searching, that order remains quite consistent between pictures or when making different observations on subsequent presentations of the same picture. Their view got its impetus from Parker (1978) who in turn elaborated eye movements into Neisser's (1976) interactive perceptual cycle model. In essence, there are five stages to the revised model. First, *extraction* of the broad view or gist. The information extracted follows the given visual acuity function and the expected complements provided by the periphery and fovea. That is, objects in the region of poor acuity are noticed but are generally not seen clearly or identified. Second is *comparison,* where recognition or expectation dominates the perceptual process and identifies incongruence or lack of correspondence. Third is *guidance,* or decision of where to look next based on the data accumulated during comparison. Also, *time* added allows for additional areas to be viewed that had not been previously scrutinized so that required *decision processes* can act on the most complete set of data.

For practical purposes the model effects itself with the following viewing characteristics: (a) subjects exhibit a consistent but not invariant scanning order; (b) subjects switch fixations to changed objects; (c) subjects respond to missing objects without fixating a previously occupied blank space (no elaboration on how this occurs or how frequently); and (d) subjects frequently pass a changed object then return to it (a restatement of the *ah ha* phenomenon without elaborating on the dynamics or frequency).

The data reported in this chapter are directed at global issues regarding scan-pattern characteristics, but also address four specific issues: First, the contribution of the viewing time to recognition; second, the qualitative changes in response as a function of time, which will be taken to reflect the contribution of successive fixations; third, the essential nature of the 2° critical window and its contribution to recognition of complex scenes; fourth, the similarity of scan patterns within and between individuals as reflecting either a cognitive strategy (which for all purposes is likely to remain unknowable) or direct correspondence to stimulus bound qualities.

THE EXPERIMENT(S)

Procedure. The task involved detecting small differences in otherwise identical pictures. Subjects were instructed that they would first be shown a set of slides for their inspection and would subsequently be shown a second set of slides each of which would require a decision as to whether it was totally new, the same as before, or different in some way from before. Subjects were then presented with a practice inspection slide for 8 sec followed by a modified version of that slide. If no difference was detected by the subjects the experimenter pointed out the differences by turning back to the previous version of the picture. Following the practice, the subjects viewed 16 inspection slides in succession, exposed for 8 sec each.

For the recognition test phase of the experiment, subjects were shown a practice slide to familiarize them with the exposure duration and 20 subsequent slides. These groups viewed these slides tachistoscopically at experimenter-controlled exposures of either 50 msec, 250 msec, or 500 msec, while two subject-controlled groups viewed the slides and responded as quickly as they could or took their time to decide, depending on testing condition.

Subjects in the tachistoscopic exposure groups were instructed that after each identification slide was exposed they were to write down their response as "same as before," "never seen before," or "different." If their response was "different," they were also to write down what they thought to be different about the picture. Adequate time was provided, following each exposure, for subjects to respond.

Subjects in the subject-controlled groups were tested individually. The task, stimulus materials, and procedure were the same as described above with two exceptions. Unknown to the subjects, eye movements were monitored during the 8 sec inspection phase and the recognition phase, and responses were made verbally to the experimenter. After the subject was seated in a viewing studio, the video level of the oculometer was adjusted to the pupil-iris contrast of that subject. Following this, a small number of eye fixations were collected while the subject's attention was being deliberately directed toward each of several known points on the subject's projection screen, thus allowing the eye position to be defined in terms of known (x,y) coordinates within the stimulus material. This "calibration" procedure was accomplished while the subject viewed 5 slides on picture search, number search, and puzzle mazes. The entire process took from 1 to 3 min and led directly into the specific experiment as though a continuation of the same task. The subject was never aware of more than the visual task at hand being performed.

Materials and Apparatus.   Black and white pictures of paintings, taken from the Meiers Art Judgment Test (1940) and Meiers Aesthetic Perception Test (1962), were made into 35 mm slides and shown from a Kodak Carousel projector (Model 860H).

Of the 20 recognition slides, 8 were unchanged ("same as before"), 8 slides contained modifications ("different") and 4 slides were completely new ("never seen before"). Of the 8 slides containing modifications, 4 slides involved changing the spatial coordinates of an object (translocation) within the painting, 2 slides involved changing the orientation of an object, 1 slide involved the substitution of one object with a similar one and, 1 slide involved both translocation and substitution of two objects as well as the deletion of a third object. For purposes of analysis all types of changes will be collapsed as no systematic differences were found between them.

The subjects in the tachistoscopic exposure groups sat in six rows facing the projector screen. The first row was 3.7 m from the screen and the other five rows were at intervals of 1.1 m. The projected images were approximately 80 cm high and ranged in width from 80 cm to 120 cm subtending visual angles of approximately 13° vertically and from 13° to 19° horizontally for the first row of seats. For the last row of seats, the images subtended angles of approximately 5° vertically and from 5° to 8° horizontally. No effect of size was found and therefore will not be further discussed. The exposure of the slides was controlled by a decade interval timer (Hunter, Model IIIC) operating a shutter (Gerbrands, Model G1166) attached to the projector lens.

The subjects in the two eye movement conditions sat comfortably in an armchair approximately 1.75 m in front of a polarized, rear projection screen set into one wall of a small viewing studio. In another room, a Kodak Carousel slide projector with a manually operated shutter, projected the slides onto the rear projection screen. The projected images were 60 cm high and ranged in width from 60 cm to 80 cm thereby subtending visual angles of approximately 19.5° vertically and from approximately 19.5° to 26° horizontally.

The subject controlled the opening and closing of the shutter on the slide projector with the use of a remote, handheld pushbutton. The experimenter controlled the slide projector, presentation rate, and inspection phase exposure time. The experimenter and the subject communicated verbally by microphone.

Coincident with the collection of verbal, behavioral data from the subject, the right eye was covertly monitored at the rate of 60 times per sec with an eye movement monitoring device (oculometer). The oculometer camera was concealed in what appeared to be a speaker box located directly beneath the projection screen. The subject, the experimenter and control system, and the projector and camera were in three separate rooms. A fuller description of the oculometer apparatus was presented by Lambert, Monty, and Hall (1974) and Karsh and Breitenbach (this volume).

Subjects. Three classes of 21 students in a beginning Art History course at Harford Community College, Bel Air, Maryland, served as subjects in the three tachistoscopic conditions, while 25 other volunteers from the same school served in the two eye movement monitoring conditions.

RESULTS AND DISCUSSION

Four issues are of particular concern: First, the importance of exposure time to recognition; second, the contribution of multiple eye movements to recognition; third, the importance of a 2° target area window in guaranteeing recognition; and fourth, the role of scan patterns as either reflections of the stimulus array, critical elements or the viewer's style. Each of these issues is addressed successively.

Exposure Time. The data for correct responses are shown in Table 1 while their complements for errors are shown in Table 2. The left portion of Table 1 details specific characteristics of Different responses while the right side allows comparison of *Same* and *Different* total correct responses. EMA is the speeded eye movement task while EMB is the relaxed response eye movement task. Since a priori considerations were aimed at detecting differences as a function of exposure duration, hence the addition of eye movements, contiguous groups and specific effects were tested by *t*-tests and where distributional concerns appeared by Mann-Whitney and Wilcoxon nonparametrics. Only those differences found significant are noted by asterisks appearing between components tested.

No change is evident for Different proper-reason responses up to the EMA condition. Tachistoscopic exposures during test, including the 500 msec, can be considered to reflect acquisition of "gist" with little specificity of difference available to the response process. During EMA where approximately seven fixations occur (cf. Table 3), more *qualitatively* accurate reasons for difference judgments are given. That is, response change is accomplished not with increased *quantitative* accuracy as would be reflected in total correct, but with more refined responses. *Quantitative* accuracy for detecting difference does not significantly increase until longer viewing time is available as is evidenced in the summary column for different–any or no reason– in the EMB condition.

TABLE 1
Mean Number of Correct Responses Per Subject

	Exposure Time	Different Proper Reason Only	Different Wrong Reason	Different No Reason	(8 Pics) Different Any or No Reason	(8 Pics) Same	(4 Pics) New Never Seen Before
E X P E R I M E N T E E R (PACED)	50 msec N = 21	1.2 (15%)	1.1 (14%)	0.9 (11%)	3.2 (40%)*	5.0 (63%)	3.8 (95%)
	250 msec N = 21	1.1 (14%)	1.3 (16%)	0.8 (10%)	3.2 (40%)*	5.5 (69%)	3.8 (95%)
	500 msec N = 21	1.4 (18%)	2.0 (25%)	0.6 (8%)	4.0 (50%)*	5.6 (70%)	3.8 (95%)
		*	*			*	
S U B J E C T (PACED)	EMA 1.668 sec N = 15	3.0 (38%)	1.1 (14%)	0.2 (3%)	4.3 (54%)*	6.8 (85%)	3.9 (98%)
					*		
	EMB 4.437 sec N = 10	3.7 (46%)	1.7 (21%)	0.0 (0%)	5.4 (68%)*	7.2 (90%)	3.7 (93%)

* = $p < .01$

TABLE 2
Mean Number of Incorrect Responses/Subject

		Exposure Time	Different Answered Same	Same Answered Different	Different Or Same Answered New
E					
X		50 msec	3.6 (45%)	2.3 (29%)	1.7 (11%)
P		N = 21			
E	P				
R	A				
I	C	250 msec	4.0 (50%)	1.7 (21%)	1.3 (8%)
M	E	N = 21			
E	D				
N					
T		500 msec	3.2 (40%)	2.0 (25%)	1.1 (7%)
E		N = 21			
R					
				**	
S		EMA			
U	P	1.876 sec	3.1 (39%)	0.9 (11%)	0.9 (6%)
B	A	N = 15			
J	C				
E	E		*		
C	D	EMB			
T		6.425 sec	2.0 (25%)	0.7 (9%)	0.7 (5%)
		N = 10			

* = $p < .05$
** = $p < .01$

Assuming "gist" to be the predominant determiner of the low number of correct *Different* responses, it can also account for the lack of improvement in the *Same* responses through 500 msec. If all the information necessary to be specific about a difference is not present, the subject is likely to respond *Same,* and "gist" is not likely to contain specific information necessary to make a *Different* decision. Enough added information seems to be available at EMA durations to add specificity, but the longer viewing does not increase the likelihood of more quantitative accuracy for *Differents.* In general, these data support the Loftus (1981) findings on the accumulation of information within and between fixations as a function of time available. That accumulation is taken to be a direct contribution of eye movements that is necessary for checking specifics of the scene and the duration of exposure must provide enough time for at least multiple eye movements.

TABLE 3
Means Per Correct Response

Mean Exposure Time	Measure	Different Proper Reason Only	Different Wrong Reason	Different No Given Reason	Different Any or No Reason	Same	New Never Seen Before
EMA 1.668 sec N = 15	Number of Fixations	7.5	6.7	5.3	7.2	5.6	3.2
	Exposure Time (sec)	2.288	2.117	2.122	2.237	1.738	0.928
	Fixation Duration (sec)	0.241	0.285	0.361	0.258*	0.245**	0.237
EMB 4.437 sec N = 10	Number of Fixations	13.6	16.6	0.0	14.6	15.1	6.7
	Exposure Time (sec)	4.518	6.171	0.0	5.038	5.104	2.260
	Fixation Duration (sec)	0.293	0.326	0.0	0.303*	0.281**	0.287

*$p < .05$
**$p < .01$

202

TABLE 4
Means Per Incorrect Response

Mean Exposure Time	Measure	Different Answered Same		Same Answered Different	Different Or Same Answered New
EMA 1.876 sec	Number of Fixations	6.0 (N = 14)	*	8.3 (N = 9)	4.4
	Exposure Time (sec)	1.800		2.701	1.338
	Fixation Duration (sec)	0.246**		0.301	0.247
EMB 6.425 sec	Number of Fixations	20.3 (N = 10)		19.4 (N = 5)	11.1
	Exposure Time (sec)	7.042		8.724	3.883
	Fixation Duration (sec)	0.291*	*	0.379	0.297

* = $p < .05$
** = $p < .01$

Eye Movements. Tables 3 and 4 show eye movement data for the EMA and EMB conditions. The data in Table 3 are shown for descriptive purposes only, as no within or between conditions proved significantly different, evidencing large variances in the data. Due to increased viewing times between conditions, the number of fixations and exposure time means reflect that time was used when allowed. However, from Table 1 it can be seen that added time provides marginal payoff for the subject.

The same/different response literature details that detecting any change would allow the subject to report a *Different* response, but *all* change possibilities must be examined for a *Same* response. On average 1.6 fewer fixations were needed during EMA for more correct *Same* than *Different* responses. Though the reason for those fewer fixations is not immediately known, it may also be related to the "gist" type response bias described above. The trade-off in number of same fixations benefits the EMA conditions whereas more fixations are needed to enhance the accuracy level of the different responses. Such a trade-off of 7–10 added fixations to enhance accuracy is hardly seen as a contribution, but may provide some insight into consolidation or chunking processes that reduces the 230,000 daily fixations to a manageable number of memorial events.

Of considerable theoretical, though low statistical interest is the elevation of fixation durations in the EMB condition. It is as though the subjects "decide" that even though they can make more fixations because they have "unlimited" time, they are perfectly willing to make longer fixations in order to take a better look at what they are viewing within a fixation as well (cf. Julesz, 1971). That trade-off may prove to be the most essential contribution of eye movements to performance. The picture discriminations required were very difficult and the flexibility available to the subject to modulate fixation parameters permitted more precise determinations of differences in the scenes. The zeros in the *no reason given* column of Table 3 reflect more specific responses—here embellishment is a contribution. Table 4 shows a significant increase in the number of fixations for incorrect responses made to *Same* versus *Different* slides. For EMA and EMB, fixation durations increased for *Same* errors compared to correct same responses. Much of that within fixation time seems to be due to uncertainty of response—another embellishment to eye movement processing. In both Tables 3 and 4 the "new, never seen before" slides were distractors and not entered into any analysis.

2° Fixation Window.   Nelson and Loftus (1980) proposed a critical 2° fixation window that was essential to recognition. That is, they claimed that a fixation had to be within at least 2° of the target to notice a change and report it. Certain procedural differences exist between their studies and the data presented here. First, they allowed free viewing during the test phase and exposed the inspection slides for 750–3000 msec. Second, no mention was made of the magnitude of the changes between elements on pictures during test and inspection. Third, they presented the original and the variation simultaneously at test. Fourth, they measured performance as a function of original exposure time—a methodologically formidable task exists for getting reliable fixations at 750 msec from any recording system, and the "ugly" system described by Loftus (1979) is no more error-free than any system. Granted there are response process problems, in that occasionally subjects will look but not see, but the assumption of a 2° window seems reasonable especially in view of visual acuity constraints.

This issue is addressed by the data in Tables 5 and 6. Table 5 shows the data from the six fastest responding subjects in EMA (all of the longer viewing subjects viewed the target or altered areas). In most cases the variations in slides were multiple though frequently subtle. The summary at the bottom of Table 5 shows that for those viewing *within* the 2° window of the changed object(s), there is a higher chance of missing the item or not detecting a change. For the 15 *no look* test occurrences, there is an equal likelihood of responding correctly so that, for these data, the 2° critical window hypothesis is untenable.

TABLE 5
Recognition Profile in EMA with 2° Fixation Window

Slide	Inspection		Test			Correct	Incorrect
	Look	No Look	Location Old	New	No Look		
19	6(2)*		4	4(2)		1	3
					2	2	0
21	6(1)		5	1(1)		2	3
					1	1	0
23	6(2)		3	5(2)		2	3
					1	0	1
27	6(2)		4	4(2)		2	2
					2	1	1
31	6(shading)		6(shading)			2	4
					0	0	0
33	6(3)		3	3(3)		1	2
					3	0	3
35	6(1)		2	1(1)		1	2
					3	1	2
36	6(4)		3	3(4)		1	2
					3	2	1

Fastest 6 of 15 subjects

* parentheses is number of
different items in picture

TEST: Average Reaction Time .570 sec
Average No. of Fixations 2.3
Average Fixation Duration .230 sec

Summary			
	Total	Correct	Incorrect
No look	15	7	8
Both old and new look	25	9	16

Table 6 presents a summary and comparable set of data for EMB. All of the subjects looked at the changed object (within the 2° window) during both inspection and test but performance was far worse than perfect. The problem is that given what seems to be a minimal amount of time, like 4–5 sec, subjects are able to make 15–20 fixations and view *all* areas on the picture that have contours, shading, semantic interest, etc., but the level of information taken in during those fixations is not necessarily qualitatively ac-

INSPECTION   TEST

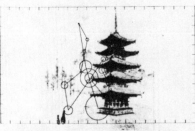
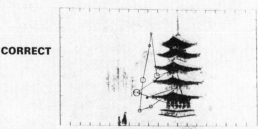

CORRECT

SUBJ 1   SLIDE 1   REACTION TIME 8.900   SUBJ 1   SLIDE 2   REACTION TIME 5.567
MEAN FIX. DUR. .678   NO. FIX. 13   MEAN FIX. DUR. .300   NO. FIX. 15

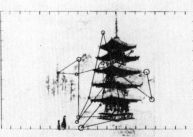
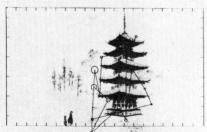

CORRECT

SUBJ 2   SLIDE 1   REACTION TIME 9.200   SUBJ 2   SLIDE 2   REACTION TIME 5.233
MEAN FIX. DUR. .316   NO. FIX. 26   MEAN FIX. DUR. .266   NO. FIX. 18

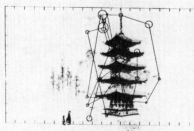
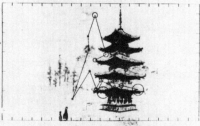

INCORRECT

SUBJ 3   SLIDE 1   REACTION TIME 9.283   SUBJ 3   SLIDE 2   REACTION TIME 6.567
MEAN FIX. DUR. .322   NO. FIX. 25   MEAN FIX. DUR. .336   NO. FIX. 18

**EYE MOVEMENT PATTERNS (OF THREE SUBJECTS) FOR
PAIRS OF INSPECTION AND TEST PICTURES:**

TEST PICTURES ARE IDENTICAL TO INSPECTION PICTURES

FIG. 1.   Eye movement patterns (of three subjects) for pairs of inspection
and test pictures: Test pictures are identical to inspection pictures.

206

TABLE 6
Recognition Profile for 10 Subjects in EMB
with 2° Fixation Window

	Inspection		Test				
		No	Location		No		
Slide	Look	Look	Old	New	Look	Correct	Incorrect
19	10(2)		10	10(2)		1	9
21	10(1)		8	10(1)		6	4
23	10(2)		3	10(2)		6	4
27	10(2)		9	10(2)		10	0
31	10(shading)		10(shading)			8	2
33	10(3)		10	9(3)		5	5
35	10(1)		10	5(1)		7	3
36	10(4)		6	10(4)		10	0

TEST: Average Reaction Time 4.71 sec
Average No. of Fixations 13.8
Average Fixation Duration .293 sec

Summary		
Total	Correct	Incorrect
80	53	27

curate enough to base decisions upon as can be witnessed by the fact that only 66% accuracy exists in EMB. We feel that when specific area limits are placed upon fixation locations even within the framework of recognized acuity ranges, little or no correspondence between their location and picture recognition is evident, and therefore the meaningfulness of those fixations must be considered as embellishments to the recognition and decision processes until additional data renders this conclusion untenable.

Scan Pattern Characteristics. Stark and Ellis (1981) provided a strong argument but very little substantiation of the cognitive schema determining the individual scan pattern. We are also able to address that issue with the data from the present experiment.

Figure 1 presents data from three subjects viewing identical inspection and test slides. Slides were exposed for 8 sec during inspection and for as long as the viewer chose to take (as in EMB) to respond during test. During inspection, subject 1 elicited a few long fixations (duration represented by size of the circle (and repeated inspection of the same regions when viewing during test, and then correctly responded to the identity of the picture, generally confirming Stark and Ellis' cognitive schema model. Subject 2 made many more fixations than subject 1 and more than was made during test, but still responded correctly even though his viewing area was more restricted. Subject 3 scanned the scene during inspection, scanned a much narrower area to the left during test, and erred in his response of "there was no fence the first time." The fence was there both times and it was viewed directly during inspection, but not within 2° during test. Some correspondence can be seen in the scan of the left side of the pagoda.

Figure 2 presents a view of data from pairs of *Different* stimuli. All three subjects search what seems to be the important elements of the scene during inspection, showing comparatively low variability, but perhaps idiosyncratic fixation durations. Subject 4 makes a few fixations of moderate length during test and "looks at" the location (dotted form) of the previous position of the woman in the boat, perhaps to note its absence, and responds correctly. Subject 5 performs similarly with more but shorter fixations and responds correctly as well. Subject 6 makes a moderate number of fixations with durations comparable to inspection, but other parts of the scene are viewed than the previous location and the search results in an error. During test a good imagination would be hard pressed to recognize correspondence between subjects or for that matter within subjects. Just as likely could be the inclusion of examples of a scan pattern showing the subject viewing the changed location and missing the response or not viewing the changed location and correctly responding, pointing out that attentional and response probabilities are equally likely to contribute to a correct response as are fixations.

Though searching for correspondences in these patterns is compelling in its own right, our mathematical assessments have proved futile to this point, as have our visual inspections. It is nice to know that to this point we can substantiate any theory of viewing pictures on the basis of scan patterns, which in effect means we can substantiate none.

SUMMARY AND CONCLUSIONS

Understanding pictures may be a lot easier (cf. Nodine & Fisher, 1979) than understanding how people look at and remember pictures. Though understanding pictures involves description and analysis using abstract "metrics" of liking or disliking, good form or poor form, buying or not buying, etc., and the metrics involved in understanding how people look at

INSPECTION   TEST

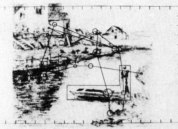
CORRECT

SUBJ 4   SLIDE 3   REACTION TIME 9.017
MEAN FIX. DUR. .306   NO. FIX. 26

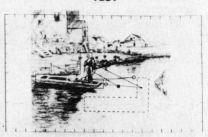

SUBJ 4   SLIDE 4   REACTION TIME 3.517
MEAN FIX. DUR. .348   NO. FIX. 9

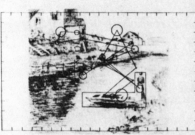
CORRECT

SUBJ 5   SLIDE 3   REACTION TIME 9.017
MEAN FIX. DUR. .450   NO. FIX. 18

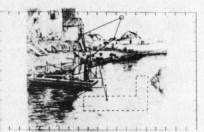

SUBJ 5   SLIDE 4   REACTION TIME 3.667
MEAN FIX. DUR. .190   NO. FIX. 16

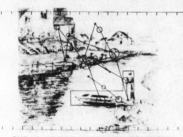
INCORRECT

SUBJ 6   SLIDE 3   REACTION TIME 9.200
MEAN FIX. DUR. .410   NO. FIX. 20

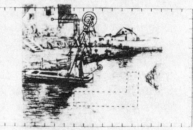

SUBJ 6   SLIDE 4   REACTION TIME 7.000
MEAN FIX. DUR. .424   NO. FIX. 15

EYE MOVEMENT PATTERNS (OF THREE SUBJECTS) FOR
PAIRS OF INSPECTION AND TEST PICTURES:

TEST PICTURES ARE MODIFIED VERSIONS OF INSPECTION PICTURES

FIG. 2.   Eye movement patterns (of three subjects) for pairs of inspection
and test pictures: Test pictures are different from inspection pictures.

pictures has become quite concrete, it is limited by state-of-the art scientific procedures.

The measurement technique and algorithm determine the accuracy and precision of eye movement measurement, but the frequent occurrence of what appears to be a completely idiosyncratic, unrepeatable eye movement pattern delimits the availability of appropriate models to describe the data. Subjects can complicate the issue further in their willingness to suffer through successive three minute viewings of the same static scene as Yarbus' subjects did, while at other times they show surprising accuracy in recognition while viewing a scene one time for 50 msec. It is quite uncertain that the 1:60 exposure duration number ratio (50 msec vs. 3 min) carries over to a metric of identity or recognition enhancement. What does seem apparent is the amount of misunderstood and possibly epi-phenomenal events that occur when subjects view pictures.

Stark and Ellis (1981) created an interesting extention of Parker's (1978) notion of a cognitive strategy that sets the sequence of the scan path. Unfortunately, few data support those notions. In fact, aids to memory consolidation are picked up without eye movements, much less the scan path's organization. What is reflected in the scan path, though, is a correlation of the fixation's location with high information areas of the picture *without* regard to sequence, and then pushed to extremes as with Yarbus' subjects, the reflected cognitive process may be as simplistic as, "It's there, so I'll look at it," and "If I look at it enough maybe I'll remember it."

When, as we have done, large numbers of subjects are scrutinized during recognition, it becomes possible, e.g., Figs. 1 and 2, to support *any* hypothesis under the sun by selectively partitioning sets of data. Whether based on notions of frequency, location, viewing time, similarity-dissimilarity—we support it *all* and thus we support *none*, yet grouped analysis provides even fewer meaningful answers. Likewise, the role of eye movements is misunderstood when faulty assumptions—like the 2° critical window, are gleaned from the data. Because along with it are other implicit notions like—people will look at anything if shown, continue to look as long as shown, and consequently look at *everything*. Everything then falls within 2° of some fixation and yet errors are made of both omission and commission, permitting conclusions like—given enough time viewers look at everything, see most everthing but tend to tell you what they think you want to hear.

III.4 Hierarchical Organization of Eye Tracking Movements

Didier Bouis
Institut für Informations
University of Karlsruhe, German Federal Republic

Gerhardt Vossius
Institut für Biokybernetik
und Biomedizinische Technik
University of Karlsruhe, German Federal Republic

The control of eye movements has been the object of research for more than 100 years. Engineers, psychologists, neurophysiologists, and others have been attempting to understand the underlying mechanism of this control. Generally it is considered to be an automatic system that provides consistent output for a specific input. We will show here that this automatic mechanism forms only the lowest part of a hierarchial control organization. The goal of this organization is to get a higher efficiency by adapting the whole system to the actual input conditions.

METHOD

For our experiments we needed a very precise eye movement measuring method with high resolution, high speed, no contact with the eye, and a low price. As none of the commercially available devices could match these characteristics, we developed a device having a resolution of 5 min of arc, a measuring range of $+15$ in both (x,y) directions and a maximum linearity error of 1% of the full scale. The output is electronically lowpass filtered at a 100 Hz limit frequency (Bouis, Baude, & Vossius, 1975).

In order to obtain reproducible data we have to devise a number of experiments where environmental conditions could be kept under control. For this reason we placed subjects in a dark room with instructions to follow, with their eyes, a light slit moving on the wall in front of them. The position of this slit was controlled by a computer as was the position of the eye, which for test purposes, was fed back on the position of the light slit (target). This experimental set-up is very flexible and can be used for any type of experiment related to eye movement control.

RESULTS

Regarding the control of eye movements, imagine that a hunter is tracking an animal with his eyes. His brain must continually direct his eyes to the animal. Let us suppose that the brain computes only the position of the animal relative to the eye and that in order to do so it needs 120 msec. In this case it can only direct the eye to where the animal was 120 msec earlier. It may never direct the eye to the target. This is why nature has chosen another way. The brain precisely computes the speed of the target relative to the eye and then provides the correct speed to the eye so that the distance between target and eye position is stabilized, then it corrects for that position.

So far most researchers have assumed that there are two controls; one for the slow eye movements, which controls the speed of the eye, the other for the saccades, which controls the position of the eye. From the beginning, our work was based on the assumption that the two systems could not possibly work independently of each other as this would cause a mutual disturbance. If for example, the saccadic system ordered the eye muscles to make a jump of 5° to the right, the slow eye movement pursuit system would see the target going fast from right to left, and it would measure the speed wrongly. So far, it was generally assumed that the pursuit system was capable of eliminating by itself, all the target jumps it sees. To disprove this hypothesis, we experimented with jumping targets. We found that the slow pursuit system sees no difference between a saccade made by the eye and a target jump. Because a saccade does not provoke a change in the eye speed, it follows that a target jump must have no effect on the speed of the eye. Data from such an experiment are shown in Fig. 1.

In the speed diagram it can be seen that 120 msec after the target jump the eye speed begins to have an overshoot or undershoot in the direction of the target jump, and we found that it is proportional to the size of the target jump. In another series of experiments we found that during a saccade the input of the speed system is blocked. Those results show that the control of the slow movement cannot discriminate a saccade by itself; it has at least to be informed by the saccadic branch that a saccade occurs.

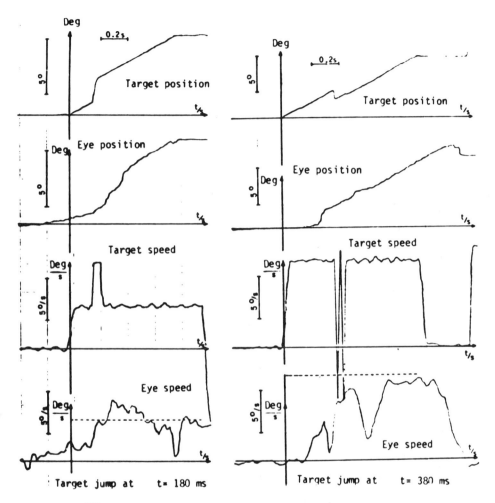

FIG. 1.   Effect of a target jump on the eye speed regulation. Size of the target jump: 4.5°.

To find out whether the slow movement system sends any information to the saccadic system, we carried out the following experiment using continuous target movements, with sudden changes of speed (Fig. 2). We found that if the changes occurred more than 180 msec before the saccade, this saccade will be a successful one, i.e., at its end the eye is on target. Changes in speed between zero and 120 msec before the saccade have no influence on its size. If the saccade occurs between 120 and 180 msec after the speed variation, the eye looks in a direction between the former and the new target pattern. These results show that the relative speed is used for the determina-

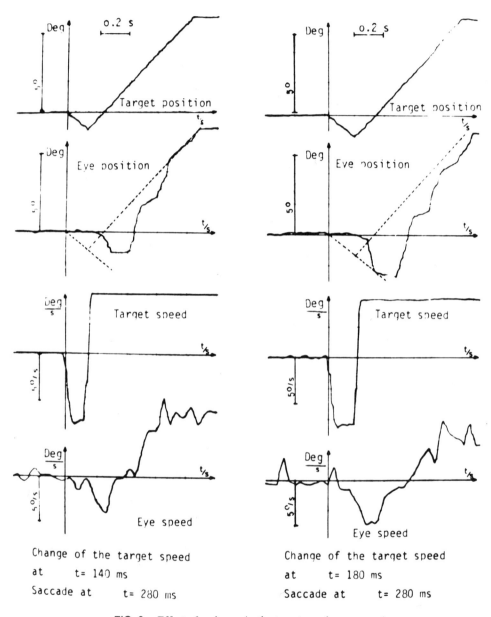

FIG. 2.   Effect of a change in the target speed on a saccade.

tion of the size of a saccade. It is computed over a 60 msec period ending 120 msec before the onset of the saccade.

Comparing experiments where the target pattern included large speed changes with others without those changes, we found that the saccade was blocked and postponed until 180 msec after the speed variation. If the variation occurred between 120 and 180 msec before, a saccade usually happened in the other experiments. Apparently in this case the controller prefers to wait until it has measured the new relative speed precisely. This is identical to the *hold* effect we found in the continuous system.

Those two systems working together and blocking each other form the lowest level of the organization of eye movements. If the brain does not wish this mutual blocking of the two systems to reduce efficiency, it has to give priority to one over the other. This hypothesis can be illustrated by two examples.

1. Let us imagine that the error in the eye speed is large while the position error is small. Correcting the position through a saccade may be very inefficient because a large speed error may mean that the computation of the speed was wrong, and then the size of the saccade will be computed by using wrong data. If the saccade occurs, the slow pursuit movement system will be blocked and cannot correct the speed of the eye.

2. If we suppose that the speed error is small and the position error is large, a change of the eye speed may reduce the efficiency of a saccade. If there is no correction of the speed but a saccade is initiated instead, the position error will be reduced to nearly zero, and we can anticipate it will stay small.

Therefore it is necessary at each moment for the brain to decide which of the two controls—saccade or slow movement—should be given priority.

We tried to express this assumption in the forms of a model. In order to decide optimally which of the two, i.e., the continuous or the saccadic control, must have priority, the brain needs to anticipate which will be the more efficient for the coming period of time. We named this period the prevision time T.

To make the mathematics of the model solvable, we made the following simplifications: Every saccade precludes an efficient correction of the relative target eye speed, therefore this one will stay constant over the prevision time. If priority is given to the continuous control of the movement, the speed will be corrected, but no saccade will happen within the prevision time. We shall use the following definitions:

$t = 0$: Beginning of the saccade.

T_1 : Time measured from $t = 0$, where the speed will be corrected, if no saccade occurs.

T :   Prevision time, measured from $t = 0$

E :   Error in position at the beginning of the saccade.

S :   Size of the saccade.

V :   Speed of the target relative to the eye.

E_2 :   Error at the moment where the conditions leading to the release of a saccade are fulfilled.

T_2 :   Time between the moment where the conditions leading to the release of a saccade are fulfilled and the beginning of this saccade.

F_V :   Previsible mean square value of the error over the Time T, if the speed is corrected.

F_S :   Previsible mean square value of the error over the Time T, if a saccade is done.

$$F_V = \frac{1}{T} \left(\int_0^{T_1} (E + V \bullet t)^2 \, dt + \int_{T_1}^{T} (E + V \bullet T_1)^2 \, dt \right) \tag{1}$$

$$F_S = \frac{1}{T} \int_0^{T} (E + S + V \bullet t)^2 \, dt \tag{2}$$

Assuming that the saccades are optimal, F_S is minimal.

$$\frac{dF_S}{dS} = \frac{d}{dS} \left(\frac{1}{T} \int_0^{T} (E + S + V \bullet t)^2 \, dt \right) = 0 \tag{3}$$

$$\frac{dF_S}{dS} = \frac{1}{T} \int_0^{T} 2(E + S + V \bullet t)^2 \, dt = 0 \tag{4}$$

$$2 (E + S) \, T + V \bullet T^2 = 0 \tag{5}$$

$$S = -\frac{V \bullet T}{2} - E \tag{6}$$

Replacing S in the expression of F_S by its equivalent, we get:

$$F_{SM} = \frac{1}{T} \int_0^{T} V^2 \left(t - \frac{T}{2} \right)^2 \, dt \tag{7}$$

A saccade must be done if:

$$F_{SM} < F_V \tag{8}$$

$$\frac{1}{T} \int_0^T V^2 \left(t - \frac{T}{2}\right)^2 dt < \frac{1}{T} \left(\int_0^{T_1} (E + V \bullet t)^2 \, dt + \int_{T_1}^T (E + V \bullet T_1)^2 \, dt \right)$$

(9)

Making $E = E_2 - V \bullet T_2$ and solving this inequation, the conditions leading to the release of a saccade can be found:

$$- \infty \leq \frac{E_2}{V} \leq \frac{1}{tg\,\theta_1} \qquad \text{or} \qquad \infty \leq \frac{E_2}{V} \leq \frac{1}{tg\,\theta_2}$$

(10)

where $tg\,\theta_2$ are depending on T, T_1, T_2, which are three variables.

Figure 2 represents this result. When the point representative of the error of the eye position and the speed error is in the shaded part, a saccade will occur; when in the other part, the speed error will be corrected. In order to find out whether the brain really operates in this way, it must be determined which combination of errors provokes a saccade.

Young, Forster, and Van Houtte (1968), and Robinson (1973), and other authors supposed that a correcting saccade was made if the error between

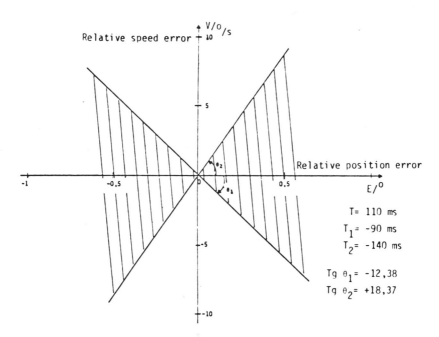

FIG. 3. Theoretical conditions leading to the release of a correcting saccade.

eye position and target position exceeded a certain limit. Wyman and Stein-man (1973) found evidence contrary to this hypothesis.

To obtain further insight into the working of the mechanism, we grouped the saccades, executed while tracking a sinusoidally moving pattern, according to their size. If the size of the correcting saccade is due to the position error, each group of correcting saccades has to correlate with a certain size of the position error. This was not the case. If the size of the correcting saccades is due to a certain size of the error and relative speed, a correlation should, and did, result.

The conditions leading to the release of a correcting saccade have to stem from the position error and the relative speed some time ahead of the actual execution of the saccade. By shaking the combination of the size of the position error and of the relative speed in various time intervals before the correcting saccades of each given group, it was found that for each group the combination of error in position and relative speed was restricted to a certain area in the position—relative speed plan at a precise time as shown in Fig. 4.

From these results it follows that there exists a certain trade-off of the size of the error in position and relative speed. In addition, this trade-off shows certain limits. No saccades occur when the combination exceeds these

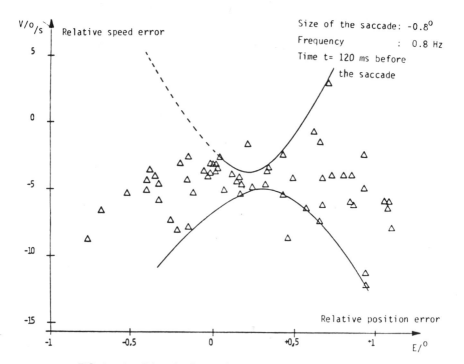

FIG. 4.   Conditions leading to the release of a correcting saccade.

limits. In this case the saccadic system is blocked; the regulation of the movement is done solely by changing the tracking pattern of the smooth pursuit system. Under this condition the continuous controller has priority. As long as the combination of the errors stays in the given limits, the priority for correcting error is given to the saccadic branch.

These results are very similar to those obtained theoretically, and confirm that the second stage of the hierarchical control of eye movement is a priority distributor system. Those first and second stages are in turn under the control of higher centers. Vossius (1972) shows that the parameters of the saccadic system can be changed. We (Bouis & Vossius, 1978; and Vossius & Werner, 1969) have previously shown that almost all the parameters of the speed control system also can be changed. The time between the conditions leading to a saccade and the saccade itself can be changed also. To demonstrate this, we carried out experiments where we fed back the saccades to the position of the target. This means, for example, that with a feedback of $+0.5$, while the eye effects a saccade of $2°$, the target makes a jump of $1°$ in the same direction as the saccade. Here again the eye has to follow a sinusoidal movement.

Again as before, each feedback and saccade size we monitor the conditions leading to the saccade and at a precise moment before selected saccades, we found that the points representing the relative movement of target and eye are located between two curves. The time between the conditions provoking the saccade and the saccade itself is given as a function of the feedback for a different saccade size in Fig. 5. When the feedback grows from 0 to 0.4 or 0.6, the time between the conditions provoking a saccade and the saccade itself is reduced and then grows again. One explanation for this result is that the brain interprets its poor performance (due to the feedback) as an error due to a too long computing time. For a higher feedback the brain may take more complex programs and change its strategy. Some of our experiments seem to confirm this assumption, but no reliable results have been found until now.

Above the three organization levels described there is a fourth one, which is able to put the three others out of function. Vossius (1972) has demonstrated that higher centers of the brain make a prevision of the future development of errors between target and eye positions. These centers then make any control inoperative and command eye movements directly.

DISCUSSION

In order to control eye movements, the brain apparently chooses a very versatile organization. The lower mechanism of this organization is formed by two branches, the saccadic and the slow movement control. Those two branches exchange information. Which of them gets the priority is decided

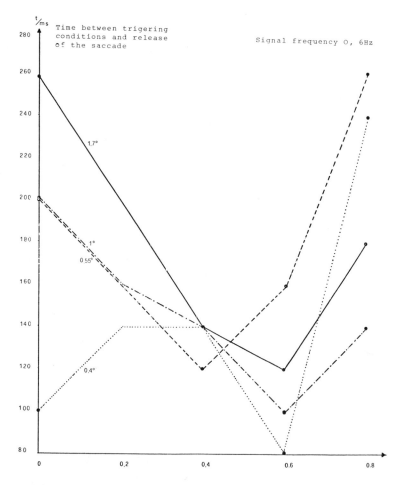

FIG. 5. Time between triggering conditions and release saccade vs. feedback factor for different saccade sizes.

on a higher level. The efficiency of these two lower levels is controlled by a third one, which, depending on this efficiency, can change almost all the parameters of the two former ones. Even higher centers analyze the regularity of the input signal and use it to give a forecast of its future movements. Those higher centers are able, when needed, to put out of function all the others and directly command eye movements.

The goal of this organization seems to be:

1. Efficiency: The system permanently adapts itself any new external conditions.

2. Rapidity: For reasons of a fast operation no complex computation is done by the lower stage of the control; rather, it works automatically. The more complex computations are done by higher centers having more time to do so.
3. Low Cost: The "more intelligent" centers of the brain are only used when needed and they may be free for other uses when not needed.

III.5 Smooth Pursuit Eye Movements and Attention in Schizophrenia and Cycloid Psychoses

Sven Ingmar Andersson
Lund University
Lund, Sweden

Early in the 20th century, Diefendorf and Dodge (1908) reported abnormalities of eye tracking in schizophrenic patients. Using a pendular target and photographing light reflected from the cornea, they noted marked disturbances of tracking both in severe and mild cases of schizophrenia (termed dementia praecox at the time). Among other psychiatric patients that they tested, only those with signs of marked deterioration showed such abnormalities. However, Couch and Fox (1934) argued that, since such tracking disturbances are not limited to schizophrenic patients, disorders of attention may represent the more central phenomenon.

Renewed interest in the smooth-pursuit eye movements of schizophrenics was generated by the work of Holzman, Proctor, and Hughes (1973) and of Holzman, Proctor, Levy, Yasillo, Meltzer, and Hurt (1974). Using electrooculography to measure changes in corneo-retinal field potential as the eyetracking of the pendulum was monitored, these authors found tracking to be inferior in schizophrenics as compared with non-schizophrenics and normals. They likewise obtained evidence for a similar dysfunction in a large percentage of close (first-degree) relatives of schizophrenic patients, leading them to argue (Holzman et al., 1974) that the dysfunction concerned represents a genetic marker. Shagass, Amadeo, and Overton (1974) confirmed the results of Holzman et al. (1973) regarding the poorer pendulum tracking performance of schizophrenics than of non-psychiatric patients and normals, but found tracking to be inferior in affective psychotics as well. Further work of Holzman and his co-workers (e.g., Holzman & Levy, 1977) suggested disorders of smooth pursuit eye movement to be associated, not only with the pathological conditions named, but also with a variety of functional psychoses and of central nervous disorders. They interpreted the tracking dysfunction to be inadequate cognitive centering which occurred despite a desire to perform the task.

Both Holzman et al. (1974) and Shagass et al. (1974) reported a lack of success in attempts to improve eye tracking performance through alerting-instructions. However, Shagass, Roemer, and Amadeo (1976) found that requiring a subject to read numbers situated on the oscillating target improved performance considerably, both for patients and for non-patients, though the differences between the two groups were not abolished in this way.

The studies of Holzman et al. (1973, 1974) and of Shagass et al. (1974, 1976) involved both the qualitative assessment of tracking performance and the recording of quantitative aspects, where the number of velocity arrests (seen as an index of the degree to which eye speed departs from target speed) represents a measure of the latter type. Details of both forms of approach have been criticized, for example by Troost, Daroff, and Dell'Osso (1974), Acker and Toone (1978), and Lindsey, Holzman, Haberman, and Yasillo (1978). The latter recommended the natural logarithm of the signal/noise ratio (ln S/N), obtained from the harmonic regression of digitized and standardized eye movement data, as being more relevant than the quantitative measure cited above.

The present study aims at comparing the pendular eye tracking performance of two main psychotic inpatient groups: schizophrenics and cycloid psychotics. The latter diagnostic category stems from the work of Leonhard (1957/1979), who describes the condition of cycloid psychosis as displaying a phasic course, where recovery after a psychotic episode may be complete. Leonhard emphasizes the importance of correct and early diagnosis of the condition, which can readily be misclassified as schizophrenia and treated inappropriately. At present the diagnosis of cycloid psychosis is widely employed within Scandinavia and several continental European countries whereas in many English-speaking countries, for example, the term cycloid psychosis is not even used and patients of this type tend, due to the similarity of various of their symptoms to those of schizophrenics, to be classified as the latter.

The work cited above on the deficits of pendular eye tracking performance in various psychiatric groups suggested it to be worthwhile to investigate the possibilities of distinguishing between schizophrenics and cycloid psychotics on the basis of measures of eye-tracking performance, which might ultimately be useful in a battery of measures aimed at the early diagnosis of cycloid psychotics. To this end a number of quantitative measures of possible relevance were selected. The pendular stimulus, which traditionally has consisted of a bob-and-string arrangement, is represented here by an electronic pendulum of constant, controllable speed. In order to investigate the possible role of attention in tracking performance, one of the two electronic pendulae utilized involves the moving light spot changing from the original color to a second color at irregular intervals.

METHOD

Recording Procedure

Each of the two electronic pendulae consisted of a string of 70 light diodes mounted in a straight line 38.5 cm in length, behind a vertical plexiglass plate. Through each diode in succession lighting up for a brief interval, and the succession reversing when the end of the string of diodes was reached, an illusion of continous pendulum-like movement was produced. The length of a cycle was 2.5 sec. Each of the diodes was controlled by a timer.

The one pendulum, termed the *sinusiodal pendulum,* displayed movement of a sinusoidal character. The other, termed the *saw-tooth pendulum,* involved the light instead ''moving'' at a constant speed, so that a graph of the movements back and forth described a (straight-sided) saw-tooth curve. The latter pendulum was equipped with a special type of light diode that could light up with either red or green light, the pendulum being programmed so that the moving spot was red most of the time but became green for short irregularly introduced intervals.

Subjects were seated 0.5 m from the pendulum, with head movement restrained by a chin support. Silver-silver chloride electrodes were placed on the outer canthi of both eyes, and a ground electrode was attached to the middle of the forehead. This electrode placement aimed at minimizing the appearance of blinks on the recordings. Eye movements were registered in the AC mode, using mingograph (M 81, Siemens-Elema, with a paper speed of 10 mm/sec) for quick visual inspection purposes and allowing the preamplifier of the mingograph to drive a Tandberg (TIR) FM tape recorder operating at a 3¾ IPS. The preamplifier was RC-coupled to balance out DC offset voltage, with a high pass filter (time constancy 2.5 sec) and a low pass filter (cut-off frequency 30 Hertz) employed for noise reduction. Calibration was carried out, just prior to the start of the task or task series for each of the two types of pendulae, through having the subject shift his gaze a number of times between the middlepoint of the pendulum and the two endpoints.

The general instructions for subjects were to follow with their eyes the movements of the pendulum. For half the subjects the task with the sinusoidal pendulum was presented first and with the saw-tooth pendulum thereafter, and for half the subjects the order was reversed. The total length of time which the pendulum was to be tracked was 60 sec for the sinusoidal pendulum and 300 sec for the saw-tooth pendulum. Subjects rested for at least 60 seconds while the one pendulum was being replaced by the other (slightly longer in a few cases due to practical considerations), instructions concerning the task that was to follow being given during this period.

Whereas the sinusoidal pendulum task involved a single (60 sec) tracking period, the saw-tooth pendulum task comprised three different tracking periods. In the first tracking period the "moving" light was red the entire time (60 sec). In the second period, which involved 180 sec of tracking and followed a 60 sec pause during which additional instructions were given, the stimulus color changed temporarily from red to green at irregular intervals. Here the subjects were instructed to press a button each time the light changed to green. The segments of the pendular movement in which the light was green, though irregularly occurring, always comprised ¼ of a total "swing" of the pendulum. Both the pressings of the button and the onset of the green segments were recorded on the mingograph, making it possible to register the times between the onset of the green stimulus and the occurrence of the button-pressing response, as well as the incidence of misses (failure to press the button when it should have been pressed) and false alarms (pressing the button at an inappropriate time). The third tracking period, which was 60 sec in length and followed a 30-sec pause, involved (just as did the first a red pendular stimulus only.

Subjects

Twenty-seven psychiatric patients admitted to the research clinic of St. Lars Psychiatric Hospital of the University of Lund for short-term therapy, as well as four non-patient controls recruited from the clinic staff, were tested. All were informed of the nature of the testing procedure and gave informed consent. The patients were a subsample of the inpatients available during a 3-month period of testing. Only patients who were judged as testable by the staff and personnel, showed no signs of organic brain disease, and had not undergone electric shock therapy for at least the previous three months were tested. Since diagnostic information was not complete at the time of testing and since a certain homogeneity of groups was aimed at, only those patients with the diagnosis of either schizophrenia or cycloid psychosis were included in the final sample of 22 patients employed in the present analysis. The sample obtained in this manner consisted of 13 schizophrenics—of which four were of a hebephrenic type (subjects 18, 19, 26, and 27), three of a paranoid (subjects 02, 05, and 11), and two of a catatonic type (subjects 14 and 15), as well as one each of the simple (subject 07), the residual (subject 08), the schizo-affective (subject 28) and the chronic undifferentiated (subject 23) types—and of 9 cycloid psychotics. As to clinical observations at the time of testing in the case of the cycloid psychotics, a marked difference was found between the cycloid psychotics 06, 17, 20, and 25, who all were described as hyperactive and the other cycloid psychotic patients, who all were described as more or less inhibited. Of the patients represented here, 9 were men and 13 women; all of the normal subjects were men. The mean age was 29.7 years for the schizophrenics (s.d. = 10.2), 27.5 years for the cycloid psychotics (s.d. = 6.9), and 29.0 years for the normals (s.d. = 5.1). All subjects had completed at least nine years of formal education. All of the patients were receiving neuroleptics at the time of testing (phenothiazine derivates or related substances). No neuroleptic or antipsychotic medication was being administered to any of the normal subjects.

Measures Obtained

Processing of the data from any given subject was carried out for each of five different 30-sec segments of the total tracking task separately, each such 30-sec segment comprising 12 cycles (or slightly more than this) of the pendulum. What is called Period 1 represents the initial 30 seconds of tracking with the sinusoidal pendulum, whereas Periods 2–5 involve successive portions of the saw-tooth pendulum task—Period 2 representing the initial 30 seconds of the first of the two red-light-only tasks, Period 3 the initial 30 seconds of the red-and-green-light tracking tasks, Period 4 a 39-sec segment of the latter task commencing 90 seconds after the end of Period 3, and Period 5 the initial 30 seconds of the second red-light-only tracking task. Since the sinusoidal pendulum was presented at the beginning for half of the subjects and at the end for the other half, Period 1 can appear in either position.

The tape-recorded signals from any given period were digitized by an ABC 80 computer at a rate of 8,200 sampling points for the 30 seconds involved. The data were saved on floppy disc and transmitted by the ABC 80 to a Univac 110/80 system at the Lund University Computer Center, where they were stored, with one file being devoted to each set of 8,200 sampling points, the value for each sampling point being in terms of the electrical voltage (V) measured at the respective point in time. Missing data (less than 5% of the total) were supplied as estimates based on the existing values.

The first step in processing these data so as to obtain summary measures indicative of a subject's tracking performance during a given period was to compute eye position P from V through solving the differential equation $dV/dt = a \cdot dP/dt - b \cdot V$, where dV/dt represents change in V over time. The validity of the measure thus obtained is based on the assumption that the value of P is always the same for the comparable point in any two cycles, and that the mean for the P values as a whole (where these can take on both positive and negative values) is 0. However, drift in the measurement equipment can occur, which can result in parts of the overall curve sagging under the mean line (which should be at the 0 level) or arching over it. Therefore, a linear correction was introduced (see the following).

The second processing step was to shorten the 30 sec recording whatever slight degree was required to obtain exactly 12 cycles, and to divide these into three segments of four cycles each. The identification of cycle length here was carried out on the basis of a preliminary Fourier analysis. The linear correction just referred to was then applied to each of the three four-cycle segments separately.

The third processing step was to perform a more thoroughgoing Fourier analysis on the series of corrected values that the previous two steps yielded. A Fourier analysis indicates how and to what degree a periodic curve of a given shape can be described as a sum of sinus functions of successively decreasing periodic length, where the periods involved are 1/1, 1/2, 1/3, 1/4, . . . , etc. of the cyclic function being studied. The sinus functions thus obtained are referred to as the 1st, 2nd, 3rd, 4th, etc. harmonic factors.

Further data processing steps, partly based on the steps just described, yielded the following summary measures of the subject's overall tracking performance during any given period:

1. The *noise/signal ratio* was calculated as the ratio between the sum of the squared amplitudes of the 2nd, 3rd, 4th, 5th, and 6th harmonics, on the one hand, and the squared amplitude of the major wave (1st harmonic) on the other. In the case of a subject's following closely the movements of the pendulum, the noise/signal ratio would be low.

2. The *number of crossings* was the number of times the two curves—i.e., the curve describing the movements of the pendulum and the curve describing the movements of the subject's eyes—crossed each other. For a subject following the movements of the pendulum closely, the number of crossings would be expected to be high.

3. The *deviation area* was the size of the area between the two curves just referred to. If the subject's eyes followed the pendulum closely, the deviation area would be low. This measure is more stable than measures based on the Fourier analysis [i.e., the measures described under (1) and (5)], in the sense that the blink of an eye does not affect this measure very much but can severely disrupt the Fourier analysis within the cycle in which it occurs.

4. The *microtremor rate* was computed as a function of the total distance which the eye traveled and the "effective" distance it covered. The *total distance, d(tot),* here is the sum of all small eye movements as measured through recording the position of the eye at 3.66 msec intervals. The *effective distance, d(eff),* is the sum of the eye movements as measured through recording the eye position at intervals which were nine times larger (33 msec). The portion of the total distance produced by microtremors is assumed to be the difference between the total distance and the effective

distance, i.e. d(tot)–d(eff). Thus, the micro-tremor rate was computed as $(d$(tot)–d(eff))/d(eff).

5. The *2nd, 3rd, 4th, 5th,* and *6th* harmonics were computed as the ratio of the respective higher harmonic factor (i.e., 2nd, 3rd, 4th, 5th, or 6th harmonic factor) to the 1st harmonic factor. These measures provided a description of the different harmonic components of the subject's wave-like eye movements in following the pendulum. It was also possible to compare the measures thus obtained with ideal values for the measures, i.e., the values the measures would take on if the subject followed the moving light perfectly. The computation of such ideal measures for the saw-tooth pendulum (Periods 2–5) yielded values of 0 for the 2nd harmonic, 0.111 for the 3rd, 0 for the 4th, 0.040 for the 5th, and 0 for the 6th harmonic.

6. The *mean reaction time* (MRT) and the *standard deviation of the mean reaction time* (SDMRT) were the mean and standard deviation, respectively, of the subject's reaction time in pressing the button when the light in the pendulum became green. The two measures were computed for Periods 3 and 4, since only during these periods did the light in the pendulum change. The reaction times in question were measured by inspection of the mingograph record.

7. *Misses* and *false alarms,* likewise obtained for Periods 3 and 4 only, were the number of times in the respective period that the subject failed to press the button when it should have been pressed (miss) or pressed the button when it should not have been pressed (false alarm).

RESULTS

Preliminary analysis of differences in the various measures between the schizophrenic and cycloid psychotic groups revealed apparent group differences, many of which, even if not statistically significant, showed a consistent direction from period to period for the five test periods involved. In order to test the hypothesis that the group differences here were of a general character, the following *within-group rank score* was obtained for each of the measures: the 22 psychiatric subjects were rank ordered, within each of the five periods, in terms of their raw score on the measure in question; for each subject the sum of the ranks thus obtained was formed; subjects were then ranked in terms of this sum, the rank of which is termed the subject's within-group rank score.

For four of the measures mentioned above, such scores yielded significant differences (Mann-Whitney U-test, two-tailed) between the schizophrenic and cycloid psychotic groups. Schizophrenics, compared with cycloid psychotics, were found to have lower *noise/signal ratios* ($p = .004$), higher *numbers of crossings* ($p = .015$), lower *deviation areas* ($p = .049$) and lower *standard deviations of mean reaction times* ($p < .001$). Thus, schizophrenics appeared to perform better than cycloid psychotics both in eye pursuit movements (first three results) and in reaction time consistency shown under the vigilance-type conditions of needing to press the button whenever the green light appears (last result). In a descriptive sense it could be noted as well that the schizophrenics as a group showed a higher *microtremor rate* than the cycloid psychotics, although this result was not statistically significant ($p = .144$). However, a more detailed analysis of the data, with consideration of the hebephrenic ($n = 4$) subgroup of schizophrenics, indicated hebephrenics to have a higher microtremor rate than non-hebephrenic schizophrenics ($p < .05$) and than cycloid psychotics ($p < .05$). The differences in microtremor rate found here were rather large, one of the hebephrenic patients, for example, showing (during two of the test periods) a microtremor rate that was approximately 2½ times that of the patient of highest microtremor rate within both the non-hebephrenic schizophrenic and the cycloid psychotic group, suggesting possible use of the microtremor rate in a diagnostic context.

The fact that, in the case of the saw-tooth pendulum, the first and last periods (Periods 2 and 5) involved red lights only whereas the two intervening periods (Periods 3 and 4) involved the repeated though irregular interspersion of segments where the lights became green instead of red, provided the basis for two difference scores (*Dif-1* and *Dif-2*), obtained for the variables (1) through (6), i.e., for all of the raw-score measures relating to eye movement performance:

Dif-1, or the difference $(2+5)-(3+4)$—where each number refers to the value of the raw-score measure obtained during the respective period—is a measure of the effect on eye-tracking performance of changing from the less attention-demanding conditions (red-light-only) to the more attention demanding (need of pressing the button whenever the lights change from red to green), where a positive score represents an improvement in performance under the more attention-demanding conditions.

Dif-2, or the difference $(2+3)-(4+5)$, is a measure of the effect of practice, a high score indicating the effect to be positive (learning or facilitation) and a low score indicating it to be negative (fatigue).

Comparing the cycloid psychotic and schizophrenic groups on the difference scores (Dif-1 and Dif-2) obtained for each of the variables described under (1) through (6) above revealed no significant or marked differences between the two groups. For both groups there was a general tendency, as evidenced by positive Dif-1 scores, for eye pursuit performance to improve under the more as compared to the less attention-demanding conditions. Such a tendency could be shown with the Dif-1 scores based on the following measures (the numbers of psychotic, i.e., cycloid psychotic and schizophrenic, subjects with positive and negative Dif-1 values, respectively, are indicated, as are two-tailed *p*-values based on χ^2): *noise/signal ratio* (20+, 2−, *p*<.001), *deviation area* (16+, 5−, *p*<.02), *2nd harmonic* (18+, 4−, *p*<.01) and *4th harmonic* (15+, 6−, *p*<.05). Improvement (+) or deterioration (−) in performance in the case of the harmonics was in relation to the ideal measures described under (5) above. In contrast with the results just cited, a deterioration of performance under the more attention demanding conditions was found with the Dif-1 scores of the *5th harmonic* (6+, 15−, *p*<.05).

The character of the improvement in performance shown by all but the last of the measures here is illustrated in Fig. 1, which presents samples of the eye tracking records of a cycloid psychotic obtained from Periods 2 and 3, respectively. As can be seen, tracking is dramatically improved when the more attention-demanding task of Period 3 is introduced, the saccades found in Period 2 being replaced by what appears at least partly to be normal smooth pursuit.

For only two of the measures mentioned under (1) through (6) did the Dif-2 scores indicate a training effect (improvement in performance in Periods 4 and 5 as compared with Periods 2 and 3), such an effect being evident for the following two measures (the number of psychotic subjects

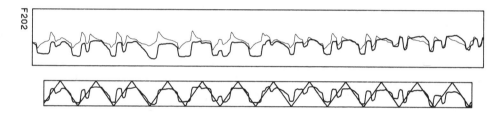

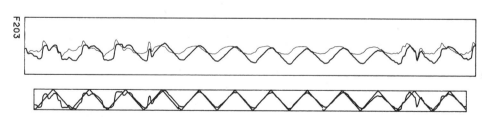

FIG. 1. An example of eye tracking records (subject 20) during Periods 2 and 3 (upper and lower 2 records, respectively). Period 2 = red lights only, Period 3 = intermittent occurence of segments where lights are green. The lower, more abbreviated record from each period has been corrected for drift and shortened to 12 cycles. Light curve = voltage, dark curve = eye position, saw-tooth curve = light (stimulus) position.

showing improvement is labeled with " + " and those showing a worsening with " − ", the p-values being derived as before): *4th harmonic* (15 + , 6 − , $p < .05$) and *6th harmonic* (16 + , 6 − , $p < .05$). On the 5th harmonic, as on the Dif-1 score, a tendency towards worsening was found, although here not significant (6 + , 14 − , $p > .05$).

In order to explore the feasibility of employing measures of pendular eye-tracking performance as elements in a diagnostic instrument of help in differentiating schizophrenics and cycloid psychotics, a cluster analysis was carried out. A cluster analysis groups individuals according to their similarity in terms of a set of variables. The variables included in the present cluster analysis represented a partly arbitrary selection of measures that were either taken from among, or were based on, those measures in the present study which yielded large or significant differences between the two groups, or revealed significant tendencies common to both groups. Seven such measures were chosen: *noise/signal ratio* (mean of the subject's scores), *number of crossings* (ditto), *deviation area* (ditto), *microtremor rate* (ditto), *standard deviation of mean reaction time* (subject's mean for Periods 3 and 4), *Dif-1 of deviation area,* and *Dif-1 of the 2nd harmonic.*

Not only the 13 schizophrenics and 9 cycloid psychotics but also the 4 normal subjects were included in the cluster analysis, the small size of the normal group not precluding its consideration here since in a cluster analysis each individual subject is compared with all the other subjects. In Table 1, the 26 subjects thus examined are listed by subject number and diagnostic category, the fact of whether a cycloid psychotic was excited (hyperactive) or inhibited at the time of testing also being indicated.

Two steps were carried out preliminary to the actual cluster analysis. The first step was to normalize the measures (over subjects) so as to transform them to a scale between 0 and 1.0 (cf. note to Table 1). Exception to this was taken in the case of subject 20, whose scores on some of the measures were outliers that were dealt with separately, being transformed to values larger than 1.0. The next step was to establish insofar as possible, on the basis of the distribution of the subject's transformed scores, three ranges for each of the measures: a normal, a cycloid psychotic, and a schizophrenic range. This provided the basis for assigning each subject points on a cycloid index and a schizophrenic index, the subject receiving one point on the cycloid index if his or her score on a measure fell within the schizophrenic range. The sums of the cycloid and schizophrenic index points respectively that each subject received in this manner formed the indices, shown in Table 1.

These indices, finally formed the basis for the cluster analysis, the results of which are presented in the form of a dendrogram in Fig. 2. Subjects are grouped in the dendogram in terms of their similarity with one another. Examination of the dendrogram reveals the following: All four of the normal subjects (nos. 29, 30, 31, and 32) fall adjacent to one another, indicative of

TABLE 1
Pendular Eye Tracking Performance Measures (Normalized), Clinical Diagnosis, and Cycloid and Schizophrenic Indices

SUBJECT NUMBER	NOISE/ SIGNAL	NO. OF CROSSINGS	DEVIATION AREA	MICROTREMOR RATE	STD. DEV. REA. TIME	DIF-1 OF DEV. AREA	DIF-1 OF 2ND HARM.	CLIN. DIAG.	CYCL. INDEX	SCHIZ. INDEX
2	.569	.336	.942	.489	.432	.804	.449	S	3	4
4	.659	.303	.641	.289	.713	.817	.426	C-	5	2
5	.559	.447	.401	.345	.551	.316	.000	S	3	2
6	.945	.291	.966	.377	.486	.000	.743	C+	6	1
7	.408	.441	.423	.415	.356	.646	.426	S	1	5
8	.388	.366	.173	.118	.551	.575	.406	S	3	4
9	.591	.453	.421	.316	.778	.563	.495	C-	4	3
11	.530	.526	.230	.248	.551	.495	.461	S	4	2
13	.573	.565	.351	.440	.551	.678	.592	C-	3	4
14	.630	.565	.432	.523	.745	.530	.689	S	3	4
15	.469	.592	.119	.264	.302	.514	.343	S	1	2
17	.616	.225	.960	.346	.486	.256	.437	C+	6	1
18	.729	.718	.503	1.000	.324	.744	.197	S	1	3
19	.876	.492	.803	.614	.799	.767	.615	S	4	3
20	2.500	.240	1.500	.373	1.750	1.000	1.250	C+	7	0
21	.404	.462	.127	.128	.421	.495	.360	C-	1	2
23	.275	.348	.287	.222	.259	.662	.387	S	2	4
24	.729	.450	.484	.427	.583	.392	.670	C-	3	3
25	.663	.216	.951	.256	.475	.571	.459	C+	6	2
26	.551	.520	.718	.887	.389	.705	.488	S	3	4
27	.368	.486	.338	.392	.259	.618	.569	S	1	5
28	.539	.658	.236	.423	.356	.476	.557	S	2	2
29	.476	.862	.021	.435	.454	.564	.360	S	0	0
30	.524	.550	.209	.397	.259	.413	.306		1	1
31	.521	.405	.302	.232	.356	.522	.313		0	1
32	.512	1.000	.022	.462	.194	.531	.383		0	0

Note. S = schizophrenic, C = cycloid psychotic (+ hyperactive, − inhibited), no clinical diagnosis = normal. Subjects in the normalization group included those listed plus five patients of other diagnosis. Some sources of subject 20 were outliers and were handled separately.

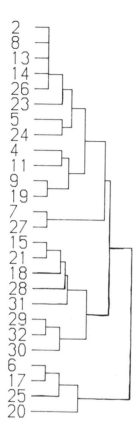

FIG. 2. Dendrogram (cluster analysis). Subject numbers are indicated.

close similarity within the present context (all have cycloid and schizophrenic index values of 0 or 1, as can be seen in Table 1). The hyperactive cycloid psychotics (nos. 6, 17, 20, and 25) form a group of their own (all are higher on the cycloid index than any of the other subjects, with values of 6 and 7, and low on the schizophrenic index, with values of 0, 1 or 2—see Table 1). The schizophrenics and the inhibited cycloid psychotics do not fall in separate groups in the dendrogram, but one can note that the two subjects with the clearest appearing schizophrenic pattern in terms of the eye pursuit performance indices (nos. 7 and 27, with schizophrenic index value of 5 and cycloid index values of 1—cf. Table 1) are both clinically diagnosed as schizophrenics.

The possibility was examined that, despite the failure of the schizophrenic and cycloid indices to effectively distinguish the schizophrenic from the inhibited cycloid psychotic patients via the dendrogram, the use of criterion values for the two indices would enable such a differentiation to be made. On the basis of the distribution of schizophrenic and inhibited cycloid psychotic patients on the two indices, a combined criterion was established according to which those patients with schizophrenic index values of 4 or more and cycloid index values of 2 or less would be tentatively classified as schizophrenics and the remainder of the patients as cycloid psychotics. Such a combined criterion was found to correctly identify 10 of the 13 schizophrenics and 8 of the 9 cycloid psychotics (cf. Table 1). Similarly, for differentiating between the two cycloid psychotic subgroups, a criterion was determined such that those cycloid psychotics with cycloid index values of 6 or more would tentatively be classified as hyperactive and the rest as inhibited. This criterion placed each of the cycloid psychotics in the correct subgroup. Finally, for differentiating patients from normals, a criterion was selected where subjects with cycloid index values of 1 or less would tentatively be classed as normal. This criterion was also completely successful, since all of the patients had cycloid index values of 3 or more. Thus, in the present study, it is possible, through use of criterion values for the schizophrenic and cycloid indices, both of which were based on pendular eye pursuit performance, to successfully distinguish between schizophrenic, inhibited cycloid psychotic, hyperactive cycloid psychotic and normal subjects in all cases but four.

DISCUSSION

The results just cited support the assumption that the distinction between schizophrenics and cycloid psychotics—largely neglected in the English-language literature—is a meaningful one and that measures of pendular eye tracking performance can be useful in distinguishing between the two groups. Further work is necessary, however, to determine what set of eye pursuit performance measures would be most satisfactory here and to assess in a larger and more representative sample what index-point ranges and criterion values should best be employed. It should be stressed that the present selection of measures for the indices was rather arbitrary and that the groups studies comprised only a small number of subjects. A discussion of possible interpretations of various of the measures considered follows.

Two measures to which objections might be raised are those concerning reaction time. One can note that the task conditions under which reaction time was measured are rather similar to those of the Continuous Performance Test, a test used to demonstrate the improvement that may occur in the vigilance performance of schizophrenics after phenothiazine drugs have been administered (cf. Kornetsky, 1972). Since all of the patients had received phenothiazine drugs or drugs similar to these, and since little is known of the effect of such drugs on the vigilance of cycloid psychotics, the possibility exists that the tendency found for cycloid psychotics to display more varying reaction time than schizophrenics may be artifactual.

A question of obvious interest in connection with such measures as those of noise/signal ratio, number of crossings and deviation area, which indicate tracking deficits of a rather obvious character on the part of the patients (cf. also Holzman et al., 1973, 1974; Holzman & Levy, 1977), is whether the deficits involved reflect central or peripheral disturbances. One can note that when the task was made more complex through instructions being given to attend to shifts in the color of the moving pendulum and to press the button when the color became green, patients' performance on these measures improved. This suggests central disturbances to lie at the basis for the deficits. The view of Holzman et al. (1974) that schizophrenics display a failure of central inhibitory control seems relevant in this connection, particularly since those authors apparently included in the schizophrenic category patients that in the present study would be classed as cycloid psychotics.

In apparent contrast to the measures just named, the patients' performance in terms of the 5th harmonic was found to deteriorate under the more complex conditions. This raises the question of what the higher harmonic measures represent. A possible answer is suggested by a detail of Fig. 1, where it can be noted in the lowermost record (which is for the more complex conditions) that the eye movements of the subject in question fail to continue on all the way to the point where the direction of the pendular movement reverses itself. Such a failure, concerning as it does only a small portion of the pendulum's total swing, could be expected to affect the higher harmonics more than the lower. That such a failure occurs to a greater extent when conditions are complex is perhaps reflective of the cognitive strain the complex conditions involve. As this tentative interpretation of the findings for the 5th harmonic illustrates, the higher harmonics may be reflective of small but meaningful aspects of task performance.

How task performance is affected by microtremor is unclear, as is the origin of microtremor, whether more peripheral (e.g., in the ocular muscles or the retina) or more central. The fact that the hebephrenic schizophrenics displayed a much higher microtremor rate than the other patients suggests at any rate the measure could be useful in differentiating schizophrenic subgroups.

As already emphasized (cf. Leonhard, 1957/1979), means should be sought of identifying cycloid psychotics at an early stage. The present findings suggest that eye tracking performance measures could be useful in this respect to aid clinical diagnosis. Such measures could also be useful in studying the phasic changes occurring in such patients during extended periods of clinical contact.

ACKNOWLEDGMENTS

The present research was supported by the Swedish Council for Social Science Research and by the Medical Faculty of the University of Lund. Special thanks are due to Robert Goldsmith for his advice concerning the manuscript, to Birgitta Rorsman for her encouragement and advice, to Ingemar Dahlstrand and Gösta Sundberg for their work in developing the data programs, to Anders Andersson and Laszlo Maroti for constructing the electronic pendulae, and to the personnel, staff, and patients of St. Lars Psychiatric Hospital in Lund who contributed their time.

Correspondence concerning this article should be sent to Sven Ingmar Andersson, Department of Psychology, Lund University, Paradisgatan 5, S-223 50 Lund, Sweden.

III.6 Eye Movements in Schizophrenics Revisited

N. Galley, M. Widera-Bernsen and H. B. Ishak
Universitaet zu Koeln and Rheinische Landesklinik
West-Germany

It is now well known and widely accepted that schizophrenic and other psychiatric patients have "abnormal" pursuit eye movements (For review see Holzman & Levy 1977). But there are several criteria in use to describe differences in eye movements of normals and schizophrenic patients. The problem is to decide whether there are several criteria of one phenomenon or several phenomena. Furthermore, what are the relationships between the several criteria in use? Which criterion best discriminates between a normal and a schizophrenic person? Some criteria are taken from the original eye movement signal, the analysis of which is very time consuming. Other criteria are taken from transformations of the eye movement signal, for example, from the eye movement velocity curve or power spectrum of the eye movement signal, the analysis of which is more economical but sometimes ambiguous, and not a popular means of describing oculomotor deficits in the neurological literature (for example: Baloh, Honrubia, & Sill, 1977; Hartje, Steinhauser, & Kerschensteiner, 1978). But deficits frequently assumes that attentional deficits play an important role for eye movement behavior for example, Hartje et al. (1978) found more saccadation in neurotic patients. Up to now there is still no convenient way to measure the attentional deficits.

Diefendorf and Dodge (1908) published registrations of eye movements in Dementia praecox patients that clearly show the staircase form of eye movements following a pendulum. As one can see in Fig. 1, the two schizophrenic patients show a nearly total absence of smooth pursuit eye movement but a substitution by saccades.

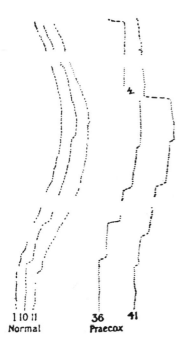

FIG. 1. Original photographic recordings of two schizophrenics (Praecox) and three normals reported by Diefendorf & Dodge (1908): "The praecox pursuits, Nos. 36 and 41, are typical. In mild cases the hesitation to adopt the pursuit-swing is less pronounced, but is regularly shown by straight lines somewhere in the pursuit."

The new interest in schizophrenic's eye movements began with Holzman, Proctor, & Hughes (1973), where the authors wrote in the abstract, "These deviations are probably referable not only to motivational or attentional factors, but also to oculomotor involvement that may have critical relevance for perceptual dysfunction in schizophrenia" (p. 179.) But somewhat later Shagass, Roemer, and Amadeo (1976) showed that manipulations of attention of the patients can improve their performance.

CRITICAL REVIEW OF THE CRITERIONS IN USE FOR DESCRIBING DIFFERENCES BETWEEN NORMALS AND SCHIZOPHRENICS

1. There are "scores for irregularity" of eye movements (Holzman et al. 1973; Shagass, Amadeo, & Overton, 1974; Keuchenmeister, Linton, Mueller, & White, 1977). These scores indicate there seems to be something wrong with schizophrenics but no descriptions of them seem adequate.

2. Holzman et al. (1973), Shagass et al. (1974), and Pivik (1979), for example, describe what would be a motoric stop. Arrest is scored when the eye velocity curve has a zero value while the stimulus is still moving. Schizophrenics have more arrests than normals. Why do they stop their eyes more frequently? Do the arrests relate to the interspersed saccades?

3. There is a score "positive velocity error" in use (Holzman, Proctor, Levy, Yasillo, Meltzer, & Hurt, 1974), when the eye velocity curve shows values high above the mean, as seen in Fig. 2c.

4. May (1979) found large saccades interspersed among the pursuit eye movement in schizophrenics.

5. Cegalis & Sweeney (1979) use a criterion "spatial error," which is given when a saccade overshoots or undershoots the target, i.e., the ending position of a saccade is far ahead (overshooting) or not reaching the actual stimulus position (undershooting). Schizophrenics have more spatial errors, but there is no qualitative information given, such as whether these are undershooting or overshooting saccades.

6. May (1979) and Cegalis and Sweeney (1979) use the criterion "saccade frequency." Schizophrenics have more saccades interspersed among their pursuit eye movements. But crucial for the value of the score "number of saccades" is the identification of a saccade, so Cegalis and Sweeney exclude per definition all saccades smaller than $2°$.

7. Lindsey, Holzman, Haberman, & Yasillo (1978) and Levin, Lipton, and Holzman (1981) use a criterion derived from the Fourier transformed eye movement signal called "signal to noise ratio," where signal corresponds to the power in the frequency band of the stimulus and noise to the power in the frequency band above. Patients show lowered signal to noise ratio or more power in the higher frequency band. Saccades are much faster than pursuit movement, so one can assume this criterion is a complex measure of more and/or larger saccades in the eye movement recordings of patients.

Which relations can be assumed to exist between these different criterions of different authors?

If one assumes that the scores "positive velocity error" and "signal to noise ratio" can be seen as complex scores of more and/or larger saccades interspersed among pursuit eye movements, four other primary scores remain: saccadic amplitude, saccadic frequency, spatial error, and eyeball arrests. What are their mutual relationships? Are they independent or correlated? What data handling is economical and most accurate as a descriptor?

If the abnormal eye movement behavior can be seen as a genetic marker for schizophrenia (Holzman et al. 1974; Holzman & Levy 1977; Holzman, Kringlen, Levy, & Haberman, 1980), it would be nice to know which score discriminates best between a control and a carrier of this genetic marker. Up to now there are only group mean values known.

In search for a causation of the phenomenon in question we must look for influencing factors: data show that manipulations of attention in patients can improve performance (Holzman & Levy, 1977). It is also known that in addition to schizophrenic patients, depressives (Shagass, Amadeo, &

Overton, 1974), elderly people (Kuechenmeister et al. 1977; Sponner, Sakala, & Baloh, 1980), Parkinson patients (Kuechenmeister et al. 1977), and other patient groups with lesions in the cortex (Hartje et al. 1978) and cerebellum for example (Baloh et al. 1977) show more saccadation, i.e., more and larger saccades in-between the pursuit eye movements. So saccadation may be seen as a neurophysiological correlate of impaired attention. Therefore, it would be interesting to manipulate stimuli enough to make normals look like schizophrenics. Assuming that distraction may be a factor, we would expect normals doing mental arithmetic while following the moving stimulus with their eyes to behave in a more schizophrenic-like manner.

Thus, we put forward the following questions:
1. What is abnormal in the eye movements of schizophrenics? Are there one or more phenomena?
2. What are the relations of the four scores (saccadic amplitudes, frequency, positional error, and eyeball arrests) to each other?
3. What is the best discriminating parameter between normals and patients?
4. Are there other factors involved, for example which influence has stimulus velocity systematically?
5. Can we make normals look like schizophrenics?

EXPERIMENTS USING A
CONTINUOUSLY ACCELERATED TARGET STIMULUS

Subjects and Methods

Subjects were 8 schizophrenic outpatients and 9 members and students of our laboratory. The average age of patients was 32-years-old (ranging from 24–35), and the average duration of illness was 3.1 years. All patients are diagnosed as paranoid-hallucinatory schizophrenic and take neuroleptic medications, but were free of symptoms of Parkinsonism. Normals were in the mean 30-years-old (ranging from 23-40).

Patients and normals had to follow a first slowly then accelerated moving light spot with their eyes. The spot moved on an oscilloscope horizontally over 20° at a distance of 80 cm. The light spot was accelerated from a slow velocity of 0.1 c/s (= cycles per second) to a relative fast velocity of 1.2 c/s in 2 minutes. We used a sinusoidal and triangular time function of the stimulus velocity, and made two trials with the patients and three with the normals. During the middle one, the normals had to do mental arithmetic. The head of the subjects was stabilized by a chin rest and a forehead front plate. Horizontal eye movements in the normals were recorded as Electro-oculogram (EOG), using Ag-AgCl-Electrodes and special EOG-amplifiers (0–200 Hz bandwith), which allowed compensation for slowly shifting electrode potentials. Eye movement of schizophrenics were recorded with AC-coupling amplifiers (Tektronix TM 504 0.1–300 Hz bandwidth). Eye movement signal and stimulus signal were recorded on tape (PCM tape 8 K 60 from Johne & Reilhofer, 0–200 Hz bandwidth), and off-line analyzed with a computer (Nicolet Med–80). Signals coming from tape were digitalized (666 points/sec) and by visual inspection (see Fig. 2) using an interactive computer program we identify coordinates of time and space of every interspersed saccade in relation to the correspondent they are 0.3–1.0 angular degree depending on the noise in the EOG signal (mostly frontal Theta-EEG).

Figure 2 shows the pursuit eye movements of a normal subject following a slowly (Fig. 2a) and a moderate (2e) moving light spot. In between the pursuit eye movement curve there are interspersed saccades (in Fig. 2a) numbered from 1 to 6. When the stimulus goes faster (2e), saccadic amplitudes and saccadic frequency increase. In this manner we got information about saccadic amplitudes, saccadic frequencies, and phase relations of some 800 saccades of each subject. These phase relations were calculated in angular degrees because the space coordinates correspond directly to the time relations, and are useful for our purpose to get information about the foveal following area (see below). The beginning position relative to the actual stimulus position was found in our equipment to be ±1 angular degree. In Fig. 2e one can see that the ending position of a saccade anticipates a future (f) position of the target, while beginning positions lag behind (b) the target. Sometimes saccades are corrective (c), which match fovea and target. The pursuit movement is frequently slowed down (s) or arrested (a), which is difficult to discriminate. That is why we do not score slowing numerically correlated to compensate the distorting effect of AC-coupling amplifiers.

Results

In schizophrenics as well as in normals, the mean saccadic amplitude of the interspersed saccades among the pursuit eye movement shows a systematic increase when the stimulus moves faster. But schizophrenics show larger saccades than normals, for highest stimulus velocities they show somewhat smaller saccadic amplitudes. So their operating range is smaller than that of the normals. All subjects show a systematic increase in their saccadic frequency, i.e., their mean number of interspersed saccades per second, when stimulus velocity increases. Though schizophrenics never show higher saccadic frequency than normals, a decrease is found for higher stimulus

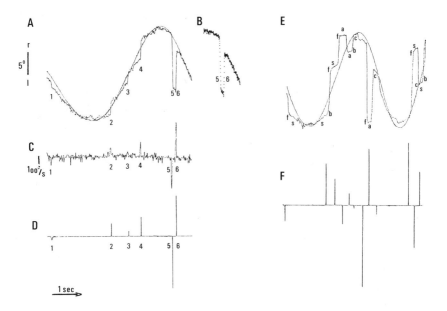

FIG. 2. (a) An eye movement signal (EOG) overlayed the stimulus movement of a normal subject during a slow stimulus velocity. (.2 Hz). One can
see that in between the pursuit eye movement there are interspersed saccadic
eye movements (numbered 1–6). (b) The point plot gives a more realistic view
of what the operator sees on the computer oscilloscope. Every point has a 3
msec time delay to the next so the operator has a good view of the eye movement velocity. (c) The eye velocity signal (won by differentiation of the eye
position signal) allows a rather crude identification of the saccades. As the
reader can imagine false positive and false negative identification should occur, if one works only with this signal. If the eye movement signal is noisy,
which is typical for the EOG, and one uses a higher sampling rate for detecting saccades, one has lost the slow velocity information, for example, the
zero condition, i.e., the eyeball arrests. (d) The saccades identified through
an interactive computer program. (e) The same normal person whose on a
moderate stimulus velocity (.3 Hz) much more and bigger saccades. The pursuit eye movement is either slowed (s) down or arrested (a), if there is a certain distance between eye axis and stimulus. The spatial relations between
saccades and stimulus are characterized by either a lagging behind (b) position of the onset of a saccade or the ending position is correct (c), matching
the stimulus position. Often the ending position goes to a future (f) position
of the stimulus. (f) Identified saccades of 2e are more and bigger in the slower
stimulus condition.

velocities. Again the operating range is slightly smaller for schizophrenics.

Figure 5 shows the mean beginning (B) and ending positions of an interspersed saccade of a normal (N) subject relative to the stimulus position.
It shows that the average saccade begins for a slowly moving stimulus as the
eye exhibits a zero lag to the stimulus but ends in front of the stimulus. For
higher stimulus velocities the beginning shows additional lagging behind the

stimulus (these phenomena can also be seen in Fig. 2e indicated as f and b), but the ending of the saccade in every case is in front of the stimulus. Therefore "corrective saccades" are mostly saccades that anticipate future positions.

Figure 6 shows the correspondent values for schizophrenics (the first three pairs of values indicated with crosses are numerically corrected for distortion from AC-coupling). There is the same tendency for the beginning of a saccade: the faster the stimulus, the more the beginning position lags behind it. But the ending positions lie much farther ahead of the stimulus than in normals, and if we assume there is a shadowed area which is the

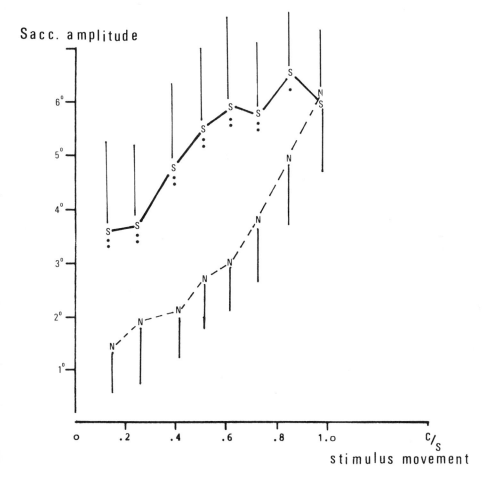

FIG. 3.   Mean saccadic amplitudes for schizophrenics (S) and normals (N) increase when stimulus velocity increases. Schizophrenics show bigger saccades for the slow moving stimulus but not for higher stimulus velocity. The vertical lines represent the standard deviations of the individual mean values of the subjects. ‡: significant on the 5% level, ‡‡: on the 1% level.

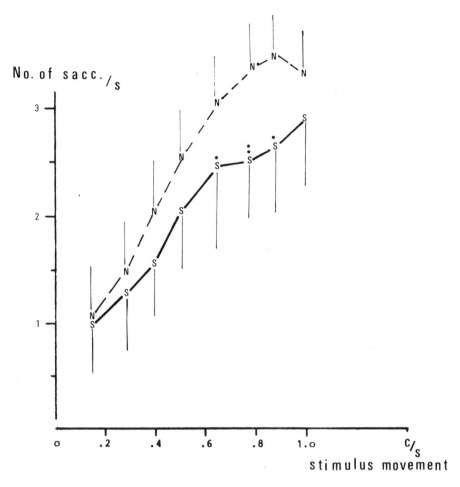

FIG. 4.   Mean saccadic frequency increases with increasing stimulus velocity less in schizophrenics than in normals.

border of the foveal following area, all but one value lie outside this area.
Contrary to the schizophrenics, all target positions of the saccades of the
normals lie inside this area.

In search of the best discriminating parameter between a schizophrenic
and a normal, we calculated individual regression lines of each subject's
mean saccadic amplitudes. As shown in Fig. 7, each initial value of a
schizophrenic lies above all normal ones. Less clearly discriminating is the
slope of the mean saccadic amplitude over stimulus velocity: two
schizophrenic curves (subjects 6 and 7) are in the range of the normals. The
correlation coefficients of the initial values and the slopes are highly

negative for both groups ($r = -.82$ for normals, and $r = -.83$ for schizophrenics) indicating a common factor for slope and initial value.

The correlation coefficients between saccadic amplitude and saccadic coefficients between saccadic amplitude and saccadic frequency in Table 1 show, for both groups, moderate positive values in the slow velocity range indicating that saccadic amplitude and frequency are loosely coupled, confirming what has become well known in the literature for tasks like reading (Bouma & Voogd, 1974). The values become negative for an increasing stimulus velocity, which means there is a ceiling effect: amplitude frequency cannot exceed the constant stimulus amplitude, so one dimension can only increase at the cost of the other.

While searching for factors that influence eye movement behavior, we assumed distraction tasks like doing mental arithmetic would cause im-

Position of sacc.-stimulus

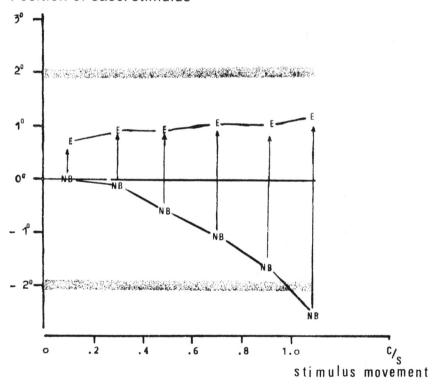

FIG. 5.   Mean values of the relative saccade positions beginning (B) and ending (E) for normal persons (N). The beginning positions show an increasing lagging behind when the stimulus velocity increases. The ending positions are remarkably constant nearly 1% in front of the stimulus. The shadowed area indicates the assured borders of the foveal following area.

Position of sacc.– stimulus

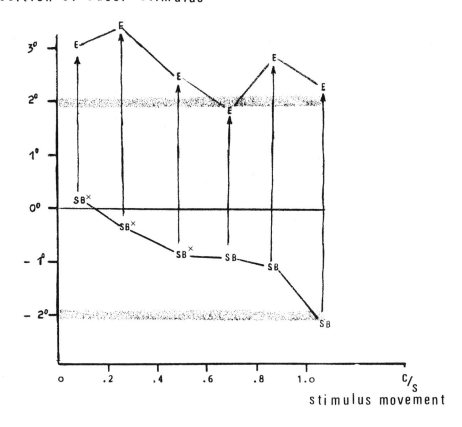

FIG. 6.   The correspondent mean values for schizophrenics (S) show the substantially greater anticipation of their ending (E) positions. All but one lie outside the assured foveal following area. In the beginning (B) positions, there are no differences from the normals. (The first three pairs of values indicated with a cross are numerically corrected for distortion from AC-coupling the patients' eye movement signal.)

paired performance in our normals. But Fig. 8 shows that saccadic amplitude in distracted normals show a small insignificant trend in the opposite direction.

DISCUSSION

Schizophrenic patients show poorer performance than normals following a slowly moving target (0.2–0.5 c/s) with their eyes, because their larger interspersed saccades go far ahead of the stimulus position, thereby increasing the probability of falling outside the foveal following area. The findings of larger saccades interspersed in the pursuit eye movements confirms the findings of May (1979). At the same time it proved to be the best discriminator between schizophrenics and controls. Because large saccades are faster than smaller ones, we assume that there were some saccades which were scored as "positive velocity errors" and "decreased signal to noise ratio." By using a continuously accelerated target we found additional effects: higher stimulus velocity patients show saccades similar in size to controls, which seems to rule out the possibility that saccades of schizophrenics are simply hypermetric.

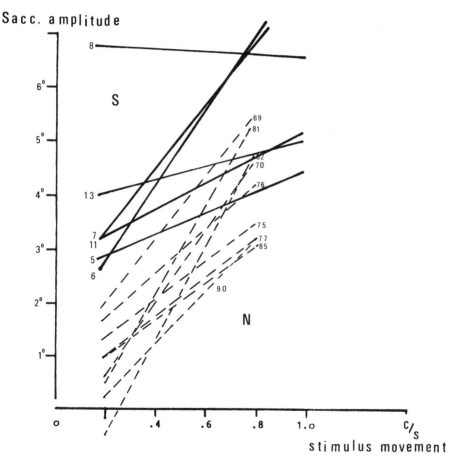

FIG. 7. Individual regression lines for all subjects' mean saccadic amplitudes show two possible discriminating factors: All initial values of the schizophrenics (S: Subjects 5, 6, 7, 8, 11, 13) lie above the normals (N: Subjects 69, 70, 75, 76, 77, 81, 82, 85, 90). And here two patients (Subjects 6, 7) show slopes in the range of the normals.

TABLE 1

| | Stimulus Frequency | | | | | | | |
	.18	.30	.42	.54	.66	.78	.90	1.02
Correl. coefficients								
Normals	.41	.54	.06	.07	.33	− .24	− .49	− .31
Schizophrenics	.38	.57	.14	−.19	− .66	− .83	− .77	− .90

Normals show a greater operating range for saccadic amplitude as a function of stimulus velocity and therefore a steeper slope. The flatter slope for schizophrenics does not prove to be a useful discriminator because two of six patient's curves fall inside the slopes of the control persons (Fig. 7). The correlation between the initial values of the saccadic amplitudes with the slope of the ongoing curve is high for both groups, i.e., both seem to have the same causative factor. This factor would allow one subject to look with large saccades at slowly moving targets and with less decreasing saccadic amplitudes when the stimulus accelerates, and the pattern could change for another subject.

One problem is that our patients took neuroleptic medications. We therefore can't rule out the possibility of drug effects, but the observations of Diefendorf and Dodge (1908) and the data of Holzman and Levy (1977) speak against an important influence of neuroleptic medications.

There was no difference in saccadic frequency for patients or normals for slow stimulus velocities. The higher the velocity the more saccades are seen in both groups. Again the operating range for the increasing saccadic frequency is smaller for patients. May (1979) and Cegalis and Sweeney (1979) reported a higher saccadic frequency in schizophrenics. This inconsistency in the data may be resolved by different threshold values for detecting small saccades: Because patients have larger saccades, there are more detected and the normal's small saccades are not always detected. For example, Cegalis and Sweeney excluded all saccades smaller than 2°, and those were by far the most (see Fig. 4)! Using the electro-oculogram "saccadic frequency" becomes less of a problem because detecting a small saccade by this method includes values from 0.3-1 angular degree. Because we got values for only six patients, there may be a higher saccadic frequency in some patients, but we are still able to say that it is not a good discriminating value. The smaller maximal values of patients fit their reported increased reaction times well (Zahn, Rosenthal, & Shakow, 1961) and are possibly caused by a common factor.

When examining saccadic eye movements' spatial and temporal characteristics in conjunction with stimulus movement, we found that schizophrenics show more anticipation of ending positions than normals, but about the same for originating positions. [Therefore, we feel we can exclude the possibility that schizophrenics' lagging behind the target is evidence of a deficit in the pursuit movement system only in velocity levels.] Therefore, our final interpretation seems compatible with current neurophysiological interpretation of schizophrenic behavior: The schizophrenic lacks a task related tonic inhibition of irrelevant behavior (Flekkoy 1980), for example, spontaneous saccadic amplitude. Normals can adapt their saccadic amplitude to the ongoing task. If the task relevance is

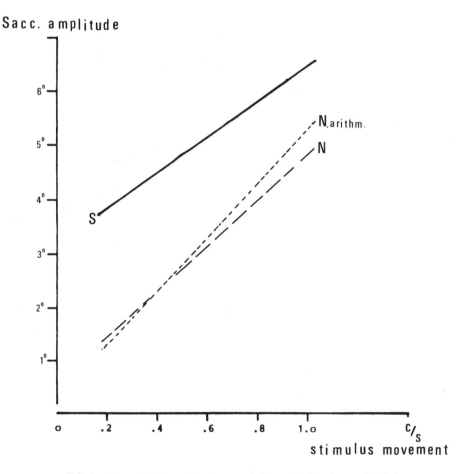

FIG. 8.   Regression line of the mean saccadic amplitudes of normals (N) doing mental arithmetics (N, aritha.) shows no assimilation to the line of the schizophrenics (S). On the contrary, one can see a small (insignificant) trend in the opposite direction: a smaller initial value and a steeper slope.

elevated by realerting procedure (Shagass et al. 1976, Holzman & Levy 1977) or by addition of a cue to the redundant moving stimulus (Shagass et al. 1976), saccadic amplitude is reduced for a while.

ACKNOWLEDGMENT

We thank Miss A. E. Dott for technical assistance, and Mrs. R. Nawrocki for reading the English version of the manuscript.

IV COGNITIVE PROCESSES AND READING

INTRODUCTION

This section is primarily concerned with macroprocesses like understanding reading and problem solving. These clearly differ from the point by point precision of microprocesses (cf. Rayner, 1983, for more detail), but also are likely to be more clearly related to understanding text. Although the first chapter by the Groners is not directly aimed at reading per se, it does address higher order cognitive processing that is as likely to occur in dynamic reading as in other hypothesis testing tasks like those described. They do a credible job at predicting performance in their most sophisticated model variant as a function of frequency distribution of eye fixation path length, error probability and solution times. This approach is somewhat unique in that it examines other than perceptual operations involved in problem solving including understanding, strategy setting, searching for good alternatives and evaluation.

Krause, Fassl, and Wystotzki provide a rather unique and intriguing examination of higher order cognitive processing. They recognize the problem of trying to understand the nature of internal representations and attempt to make these more external by comparing text with text and pictures. When similarities and differences are recognized their next step is to examine fixation dynamics, recorded while subjects solve transitive inferences, in order to better understand the symbolic distance effect. Somewhat counterintuitively they find that the smaller the inference comparison distances, the greater the response time. Although they attribute this to a greater processing load, they remain unclear about the cause. It may be that little consolidation of the inference propositions is possible for small distances, therefore assessment is quite direct, whereas with larger distances the propositions are more consolidated in memory and disparent statements are more readily discovered by memorially checking summary propositions. As with the authors' alternative, this one is also speculation.

In chapter IV.3, Heller and Müller examine the relationship between saccade size and fixation duration. By varying the meaningfulness of the text and spatial extent of the preceding and critical word, they show that fixation durations increase when spatial extent increases from $2.5°$ to $6.5°$ but no change occurs thereafter. That effect is limited to meaningful text because when text represents a 0–order approximation there is little or no increase found at $4.5°$. They include a discussion of a "physiological refractory period," "minimal pause time," and the "prior movement effect" as well as comments on peripheral preprocessing which may be more relevant—remember the "tunnel vision effect."

In chapter IV.4, Shebilske and Fisher discuss and demonstrate first, the criticalness of defining a fixation in terms of data sampling and extent, and second some of the macrolevel characteristics, e.g., reader flexibility, evidenced when reading extended discourse. Specifically, these authors recognize some of the dangers in allowing global and unspecific definitions of fixation or gaze duration, as evidenced in Just and Carpenter (1980), to distort the resultant understanding of reading text and how that can bias the resultant model. From the data described it is shown that readers do not come close to fixating every word while reading. In addition, eye movement dynamics are changed as a function of the reader's perceived importance of the section of the passage.

In the final chapter of this section and volume, Huber, Lüer, and Lass examine eye movements of aphasics reading text. They take exception to the more traditional approach of error analysis and measure eye movements in order to get a more "direct" metric of linguistic processing. Their sentence construction analysis examined actor phase, word category and sentence structure variables for differences between normal and aphasic performance. They found that there was a high correlation between the eye movements of the controls to the subsequent linguistic statement, but such a correlation for the aphasics did not present itself. For the aphasic, content held priority over linguistic adequacy.

Dennis F. Fisher

IV.1

A Stochastic Hypothesis Testing Model for Multi-term Series Problems, Based on Eye Fixations

Rudolf Groner and Marina Groner
University of Bern, Switzerland

INTRODUCTION

In recent years an increasing trend can be observed to utilize eye movements as an empirical basis for models of cognitive activity (for numerous examples see Monty & Senders, 1976; Senders, Fisher, & Monty, 1978; Fisher, Monty, & Senders, 1981; Groner & Fraisse, 1982).

In this chapter we will try to demonstrate that it is especially promising to use mathematical models in order to make the underlying assumptions transparent and to arrive at strong behavioral predictions. More specifically, it can be argued that probabilistic models are especially well suited to take into account the uncertainty inherent in the search for a solution in a given task. This view is reflected by the assumption that an important part of the thinking activity can be considered as *hypothesis testing behavior.*

Such a conceptualization can be traced back to Dewey (1933) and Claparède (1933) among several early formulators (for a historical review see Chapter 1 in Groner, 1978). These attempts have in common a very broad usage of the term *hypothesis* in a wide variety of tasks. Another tradition (e.g., Restle, 1962; Falmagne, 1970; Millward & Wickens, 1974) goes back to cognitive theories of discrimination learning. This work is entirely restricted to the concept identification paradigm, but formalization of the assumptions allows a better empirical test than the earlier hypothesis theories.

Our approach tries to combine some of the advantages of both traditions. Again, formal models are used, but in addition to concept identification, which we have analyzed before (Groner, 1978; Groner & Groner, 1982), we concentrate here on multiterm series problems. An example is given in Fig. 1. The task is to establish an ordering of the terms, given a set of premises, e.g., statements about the order relation between two terms. The formalization allows a systematic and critical test of different model variants on the basis of actual data, a possibility extensively explored by Groner and Groner (1982).

Finally, in addition to the traditional behavior measures like solution latency, error frequency, trial of last error, etc., eye movement data are analyzed to obtain more information about the visual information pick-up of the subject and its relation to the current task. Used in this way, eye movements provide a continuous stream of data that is closely related to the underlying information gathering strategies of the subjects.

As will be seen below, the models proposed consist of two parts: an information processing part that is deterministic in principle and provides a computationally sufficient mechanism for generating the solution, and a hypothesis selection part that is described in probabilistic terms.

ASSUMPTIONS ABOUT THE ROLE OF EYE FIXATIONS

The first assumption seems almost trivial: The task must be performed under such experimental conditions that eye movements have a real *functional* significance, e.g., the access to the information should require an eye fixation. This condition limits experimental presentation to the visual sense modality. In order to interpret a fixation as an attentive response to some information in the display, it is necessary to separate the informational units on display by a distance that exceeds the functional visual field. Care should be taken to exclude the possibility that peripheral visual processing alone would allow sufficient access to the stimulus information.

Such an assumption would, up to this point, explain the usefulness of at least the first fixation on every informative part of the display. There would

Sam is taller than Bill	Sam is taller than Jack
John is taller than Jack	Sid is taller than Jack
Fred is taller than Jack	Sid is taller than Bill
John is taller than Sam	Fred is taller than John
Jack is taller than Bill	Sam is taller than Sid

FIG. 1.   An example of a six-term series problem as presented to the subjects. The grid refers to those areas analyzed as a single gaze.

be no need for any following fixation if the information of the first fixation has been stored in the subject's memory. However, if we assume that subjects attempt to reduce their memory load, it would be reasonable to assume that they will not store that part of the information which is permanently available from the stimulus display. Such material would be taken in when it is needed in the course of the solution process. In such a case, the stimulus display would serve as an external memory store, accessible by means of eye movements.

This point has been tested empirically (Groner, 1978, p. 121) by removing the information after the subject had read it at least once, but not yet solved the problem. Even with a very simple problem involving only three informative statements (which would have been recalled easily, if the subject would have attempted to store them), only 13% of the subjects were able to solve the problem.

Therefore, it is reasonable to conclude that consecutive eye fixations on the same display unit bear some functional significance. Of course, it is still doubtful to assume an equal functional value for every single fixation. Unless subjects close their eyes or look at some part of the environment outside the stimulus display, the eye will be found to point somewhere. In our approach, we assign a function to every fixation within the stimulus display. As will be seen later, however, great differences in function are assumed.

Since subjects do not know the location of the relevant information in advance, they first must find it. Therefore two classes of eye movements can be distinguished, *scanning fixations* associated with the stimulus search, and *processing fixations,* which are supposed to take place after the relevant information has been found and is used for solving the problem. This distinction was empirically tested in several experiments (Groner, 1978, p. 123–130) where the subject's hypothesis was under the control of the experimenter. We found that under suitable experimental conditions the two classes of eye fixations can be well distinguished by just considering the *duration* of the fixation (scanning consumes about 100–200 msec—processing is in the range of 300 msec and longer). Furthermore, we found that during processing the eye rarely moves, but remains in the position of the last fixation. This result is by no means trivial, since the phenomenon of lateral eye movements (Day, 1964; Bakan & Shotland, 1969) would lead to different expectations. Apparently, it is important for lateral eye movements to appear when the stimulation is acoustic.

Before turning to the detailed description of the model, we should clarify the level of resolution the model holds for predictions. In a first stage of the analysis a somewhat coarse screen is preferred, in order to avoid unnecessary intricacies. Therefore, a statement like "Sam is taller than Jack" (see Table 1) was chosen as an inseparable informational unit, and consequently a fixation is defined as *the time spent by the eye anywhere within this unit.* Instead of defining a fixation as an intersaccadic period of relative rest, the external size of the informational unit constitutes the frame of a fixation. In terms of Just and Carpenter (1976), such a location constitutes a "gaze," but here we will use the word fixation synonymously.

A HYPOTHESIS TESTING MODEL FOR MULTI-TERM SERIES PROBLEMS

This section gives an informal treatment of the general hypothesis theory. A more elaborate and formal presentation can be found in Groner and Groner (1982) where hypothesis theory has been formalized in set-theoretical terms.

The central characteristic of hypothetical reasoning is *anticipation*: something is tentatively assumed and, if possible, consecutively tested through some observations in the reality. We call a hypothesis *compatible* if its prediction is in agreement with reality. The compatibility condition for series problems can be stated as follows:

> Let c_i be a term, here represented by a first name, to which an ordinal position
> m should be assigned, e.g., any of the following: "tallest," "second-tallest,".
> .., "smallest." Then the hypothesis $c_i = n$ is compatible with a set of premises
> if there exists no c_k such that c_k is larger than c_i, unless the particular c_k has
> already been assigned to a preceding ordinal position m.

As will be noted, this compatibility condition is recursive in the sense that the order generating process starts with the largest and ends with the smallest position. The only alternative possibility is to reverse the order of processing beginning with the smallest and ending up with the tallest. This also implies the requirement to store in memory all preceding terms which have already been assigned to a position. However, the model is still open to a number of terms being simultaneously tested and to the memory for previously falsified hypotheses, etc. In this way it is possible to systematically construct a set of models that we call *model variants*. In the following we examine in more detail two model variants that are applied to the six-term series problem of Table 1.

First Model Variant (HTM)

The first model variant assumes a process of hypotheses testing with minimal memory load (= HTM). Figure 2 gives the sequence of operations as proposed by this model variant.

To begin, a premise is read and the term that is the grammatical subject is chosen for the hypothesis about the first position (Huttenlocher, 1968).

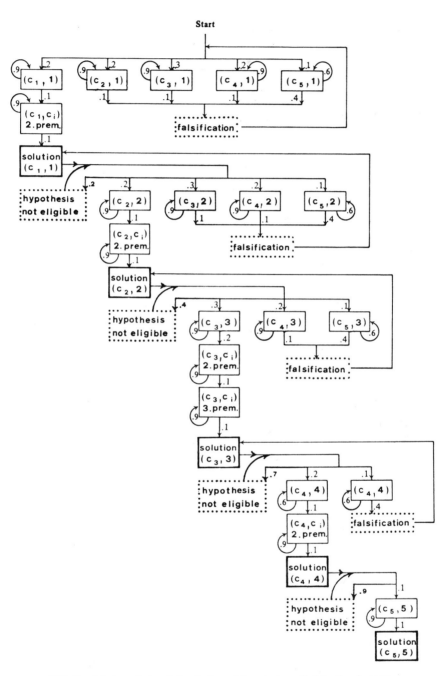

FIG. 2. Markov chain of the first model variant applied to the six-term series problem from the start up to the fifth partial solution.

261

Since the experimental conditions provide a complete randomization of the spatial arrangement of the premises and all preferred directions are balanced, it is legitimate to estimate the choice probabilities of different hypotheses by the relative frequences of the terms serving as a grammatical subject of the premise. In our example (Fig. 1), the subject might fixate (with probability 0.2) one of the two premises concerning John (e.g., "John is taller than Sam") and therefore choose John for the hypothesis (c_2, 1) e.g. "John is the tallest." In the next step more premises are fixated in a completly random order (reflecting the assumption of no memory for a systematical search), and the same hypothesis will be maintained as long as it is comparable with the current input information. In the present example, there is only one premise ("Fred is taller than John"), falsifying the current hypothesis and it will be chosen with a probability of 0.1. After falsification the premise fixated next will again be used for a new hypothesis, but since there is no memory for previous hypotheses, it will again be (c_2, 1) with probability 0.2.

If the sampling of scanned premises is assumed to be independent, a problem arises as to whether the process will ever finish, since there will never be absolute certainty that there is not a falsifying premise hidden somewhere. Therefore, another parameter is introduced which stops the process, and it is supposed to indicate when a hypothesis will be accepted as a solution. The numerical value of 0.10 was found to be adequate. Such a probability also seems quite plausible since it predicts an average of ten more premises to be scanned until the hypothesis finally is accepted, where ten is also the number of premises being presented on the visual display. However, there is an uncertainty inherent in the process as to when to terminate the search process. It has successfully been used for predicting particular kinds of errors (Groner & Groner, 1982, section 8.1.). Now we will concentrate on the predication of the number of fixations necessary for arriving at a correct solution about the first position.

If subjects sampled the correct hypothesis by fixating the premise "Fred is taller than Jack," represented by the left-most branch of Fig. 2, they will continue the search until finding the second premise which confirms the hypothesis "Fred is taller than John," at which point they will accept the current hypothesis as a solution. This solution about the first position has to be stored for solving all remaining positions, otherwise the compatibility rule would not work.

It is easy and straightforward to follow the predictions of the second and third position in Fig. 2. With such a representation we arrive at a flow chart corresponding to a Markov chain where each block corresponds to a state which itself is directly related to an eye fixation.

Second Model Variant (HTG)

This model variant is made more efficient by replacing the independence-of-resampling assumptions with a partial dependence. First, a perfect memory for instances is assumed, i.e., no premise will be scanned more than once during the evaluation of the same hypothesis. The memory for the previously falsified hypotheses goes back only to the last falsified hypothesis which will not be resampled. Figure 3 shows the corresponding Markov chain for this model variant. The left-most branch would be activated with the correct hypothesis and would consume exactly ten fixations (i.e., the number of premises in the display). The next branch to the right would be entered if the first premise involved term c_2. After that, eight of the nine remaining premises will be irrelevant (= branch down), and only one could falsify the hypothesis (= branch to the left), and next the same distinction applies with the remaining eight premises, and so on. At the bottom of this branch, the premise scanned next might contain an eligible new hypothesis, but if c_2 is sampled again, the resampling for a new hypothesis will continue until an eligible hypothesis is scanned. The stopping problem of the first variant does not occur in the second variant, since an exhaustive search will guarantee the correct solution. This property might be considered as positive from the standpoint of problem solving efficiency, but negative with regard to predictive power, because errors could not be predicted by inherent shortcomings of the underlying problem solving strategy.

For an exact description of the solution for all six order positions, 151 states are needed, but it should be noted that under the present experimental conditions there is not a single free parameter which must be estimated.

The Prediction of the Probability Distribution of Fixation Path Lengths Compared with Data

After having derived the Markov chains where the transition through each state consumes exactly one fixation, it is an easy and straightforward matter to calculate *the predicted probabilities for different fixation path lengths*. The probability of arriving at a state S_i after n trials (= fixations), denoted by $P(S_i, t_n)$ is given by the recursive equation

$$P(S_i, t_n) = \sum_{j=1}^{N} P(S_j, t_{n-1})P(S_j, S_i)$$

where $P(S_j, t_{n-1})$ is the probability of having been in state S_j at the previous trial t_{n-1}, $P(S_j, S_i)$ is the transition probability from state S_j to state S_i (which

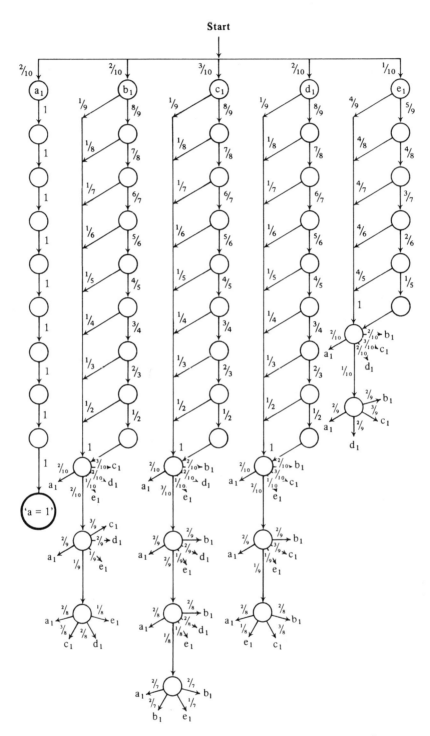

FIG. 3. Markov chain of the second model variant from the start up to the first partial solution.

is assumed to be constant over the whole process), and N is the number of states. By successively computing the sum of products for an increasing n, one obtains the probabilities that the process is in state S_i at trial t_n. Among all states, those associated with an observable event are most interesting, especially that state which corresponds to a solution.

In the following figures we present the probability mass function $p(F)$ where F (for fixation path lengths) is equal to t_n, and

$$p(F) = P(S_s, t_n) - P(S_s, t_{n-1})$$

In this way it is possible to arrive at a formal prediction of the whole probability distribution that can be compared with its empirical counterpart. In the present case it is the relative frequency of the number of fixations needed for a solution (= fixation path length). These data have been obtained by the following procedure: 16 adult subjects (volunteers recruited from a newspaper advertisement, 9 females and 7 males, age 18–57) first solved 4 warming-up items, consisting of two five-term series problems and two six-term series problems. After a short break, two more six-term problems were presented, which were identical to the one presented in Fig. 1, with names replaced and the order of premises randomized. The eye movements were recorded by means of a home-built corneal reflectance camera (Groner, Kaufmann, Bischof, & Hirsbrunner, 1974), which should guarantee a measurement error of less than 1 ° of visual angle.

Figures 4a–4h show the probability distribution as predicted by the first and second model variant compared with the empirical data. Each figure represents a partial solution concerning the tallest, the second tallest, and so on down to the fifth-tallest. According to the present model, the final position needs no special test since it involves the only remaining term. In Figures 4b–4e a very good fit between the predictions of the first model variant HTM and the data can be observed. The only exception is the first partial solution (Fig. 4.1). An aposteriori interpretation of this deviation would be that the subjects were exploring the display at the start of the task before engaging in their problem solving strategy. If we move the observed values ten fixations to the left (which would correspond to an initial scanning of all informational units on the display), the goodness of fit remains satisfactory.

It is also possible to combine all partial solutions to predict the fixation path length for the entire six-term series problem. This is done in Fig. 5. The excellent fit between the predicted probability distribution of the first model variant HTG compared with data is quite encouraging, especially if we keep in mind that there is only one free parameter involved.

This result is somewhat surprising since one would hardly expect that subjects operate on such a low efficiency level with respect to their memory utilization. At least their eye movement behavior could be predicted very

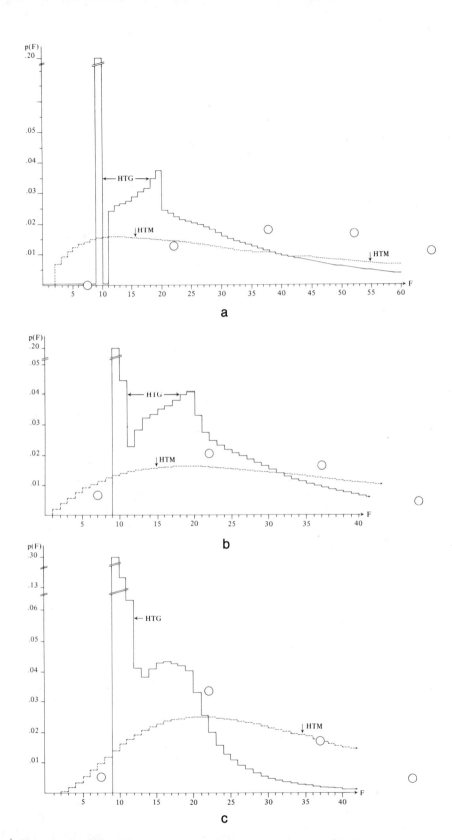

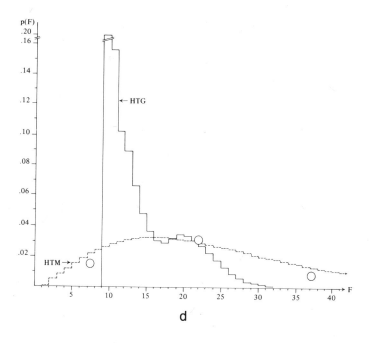

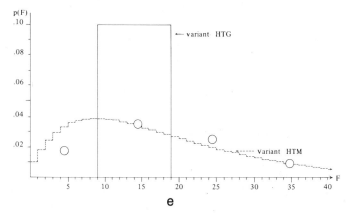

FIG. 4. Predicated probability distributions of fixation path lengths (F) for model variant HTM (dashed line) and HTG (full line). The circles represent empirical observations of 32 observations, grouped in intervals of 15 fixations. (Their actual frequencies relate to the ordinate value by a corresponding scale factor of 15). (a) First partial solution (about the largest), (b) Second partial solution, (c) Third partial solution, (d) Fourth partial solution, (e) Fifth partial solution.

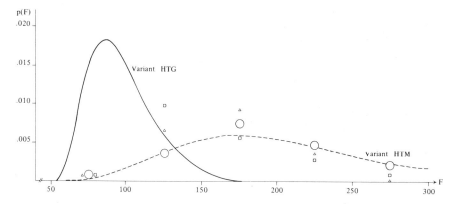

FIG. 5. Predicted probability distributions for the six-term series problem (dashed line: HTM, full line: HTG) compared with eye fixation data. The data are the number of fixations spent from the beginning up to the complete solution, and they are grouped in intervals of fifty fixations. Circles represent the observations under normal conditions. Triangles are observations under experimentally controlled hypothesis testing. Squares are observation after specific instruction for HTG (see text).

precisely by that model variant which assumes an absolutely minimal memory load on the cost of spending a large amount of gaze fixations. Of particular interest here are: (1) Do other behavioral measures also suggest the model variant HTM? (2) Is it possible to get a closer access to subjects' strategies by means of additional experimental control?

GOING BEYOND EYE FIXATIONS

The Prediction of Error Probabilities

As we noted earlier, the first model variant predicts a particular kind of error: If the search for information is unsystematic and not exhaustive, one can never be sure whether there is still some informtion to be found that could disconfirm the hypothesis, if the search would continue long enough. Any stopping rule that is necessary for providing a finite and efficient search permits the error of maintaining an incorrect hypothesis.

The probability of that type of error can be deduced from a Markov chain that is a slight modification of Fig. 1. In principle, one could deduce the probability of every error where a term, to be assigned to a later position, has been already assigned to an earlier position (e.g., "Bill is tallest" or "Jack is second-tallest"). This error will be called a type 1 error as opposed to a type 2 error (e.g., "Fred is second-tallest") which cannot be predicted without further extending the model variant. Since an exact test of each single prediction would require a very large data sample, it is useful to collect all errors within a partial solution into one category of either types 1 or 2 errors. Correspondingly, we subsume all states within the same partial solution of the Markov chain leading to a falsification into one branch.

Second, in analogy to the "verificatory" branches (leftmost in Fig. 2) the falsification branches were also extended over more than one relevant premise. The corresponding number of states in this branch is a free parameter with the last state being absorbing (which can be interpreted as a type 1 error). By applying the compatibility rule it is possible to derive predictions for type 1 errors as the limiting value of $P(S_i, t_n)$, $t_n \rightarrow \infty$. As an approximation to t_n we used the length of the longest observed fixation path.

An experiment was designed to estimate the length of the falsification branches and to test the prediction of error frequencies. A sample of 128 subjects (volunteers, mainly students in the first year) were tested with the same tasks as specified above; however, without recording eye movements. The results were categorized into correct solutions, type 1 errors, and type 2 errors. Table 1 gives the results of the experiment together with the predictions of the model. As can be seen in the last column, the number of type 2 errors, e.g. those which cannot be related to the first model variant HTM, is in general much smaller than the amount of type 1 error. It can also be noted that there is a very good fit between data and predictions. This result supports the model variant HTM as an adequate mechanism explaining different data domains.

Predicting The Solution Times for Partial Solutions

In this section latency distributions are discussed, e.g., the probability distribution of the time required for each partial solution. We started with a

TABLE 1
Error Frequencies in the Six-term Series Problem Compared with
the Predictions, including Parameter Estimates

	observed percentage of type 1 errors	*predicted* probabilities of type 1 errors	*r* (= *estimated*) number of premises searched	*observed* percentage of type 2 errors
1. partial result	.202	.200	3	-
2. partial result	.123	.154	3	.004
3. partial result	.175	.200	2	.008
4. partial result	.135	.111	2	.034
5. partial result	.111	-	-	.080
6. partial result	-	-	-	.068

Markov chain that is a modification of Fig. 2, now subsuming all states within the same (i-th) partial solution under a single state S_i. The process starts at S_1 and has always just two possible transitions, one from the current state to the next (with the interpretation of having accepted the currently active hypothesis as the partial solution and going over to the next order position), and the other the probability of remaining in the same state (interpreted as the continuation of the test with the active hypothesis). The assumption underlying the model variant HTM (lack of memory) corresponds to the main property of a Markovian process that given the process at time t, its future progress is independent of the past. When recording the solution times, only the beginning and the end of the postulated process are directly observable, which makes it necessary to subsume the finer details of the process under a single state. As a consequence, however, the problem arises of estimating parameters that have no directly observable counterpart. Furthermore, it is necessary to adapt the model to a continuous time scale.

So far the variable t (for trial) was denoting a single event in an information processing framework, corresponding to a step of a discrete Markov chain. We now change this notation and take t (for time) as a continuous variable. Let $P_i(t)$ be the probability of the process to be in state S_i at time t.

It can be proved (Groner, 1978, p. 188–191) that the probability of being in the final state is given by

$$P_N(t) = 1 + (-1)^{N+1} \prod_{j=1}^{N-1} d_j \left(\sum_{k=1}^{N-1} \frac{e^{-d_k t}}{d_k \prod_{\substack{\ell=1 \\ \ell \neq k}}^{N-1} (d_k - d_\ell)} \right)$$

The solution for $P_N(t)$ is the basis for predicting the cumulative probability distributions of the latencies. Here, $P_N(t)$ refers to the probability of having arrived at the ($N-1$)th partial solution in the time interval from the beginning of t. The parameters $d_1 \ldots d_{N-1}$ reflect the intensities of transitions on a continuous time scale. It should be noted that all intensity parameters are assumed to be different (as can be expected from the first model variant).

In order to test these predictions, an experiment (with 10 subjects, each solving 2 problems with 6 partial solutions = 120 observations) was set up with the same kind of six-term series problems as introduced earlier. Since the number of observations is too small for an adequate test of the hypothesis, the present example is more like a demonstration than a test.

Figure 6 shows the result of this experiment together with the best fitting curves. The six intensity parameters have been estimated consecutively by minimizing the chi-square of deviation and by taking the estimates of d_1 un-

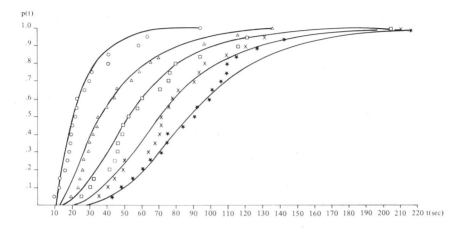

FIG. 6. Latency distributions for the six-term series problem. The empirical culmulative distribution of solution times are represented as follows: open dots for the first partial solution, squares for the third partial solution, and filled dots for the sixth partial solution. The lines represent the best fitting curves, from left to right in the order of the first up to the sixth partial solution. The parameter estimates are: $t_o = 11$, $d_1 = 0.037$, $d_2 = 0.157$, $d_3 = 0.067$, $d_4 = 0.055$, $d_5 = 0.059$, $d_6 = 0.339$.

til d_i from all earlier partial solutions as constants (= fixed parameters) in estimating the d_{i+1} of the next partial solution. In addition it was necessary to introduce a constant of 11 seconds (denoted t_o) reflecting the initial delay before starting with the actual process of problem solving. The data of the third, fourth, and fifth partial solution show an increasing tendency towards a step-like shape. Since there is a large sampling error due to the small sample size, it cannot be decided whether there is a systematic discontinuity, a tendency that could not be explained on the basis of the first model variant. Otherwise the goodness of fit between predictions and data is quite satisfactory. Without considering earlier empirical evidence this result would be relatively weak. However, in combination with the other predictions, the result reported in this section adds further corroboration to the first model variant HTM as an empirically adequate explanation of human problem solving in terms of hypothesis testing theory.

THE EXPERIMENTAL MANIPULATION OF THE SUBJECTS' PROBLEM SOLVING STRATEGY

So far subjects were completely free to choose any method or strategy to solve the multi-term series problems. Their hypothesis testing strategy was inferred indirectly by comparing the observed behavior with the prediction of formalized models. Two studies, where subjects' problem solving strategy was under direct experimental control are of interest.

In the first study we attempted to experimentally simulate the model variant HTM. Six subjects were presented with the original displays (Fig. 1) but their task was now to decide on the truth of statements given orally by the experimenter (e.g., experimenter: "John is the tallest"—subject: "False"—experimenter: "Sam is the tallest"—subject: "False," etc.). The statements of the experimenter were generated by a random sampling scheme in accordance with the probabilities of HTM. The eye movements were analyzed in the same way as before except that those periods where the experimenter gave his statement were eliminated.

The resulting distribution of the fixation path length is represented by triangles in Fig. 5. Although there seems to be a slight tendency towards shorter fixation paths under the controlled condition, the difference is not significant. The result suggests that it is possible to reconstruct the subjects' eye paths under normal conditions from that collected under conditions of controlled hypothesis testing, although this conclusion has to be taken with care because of the small sample size and the possibility of accepting the null hypothesis.

Another experiment investigated the questions of whether the subjects are fixed on an HTM-like strategy, or whether a more efficient strategy can be induced by proper instruction. For that purpose, 12 more subjects received a thorough instruction about the strategy of the second model variant HTG. They were taught to immediately select a hypothesis from the first premise encountered, and to search through the display in a systematic non-repetitive way (for a verbatim report of the instruction, see Groner, 1978, p. 167). With the exception of this instruction, all other conditions remained the same as above.

The results of this experiment are indicated by small squares in Fig. 5. Compared with the two other conditions, there is a significant decrease of the fixation path length. However, there is also a significant deviation between the observed values under instructed conditions compared with the predictions of model variant HTG. Apparently the instruction alone was not sufficient to bring the information gathering strategies of our subjects into a strict correspondence with the model variant HTG. The most striking difference is the fairly constant delay of about 20 fixations between the predictions and observations. There are at least two explanations that would account for this delay: The subjects read the whole set of premises before starting to generate or test a hypothesis, despite the explicit instruction not to do so; or possibly, the subjects made a double test, e.g., having found a solution, they looked a second time through the whole set of premises to make sure that they had not overlooked contradicting information the first time.

This experiment has shown that it is possible not only to change molecular measures of cognitive behavior like eye movements by means of instruction, but to change them in the direction predicted by a particular information processing model.

CONCLUDING REMARKS

There is a large body of literature on series problems, especially three-term series problems (for a review see Johnson-Laird, 1972), but also multi-term series problems (e.g. Potts, 1978). Most of these contributions focus on psycholinguistic factors or modes of memory representation. (For an eye movement analysis of series problems along this line see Krause, 1982, and Krause, Fassl, & Wygotzky, this volume). We will not enter this discussion here, since our approach is mainly concerned with the intermediate phases of the whole process. These include (1) understanding the task, (2) setting-up a problem solving strategy, (3) searching for relevant information, (4) evaluation of the relevant information, (5) establishing a memory representation, and (6) retrieval from memory. It should be clear that there is still ample space for work on the other aspects of the process as a whole.

However, none of the approaches mentioned above presents a formalized procedural model that allows for the prediction of entire frequency distributions from the underlying assumptions. In the realm of eye movements, we only know of one similar approach, although using another task; the work by Suppes, Cohen, Laddaga, Anliker, and Floyd (1982). By proposing a procedural model for some algorithms of arithmetic, Suppes et al. were able to make exact predictions on the distribution of fixation durations.

The main result of our studies was the finding that one particular model variant was capable of predicting the frequency distributions of eye fixation path lengths, or error probabilities, and of solution times.

Even more surprising than such a high degree of convergent validity is the specific nature of the successful model variant, which can be characterized as the minimal one with respect to the amount of memory load and, as a consequence, also with respect to problem solving efficiency (defined by the length of the eye fixation path, the amount of type 1 error, and the solution time). Certainly one would not expect a priori such a low efficiency level of human problem solving. However, we should keep in mind that our approach is strongly "molecular," i.e., the analysis of the underlying processes addresses lower units in a hierarchical organization than the usual approach dealing with solving protocols aloud where more efficient heuristic principles have been postulated (e.g. Newell & Simon, 1972).

One can speculate that the primary reason for the apparent inefficiency on a lower level of analysis is the well known limitation in short-term memory capacity. To minimize processing load, the problem solver utilizes, as far as possible, those elements of the environment that remain constant. That part of the information which remains accessible from the outside world will not be even temporarily stored but will be read in at the moment when it is necessary. In this way, the visual display serves as an external memory device for the problem solver. Implicit in this interpretation is the assumption that eye movements are inexpensive for the problem solver, since he not only fixates the same input unit several times but even must start a search in order to find it. However, due to the speed of saccadic eye movements, this extensive search process can still go on without interrupting the much slower execution of the higher level processing. Thus, the time course of human information processing seems to be well balanced with respect to its different components. It also appears that eye movements are particularly suited for an analysis of human information processing behavior in real time.

ACKNOWLEDGMENTS

This research was supported by grants of the Swiss National Science Foundation. We gratefully acknowledge the help of Franz Kaufmann and Beat Keller in running the experiments.

IV.2 Three-dimensional Orderings, Text Representation, and Eye Fixation

W. Krause, J. Fassl and F. Wystotzki
Akademie der Wissenschaften
Berlin, German Democratic Republic

The internal representation of a simple text can be analyzed through the construction process (Foos, Smith, Sabol, & Mynatt, 1976; Krause, 1982) or by means of task solving strategies, if hypothetical. In the case of memory scanning (Sternberg, 1969), the scanning process is known (Geissler, Puffe, & Scheidereiter, 1982) and requires a listing of elements as internal representation. Unfortunately, in the case of transitive inference, the inference processes is not known, but usually a symbol distance effect is observed. Though many researchers interpret this effect through linear orderings as internal representation, no conclusive data are yet available. For that reason we feel it is impossible to conclude anything about the internal representation from the inference process. Therefore we use two methods of converging operation in order to analyze the internal representation of a simple text:

a. We transform the assumed internal representation into an external representation and compare the reaction time of answering questions between two series:
   1. Subjects were given text only.
   2. Subjects were given text and picture about text.
   In the case of similar reaction time distributions, we can conclude that the internal representation is similar to the external representation.
b. We analyze the solving strategies of transitive inferences by means of eye fixation measurements in order to get some explanation of the symbolic distance effect.

THE INTERNAL REPRESENTATION OF
ONE-DIMENSIONAL ORDERINGS

Many papers in the field of reasoning about texts deal with comparative sentences (e.g., "A horse is larger than a collie") and declarative sentences (e.g., "A collie is a dog"). Thus the performance on real linear orderings and on artificial set inclusion relations were investigated (Potts, 1972, 1978; Griggs, 1976; Frase, 1969, 1970). Only the adjacent pairs were presented, but subjects were tested for their knowledge of all the pairs. Because the relations are transitive, statements about remote pairs can be deduced. Interestingly enough, even though the remote pairs were never presented,

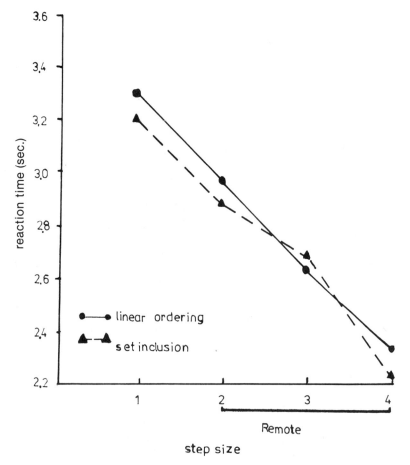

FIG. 1.   Reaction time (sec) as a function of remoteness (step size) for linear orderings and set inclusion relations according to Potts (1978).

reaction time on the remote pairs was shorter than on the adjacent pairs.

The most widely accepted interpretation for the distance effect obtained with linearly ordered information is that proposed by Moyer (1973). He argues for the existence of an "internal psychophysics" whereby subjects store actual perceptual representations of information. Potts (1972, 1978) extended this position to account for his work on linguistically derived artificial linear orderings. He argues that subjects arrange the terms of the orderings along an *internal interval scale* and that the greater the distance separating those two terms on the scale the easier it is to compare them. With this interpretation, linear orderings and set inclusion relations are striking examples of how information is integrated. More exactly, they demonstrate how a text can be transformed into a cognitive structure in the sense of an imagery as internal representation.

THE INTERNAL REPRESENTATION
OF THREE-DIMENSIONAL ORDERINGS

In our investigation we examined the *generalizability* of text transformations into cognitive structures. The above described results are restricted to paragraphs that employ transitivity. The transitivity allows remote pairs to be deduced and a "line" representation to be constructed. The question is whether subjects could construct a cognitive structure with the property of simplifying the solving process if a text containing a *three-dimensional ordering* is to be comprehended, that is, if a text includes different types of relations *without employing transitivity*.

The problem is important from the standpoint of cognitive psychology as well as from that of articial intelligence. In the case of cognitive psychology, generalization of linear order results to three-dimensional orderings seems crucial. In this case of artificial intelligence, it is important to know which kind of representation causes the most simplified procedure.

As mentioned above, we use two methods to analyze the internal representation. First of all, we assume that a simple text is internally represented as a cognitive structure. Starting from this idea we (re)transform the assumed internal representation into an external structure. If we observe the same reaction time distribution in the text situation and in the structure situation, then we assume that the supposed structure is similar to the internal representation.

The second method aims at analyzing the reasoning process itself. By means of eye-fixation measurements we try to corroborate Moyer's interpretation of the symbolic-distance effect. It is our intention to establish that the decrease of reaction time as a function of remoteness can only be explained if a cognitive structure as internal representation is assumed.

THE ANALYSIS OF THE INTERNAL REPRESENTATION THROUGH COMPARISON OF REACTION TIMES IN TEXT AND STRUCTURE (OR PICTURE) SITUATIONS

In our investigation, we used texts with different relations between terms. Subjects learned a series of paragraphs, each describing a three-term, a four-term or a five-term series problem. A sample paragraph is given below:

$$
\begin{array}{ll}
 & \text{L ist hoher als R.} \\
 & \text{M ist vor R.} \\
 & \text{Y ist vor M.} \\
 & \text{G ist neben Y.} \\
 & \text{S ist tiefer als G.} \\
\text{That means:} & \text{L is higher than R.} \\
 & \text{M is in front of R.} \\
 & \text{Y is in front of M.} \\
 & \text{G is beside Y.} \\
 & \text{S is deeper than G.}
\end{array}
$$

Subjects were instructed to imagine the letters as elements or points in space. After comprehension of the text, subjects were asked to answer questions concerning the text

1. by means of memorizing the comprehended paragraphs and
2. by means of a given picture as demonstrated in Fig. 2.

For example:

Is Y in front of R?   (2 "inference steps").

The elements denoted by letters (e.g., "R") were linked with different relations such as "higher than," "deeper than," "in front of," "behind," and "beside."

Based on the assumption of rules or axioms of concatenations between single sentences, we are able to formulate two hypotheses about the inference process in memory, similar to linear orderings.

1. Subjects store the single sentences and do not store deducible information. Inferences are drawn only when required by a test on the information. The time to answer the question *increases* with an increased number of inference steps which are necessary for answering questions about remote pairs.

2. The other assumption is that—when generalizing linear orderings—the single sentences are integrated into a three-dimensional order dur-

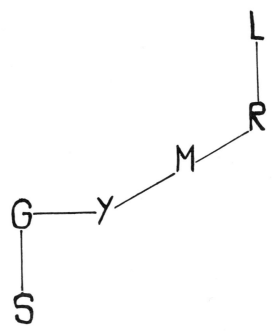

FIG. 2. Picture representation of text given above.

ing the acquisition of information. We assume that this three-dimensional order is similar to an image and designate this as a cognitive structure. If we suppose that the retrieval process about this cognitive structure is the same observed in the case of linear orders, then we expect the reverse relationship between reaction times as compared with hypothesis (1). The reaction time should be *decreased* with the increased number of sentences or step size. This effect is the so-called symbolic distance effect (Moyer, 1973; Potts, 1978).

Figure 3 shows the averaged reaction times for three-, four-, and five-term series problems as a function of step size or remoteness. This result corroborates the integrations hypothesis. Subjects are able to integrate sentences with *different* relations between terms into a three-dimensional order. Obviously this integration process is restricted neither to one-dimensional orderings nor to transitivity.

What kind of internal representation was constructed in our experiment? We started from the assumption that a cognitive structure is internally represented. Then we compared two experimental conditions. In a first condition, subjects were given the text only and in the second subjects were given the text together with a picture about it (Fig. 2). In the first situation,

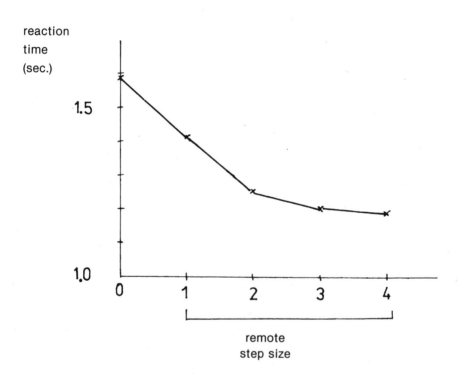

FIG. 3. Reaction time (sec) as a function of remoteness for three-dimensional orderings with 30 subjects. Subjects have to answer questions using an internal representation of a text. The data are averaged from two series of three-term, four-term and five-term series problems. The adjacent points 0/1, 1/2, 2/3 were significantly different at the .05 level (*t*-test for paired observation).

subjects have to answer the question from their internal representation, whereas in the second situation, subjects answer the questions from the externally presented picture. If the functions in both situations are similar, then we believe that our assumption for the first condition was correct. (Naturally, we assume that retrieval processes in both situations are similar.)

Figure 4 shows that reaction time as a function of step size with and without a picture of the type shown in Fig. 2 (artificial information). The reaction time decreases as the number of steps sizes increases in the situation without a picture as well as with a picture. (We carried out the same experiment for realistic information and received the same results [cf. Geissler et al., 1982].) The similarity of the two curves leads us to the conclusion that the internal representation is similar to a structure as given in Fig. 2.

The result in the reaction time experiments demonstrates that integration of information is not restricted to the case of using only one type of relation. The reduction of the inference process into a simple comparison

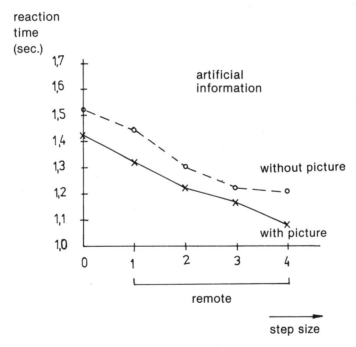

FIG. 4. Reaction time (sec) as a function of remoteness (step size) for artificial information with 30 subjects. With picture: Answering questions by means of a picture as external representation. Without pictures: Answering questions by means of an internally represented memory structure. The two curves were not significantly different at the .05 level (U-test of Mann and Whitney).

process in the case of linear orderings seems also to be relevant to the case of three-dimensional orderings.

An open question is: Why does reaction time decrease as a function of remoteness? What kind of retrieval strategies about this cognitive structure have to be assumed in order to explain the higher reaction time for remote pairs?

THE ANALYSIS OF THE INTERNAL REPRESENTATION THROUGH STRATEGY ANALYSIS OF "INFERENCE PROCESS" BY MEANS OF EYE FIXATION MEASUREMENTS

We carried out the eye fixation experiment for series (2) with 15 subjects. They were given the text with the picture (Fig. 2) about the text and were asked to answer questions by means of the fixation of the picture elements. We registered the eye fixation sequence.

First of all, Table 1 shows the number of questions, classified through different kinds of eye sequences. The situations (b) and (c) were significantly different at the .05 level (Wilcoxon-test), confirming that in most cases subjects directly compare the questioned letters and do not deduce the information.

In order to explain the time difference as a function of remoteness we classify the eye fixation sequences into different operations:

Scanning:
- fixations *before* one of the letters of the question is fixated: Fixations for location. These fixations characterize a searching process. We designate this as fixations *before comparison*.

TABLE 1
Number of Questions Classified Through Different Kinds of
Eye Fixation Sequences

a. total number of questions:	244
b. number of questions in which the questioned letters are directly fixated:	126
c. number of questions in which also other letters between the questioned letters are fixated:	53
d. number of questions in which only one of the questioned letters is fixated:	65

- fixations after the last of the letters of the question is fixated. We designate this as fixations *after comparison.*

Processing:

- fixations directly between the two letters of the question: Fixation for decision. We designate this as fixations of *direct comparison.*
- fixations between the letters of the question that do not directly compare the letters themselves. Also other letters between the questioned letters are fixated during the comparison. These fixations are a search for the next questioned letter and a test for the relation. We designate this as fixations *during the comparison.*

An example of these comparisons is given in Fig. 5. First of all, we determined the averaged number of fixations to answer a question as a function of remoteness. Figure 6 shows those data. Obviously there is no difference in the averaged number of fixations between the four situations (steps size 1 to 4). The averaged number of fixations per question is approx. 3.5 and is independent of the remoteness of the pairs. The number of fixations cannot explain the decrease of reaction time in Fig. 3.

If we assume that the increase of the reaction time in case of one "inference step" is caused by more processing in order to increase the security of decision, then we have to compare the number of fixations based on our classification. The result is given in the lower diagram of Fig. 6. We only compared the situation 1 "inference step" with the situation 4 "inference steps." In case of "direct comparison" and "after comparison" the number of fixations is equal. In case of "before comparison" the number of fixations is increased, whereas the number of fixations is decreased in case of "during comparison." Obviously subjects carried out more scanning fixations and processing time was greater than the scanning time

Question: Is L higher than Y ?

Eye fixation: Start— M — L — R — M —L — Y— G — M
|←before ——→|←— during —→|←direct→|←after —→| comparison

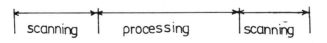

FIG. 5. Classification of eye fixations.

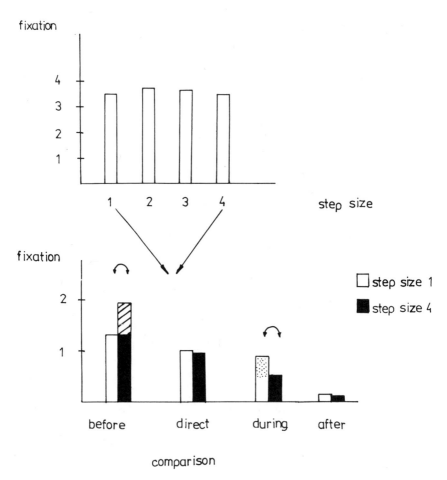

FIG. 6. Averaged number of fixations to answer a question as a function of remoteness (above) and for different fixation operations (below). The difference in case of "before comparison" is significant at the .05 level analysis of variance and Duncan test, total number of fixations: 658.

(Groner, 1975, 1978). The reduced reaction time in case of large letter or element remoteness might be caused by the reduced number of processing fixation found during comparison.[1]

Figure 7 shows the averaged frequency of eye movements for the two questions: Is L higher than M? (1 step) and Is L higher than S? (4 steps). (In the figure only such eye movements between two points were marked that showed more than 25% of the maximum frequency). In the situation "one

---

[1]Unfortunately we were not able to register the fixation times in this experiment.

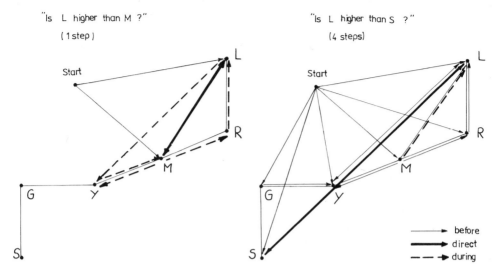

FIG. 7.   Eye movements in two situations: Is L higher than M? (1 step) and
Is L higher than S? (4 steps).

step,'' more fixations during comparison were carried out, whereas in the
situation "four steps," more fixations before comparison and fewer fixations during comparison were observed. Based on the time difference between "before" and "during," mentioned above, this fact corresponds to
the decreased reaction time as a function of remoteness.

Table 2 shows the averaged frequencies of eye movements related to one
question for the four fixation operations: before, direct, during, and after
comparison for the step size 1 and 4. Subjects needed more fixations than
minimally necessary.

Our results give us some insight into the nature of the symbolic distance
effect. The higher reaction time in the case of small distance in comparison

TABLE 2
The Averaged Frequencies of Eye Movements Related to One
Question for the Four Fixation Operations and for 1 and 4
"Inference Steps."

| | | | | | comparison | | | | | |
| | before | | direct | | during | | after | | total | |
Step size	exp.	theor.	exp.	theor.	exp.	theor.	exp.	theor.	exp.	theor.
1	1,38	1,0	1,0	1,0	0,8	0	0,2	0	3,38	2
4	1,91	1,0	0,9	1,0	0,52	0	0,18	0	3,51	2

with that of large distance is caused by more processing. This process agrees with the assumption of a cognitive structure as internal representation and disagrees with the assumption of isolated sentences as internal representation. The reason for this effect of more processing in case of small distance is unclear. One possibility is the increase of the security of the decision. But this is a speculation.

IV.3 On the Relationship Between Saccade Size and Fixation Duration in Reading

Dieter Heller
Universität Bayreuth, German Federal Republic

Hermann Müller
Universität Würzburg, German Federal Republic

At present many of the efforts in eye movement research on reading are concentrated on questions of eye movement control. To answer those questions, several control models of reading eye movements have been proposed differing according to the level of information processing activities (visual and/or linguistic) on which the eye movement control is assumed to be based. In support of the controlling function of these internal activities, experimental results are presented that account for parts of the variability in saccade size and fixation duration by demonstrating relationships between visual, syntactic, and/or semantic characteristics of the text and the eye movement pattern.

Regarding saccade size, McConkie and Rayner (1975) observed a reduced portion of longer eye movements when eliminating the word length information in peripheral vision by filling the spaces between the words. Rayner and McConkie (1976) found that saccade size is primarily dependent on the word length pattern in peripheral vision, while O'Regan (1979a, 1979b) demonstrated that saccade size is influenced by both the length of the word in peripheral vision and the length of the word being fixated currently. Moreover, O'Regan was able to show that the control of saccade size is not only based on visual word length information, but also on linguistic processing activities: With the same sentence context preceding a critical word (a "THE" or a three-letter verb ("VRB"), for instance, "HAD," "ATE," etc.) the "THE" in peripheral vision resulted in longer saccades than the

"VRB" (for instance, "THE PIG THAT GRUNTED/THE MOST WAS FRIENDLY" compared to "THE PIG THAT GRUNTED/ATE MANY BISCUITS"); this "THE-skipping" effect was stronger the more predictable the sentence structure was ("verb-type structure": "THE PIG THAT GRUNTED/THE MOST WAS VERY FRIENDLY" compared to "noun-type structure": "APPARENTLY THE LOVERS/THE GIRL KNEW LIVED IN NEW YORK").

Just as saccade size control is based on visual and linguistic processing activities, so also is the control of fixation duration. Rayner (1975) demonstrated that the fixation duration on a critical word depended on the visual features of a stimulus pattern which was displayed in the critical word position during the previous fixation (fixation $n - 1$) and which was replaced by the critical word during the subsequent saccade. That is, the fixation duration on the critical word (fixation n) was longer when there was less visual similarity (regarding word shape, external letters, etc.) between the stimulus pattern displayed initially and the critical word. This result was accounted for by peripheral "preprocessing". Peripheral processing activities also seem to be applicable to the observation reported by Heller (1976) that the first fixations on a line are longer than fixations in the middle, while the last fixation is shorter than all others.

Granted then that peripheral processing activities quite likely contribute to fixation duration, activities of processing the word being fixated currently also have an effect. While they are unconcerned about fixation duration per se, Just and Carpenter (1980) averaged and performed multiple linear regressions on durations of clusters of fixations called "gazes" on different words and showed a significant effect of the number of syllables of the fixated word (the analysis assumed a syllable-like coding process in advance): Gaze duration increased with the number of syllables ("word encoding"). On a higher level of processing ("lexical access") this analysis revealed an effect of the word frequency: The more infrequent the word the longer was the gaze duration on it. This frequency effect was especially striking for encountering an unknown word the first time ("priming effect"), but it decreased with repeated occurrence of that word ("repetition effect"). On the processing level of "case role assignment" gaze durations differed significantly according to the syntactic function (case roles, for instance, agent, instrument, verb, direct or indirect object, etc.) of the word being fixated.

Control models of reading eye movements generally assume that saccade size and fixation duration are independent eye movement components that have to be accounted for separately, even though it seems to be plausible that fixation duration should be longer if a line is read with fewer fixations, i.e. with larger saccades. However, Rayner and McConkie (1976) reported that the correlation between the amplitude of the preceding saccade and the duration of the subsequent fixation ranged from − .084 to .128, and the correlation between fixation duration and the size of the following movement ranged from − .041 to .108. Andriessen and De Voogd (1973) earlier obtained similar results.

The absence of significant correlations in the data of Rayner and Mc-Conkie (1976) may be due to not having controlled the comprehension, peripheral, and position factors. Thus, one should not expect a fixation following a long saccade to take more time than a fixation following a small saccade if the first is directed on a short, frequent, and repeatedly occurring word at the end of a line, whereas the last is directed on a long, rare, and the first time occurring word near the beginning of a line. The "independence assumption" is questioned by a study of Salthouse and Ellis (1980), who were able to demonstrate a significant effect of the amplitude of the prior movement on fixation duration, i.e., fixation duration increased by about 6 to 8 msec for each degree of the preceding saccade. Contrary to that, there was no effect of the amplitude of the following movement. Although searching for determinants of fixation duration which are also active in reading, Salthouse and Ellis did not employ a reading task, arguing that variables such as "(a) comprehension difficulty—the syntactic and semantic context in which the fixated material is embedded. (b) peripheral information—the amount and type of material in the periphery, and (c) fixation location—the direction and distance of the eyes from one fixation position to another" (Salthouse and Ellis, 1980, p. 208) generally could not be controlled in reading experiments. In their own experiments Salthouse and Ellis tried to control: (a) *comprehension factors* by presenting simple target stimuli which consisted of either two or four letters and requiring a simple decision if the target contained a vowel or not, (b) *peripheral factors* by presenting all targets within a range of 2° and separated from other stimuli by at least 3°, and (c) *position factors* by requiring the same sequence of eye movements in a given experimental block, i.e., the subjects always had to move their eyes from a starting mark to the target item and from the target item forward to an end mark.

However, requiring the subjects to fixate the target stimulus as briefly as possible and to signal the decision as fast as possible, the Salthouse and Ellis task resembles a reaction time experiment more than a reading task, and further, the findings question the conclusions drawn from sequential correlations. Our own experiment attempts to investigate those three factors in relationship between saccade size and fixation duration in a more normal reading situation.

METHOD

In addressing the question of whether there is a movement amplitude effect in reading, we constructed texts with one word on a line chosen to be the critical word. It was controlled by position, word length, external word shape, lexical activation, and syntactic function. In so doing, we intended to reduce the variability in fixation duration on the critical word, which might be due to these factors, in order to examine movement amplitude effects more accurately. The critical word was placed in the middle of the line, which allowed varying the preceding and/or the following movement without the complications that occur with movements at the beginning and the end of the line (for instance, return sweeps, corrective movements, etc.).

For the variation of the movement amplitudes we chose different distances, i.e., blank spaces between the critical word and the words immediately preceding and/or following. Deciding upon these distances required accounting for information accessibility in peripheral vision from the preceding fixation required for programming the saccade to the critical word, and the information available about the critical word that is limited to only gross visual cues that peripheral (pre-)processing is limited to. According to McConkie and Rayner (1975), this should be the case in a distance of about 3°, and 3° was also the smallest distance used by Salthouse and Ellis (1980). As saccade size in reading normal texts in a normal reading distance is seldom longer than 7° and shorter than 1°, we decided to use the following distances: 1°, 3°, 5°, and 7°. Figure 1 shows text with the critical line indicated by an arrow and the critical word underlined. The texts always consist of a minimal nine lines and one or two buffer lines at the beginning and the end of the text.

Since we did not mean to factorially combine the amplitude of the preceding and the subsequent saccade, but rather to control the size of the one, while varying the amplitude of the other, we decided that 7° be kept

```
    Mit        dem       Hut     auf      dem

    Kopf     und    dem     Stab      in    der

    Hand      zog    ich       los.    Da

    kam   ein    Wind     auf      und   riss

➤  mir      den       Hut              vom

    Kopf.   Er    flog      ins    Laub.   Ich
```

FIG. 1.   Example of text with the critical line indicated by an arrow and the critical word underlined. The texts always consist of a minimal nine lines and one or two buffer lines at the beginning and the end of the text.

constant, which is certain to exclude peripheral influences. Thus, the combinations of the prior and the following saccade amplitude were: 1°/7°, 3°/7°, 5°/7°, 7°/7°, 7°/5°, 7°/3°, and 7°/1°.

Figure 2 shows the corresponding combinations for the critical lines of the text displayed above. In order to avoid, first, that the critical word attracted the subject's attention in advance by being separated from the words to the left and right by unusually big blank spaces and, second, that the fixation duration on the critical word was altered by attention processes merely depending on the unusual spaces preceding and following the critical word, we embedded the critical line in a uniform text that was unusually spaced throughout as it can be seen in Fig. 1. Moreover, for the construction of all of the texts we admitted only two-, three-, and four-letter words that normally do not require more than one fixation and that additionally have the advantage of consisting of only one syllable (except for some four-letter words); with regard to the critical words we restricted word length more narrowly to three letters. In addition, the critical words we chose were frequent, i.e., familiar, nouns that had already been presented on a previous line. With regard to the syntactic role of the critical word, the direct-object function was chosen, which could be easily predicted, having identified the preceding predicate.

As each text contained only one critical word we constructed 7 versions of the same text, each including one of the 7 critical lines. As an example of the 7 text versions, the 7 critical lines of Fig. 2 were inserted one at a time into the line of Fig. 1, which is indicated by an arrow. We then constructed 7 texts with different contents, completing the factorial 7 texts × 7 versions.

If there is an effect of the movement amplitude on fixation duration it should appear independently of the text material being meaningful (context-bound) or meaningless (free of context). To test this prediction we con-

(1°/7°)	mir			den	Hut			vom
(3°/7°)	mir		den		Hut			vom
(5°/7°)	mir	den			Hut			vom
(7°/7°)	den				Hut			vom
(7°/5°)	den				Hut		vom	Kopf
(7°/3°)	den				Hut	vom		Kopf
(7°/1°)	den				Hut	vom		Kopf

FIG. 2. Example of the varying blank spaces between the words on the critical line. The degrees in parentheses indicate the distance between the critical word (Hut) and, respectively, the previous word and the following word.

structed another series of 7 text displays each consisting of 7 critical lines (as well as filler lines between) taken from the texts described above; i.e., from each of the 7 versions of the same text we selected one critical line and combined it with 6 critical lines taken from the other texts. These texts can be referred to as 0–order approximations according to Miller and Selfridge (1950), for, with the exception of the critical words, which always occupied the position in the middle of the line, all other words were arranged in randomly scrambled order.

In order to estimate how fixation durations are altered by the unusually big spaces between the words throughout the texts, we constructed two other text displays, normally spaced. With regard to the contents, one is identical with the meaningful text shown in Fig. 1, while the other corresponds to the randomly arranged text. The series of paragraphs consisted of 49 meaningful + 7 meaningless unusually spaced texts, and meaningful + 1 meaningless normally spaced texts.

Twenty psychology students and lecturers participated as subjects in a first experiment. In a pre-experimental session, the subjects were acquainted with the experimental set-up by reading some unusually spaced text displays for practice. Every subject was presented one version of each of the 7 meaningful texts (in random order). Twelve of the 20 subjects additionally had to read one of the 0–order approximations, which was always presented after the meaningful texts. Afterwards, the same 12 subjects were presented the two normally spaced text displays.

Three months later two of those subjects participated in a second experiment in which they had to read all the 56 unusually spaced text displays (in 8 blocks, everyone consisting of 7 meaningful and 1 meaningless text).

The Eye Movement Registration

The electro-oculographical system we used is described by Heller (this volume). It consists of ZAK-amplifiers and a 64K Kontron microcomputer with two 8 inch floppy-disks. The sampling rate was 125/s. The accuracy of the registration is in the horizontal $< 1°$ of visual angle. The texts were attached to the subject's head with a balsa wood framework that curves the text on a radius of 31 cm, i.e., 1 cm of a line causes 1.85 degree of visual angle.

RESULTS

Evaluating the fixation duration on the critical word required that our subjects were able to perform the eye movement pattern on the critical line we had intended by the special arrangement of the words. An eye movement sequence was classified to be correct if the number of saccades did not exceed the number of distances between the words and if the saccade amplitudes were similar to these distances. In reading the meaningful texts, 59% of the critical lines showed the eye movement pattern expected; in reading the 0–order approximations, 64% of the critical lines were classified to be correct. As for the two subjects who read the whole series of 56 unusually spaced texts, all critical lines were available for a more detailed analysis. Table 1 shows the main results. The individual values of the collective results (left part of the table) are based on 10 to 13 (meaningful texts) respectively 7 to 10 observations (0–order approximations), while each value of the data of the two subjects is based on 14 observations.

As can be seen from Table 1 the average saccade amplitudes do not correspond that much to the blank spaces between the words, but rather to the distances between the middle of the one word and the middle of the next one; i.e., in no case do the means differ more than .5° from these distances being about 2.5°, 4.5°, 6.5°, and 8.5° in size. Thus, from now on we will no longer refer to the blank spaces between two adjacent words, but rather to

TABLE 1
Mean Saccade Amplitude and Standard Deviation in the Critical Line.
The First Column Indicates the Distance Between the Preceding
Word and, Respectively, the Following Word and the Critical Word.
The Other Columns Show the Observed Values for the Different
Conditions. All Values are Degrees of Visual Angle.

| Distances | | collective results | | | | results of two subjects | | |
		meaningful text		0–order approximation		meaningful text		0–order approximation
1/7	$\bar{X}$	2.64	8.27	2.73	8.92	2.23	8.62	2.74	8.39
	s	.26	.59	.31	.75	.37	1.13	.56	1.12
3/7	$\bar{X}$	4.61	8.39	4.53	7.99	4.02	8.93	4.37	8.23
	s	.74	.93	.56	.93	.53	1.21	.73	.99
5/7	$\bar{X}$	6.39	8.55	6.43	8.31	6.24	8.47	5.79	8.61
	s	.31	.42	.59	.68	.64	.80	.83	1.27
7/7	$\bar{X}$	8.46	8.31	8.46	8.52	8.27	8.37	8.44	8.54
	s	.51	.64	.67	.60	.96	.98	1.12	1.17
7/5	$\bar{X}$	8.31	61.4	8.59	5.93	8.38	6.33	8.13	6.09
	s	.69	.54	.68	.81	1.03	.93	1.26	1.05
7/3	$\bar{X}$	8.73	4.16	8.42	4.54	8.53	4.65	8.04	4.42
	s	.72	.28	.90	.63	1.06	.78	.82	.49
7/1	$\bar{X}$	8.81	2.32	8.76	2.50	8.09	2.78	8.56	2.76
	s	.65	.37	.66	.23	1.08	.48	.83	.71

the distances between their middles. Neither in the collective result nor in the results of the two subjects do the standard deviations of the mean saccade amplitudes exceed the length of the three-letter words, being about 1.5°. Since these dispersions are due to the starting point and/or the landing point of the saccades not being precisely in the middle of two successive words, i.e., the deviations at two fixation points contribute to these dispersions, we can be reasonably sure that no fixations were inside the blank spaces between the words. That is especially true for the two subjects who read all the unusually spaced texts whose standard deviations are less important throughout. Thus, without any special instruction to do so, our subjects performed the eye movements we had intended by the arrangement of the words on the critical line.

With regard to the effect of the saccade amplitudes on fixation duration, two alternative predications are illustrated in idealized form in Fig. 3.

If there is an effect of the prior movement amplitude as indicated by Salthouse and Ellis (1980), fixation duration on the critical word is expected to increase continuously with the prior movement ascending from 2.5° to 8.5°. If, in addition to that, there is an effect of the amplitude of the subsequent saccade, fixation duration should decline again with the subsequent saccade decreasing from 8.5° to 2.5°. Provided that both effects are equally strong as well as additive, fixation durations on the critical word should be on one level if the combined movements preceding and following the critical

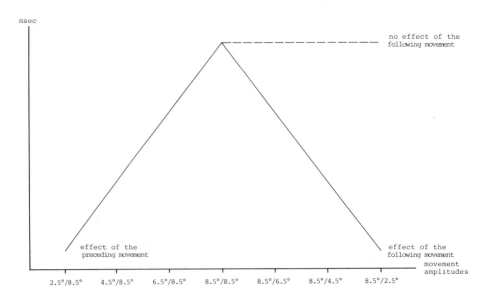

FIG. 3.   Fixation duration on the critical word depending on the amplitude of the preceding and/or following movements.

word are symmetric (for instance, 2.5°/8.5° and 8.5°/2.5°). If there is no effect of the subsequent saccade, fixation duration on the critical word should be stable at the level corresponding to the maximum size of the prior movement, while the amplitude of the subsequent saccade varies. As previously stated, one of those alternative data patterns should turn out independently of the text material being meaningful or randomly arranged.

The average fixation durations on the critical word actually obtained in our experiments are shown in Fig. 4 and Fig. 5, separately for the meaningful texts and the 0-order approximations. Figure 4 depicts the collective results of 20 subjects (meaningful texts) and further, additional results (0-order approximations) for 12 of these; Fig. 5 illustrates the results of the two subjects who read all the 56 unusually spaced texts. The means on which Fig. 4 and Fig. 5 are based as well as their standard deviations are also listed in Table 2.

Considering the data patterns obtained in reading the meaningful texts, we found a slight though clear (result of the two subjects) increase in fixation duration on the critical word with the size of the prior movement ascending from 2.5° (condition 1) up to 6.5° (condition 3). In no case can a rise in fixation duration be observed with the size of the preceding saccade increasing from 6.5° (condition 3) to 8.5° (condition 4). After having reached a maximum level with an amplitude of the prior movement being 6.5° (condition 3), fixation durations are remarkably stable, i.e., they are not affected by the decreasing amplitude of the subsequent saccade. Contrary to the meaningful texts, we cannot but describe the data patterns observed in reading the 0-order approximations as fluctuating more or less irregularly around a parallel to the x-axis, i.e., fixation durations on the critical word do not show any relationship to the varying movement amplitudes at all. In no case did we find an increase in fixation duration with the amplitude of the prior movement ascending from 2.5° (condition 1) to 4.5° (condition 2), in fact there was an opposite trend.

The collective data could not be subjected to a more sophisticated statistical analysis because too many critical lines of the individual subjects could not be classified as correct: Nearly all subjects had a part of the data missing, and if the critical line of one subject was available under one condition, it often was not under another. As can be seen already from the standard errors of the meaningful texts (Fig. 4), however, the standard errors of condition 1 (2.5°/8.5°) and condition 3 (6.5°/8.5°) as well as condition 1 and condition 4-7 do not overlap (except for condition 4). This means there is at least some evidence that condition 1 and condition 3-7 may actually differ, while there is no indication of a difference between the last. In comparison with the meaningful texts, the standard errors of the 0-order approximation do not show any evidence of a systematic difference between the mean fixation durations.

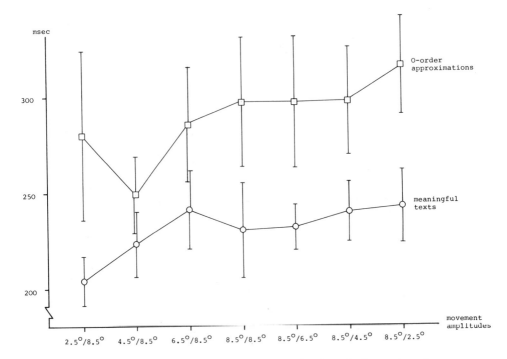

FIG. 4.   Fixation duration on the critical word and standard error depending on the amplitude of the preceding and/or following movements (collective results).

Contrary to the collective data, the data of the two subjects who read the whole series of 56 unusually spaced texts were completely available. We evaluated these data (fixation durations on the critical word) in two two-way analyses of variance (with replications) involving the factors movement amplitudes (2.5°/8.5°, 4.5°/8.5°, 6.5°/8.5°, 8.5°/8.5°, 8.5°/6.5°, 8.5°/4.5°, and 8.5°/2.5°) and critical word (7 critical words). These analyses were performed separately for the meaningful texts and the 0-order approximations, because introducing the two gradations of text meaningfulness implied the question of whether or not the fixation duration on the critical word was influenced by the movement amplitude factor depending on the meaningfulness of text material in which the critical word was embedded. The reason for including the critical word factor was that we did not want to reduce the variance in our data by having means instead of individual values as cell entries. These analyses of variance revealed a significant effect of the movement amplitude factor for the meaningful texts ($F(6,6) = 23.13$, $p < .01$), but not the 0-order approximations ($F(6,6) = 1.9$, ns). The movement amplitude factor (meaningful texts) was the only significant source of variance, i.e., there were no differences between the overall fixation durations on the critical words (critical word factor) and there was no interaction of movement amplitude × critical word. For comparing the mean fixation durations on the meaningful texts we calculated the confidence interval for the comparison differences after the Tukey method fixing the error rate per comparison to $p = .005$. As the individual comparisons showed, condition 1 (2.5°/8.5°) and condition 2 (4.5°/8.5°) differed significantly both from one another and from the remaining means, while there was no significant difference between the last. This confirms our description of the data patterns of Fig. 5 given above.

Another question to be settled in our experiments is how the overall characteristics of the eye movements change when reading text displays that are normally spaced compared to text material having unusually large spaces between the words. This change of global eye movement characteristics can be seen from Table 3, which shows the means and standard deviations for the 12 subjects, everyone having read a normally spaced version of one of the meaningful texts (MN for meaningful normal) as well as an unusually spaced version of the same text (MS for meaningful spaced)

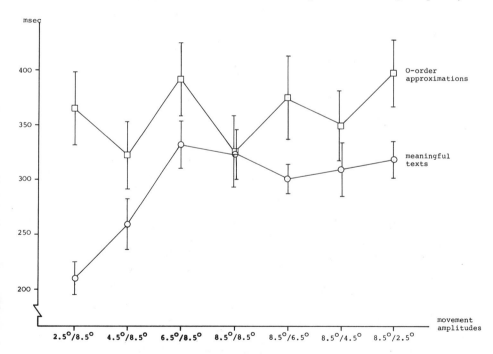

FIG. 5.   Fixation duration on the critical word and standard error depending on the amplitude of the preceding and/or following movements (result of two subjects).

TABLE 2
Mean Fixation Duration on the Critical Word in msec ($\bar{X}$) as Well as
Standard Deviation (s), Standard Error (se) and Number
of Observations (n)

		1	2	3	4	5	6	7
Condition		2.5/8.5	4.5/8.5	6.5/8.5	8.5/8.5	6.5/8.5	4.5/8.5	2.5/2.5
Collective result								
meaningful texts	n	10	12	12	12	11	13	13
	$\bar{X}$	204.00	222.67	240.67	230.00	231.27	239.38	242.46
	s	41.18	60.14	70.69	85.36	38.77	56.80	69.08
	se	13.02	17.36	20.41	24.64	11.69	15.75	19.16
0-order	n	8	9	10	7	7	5	8
	$\bar{X}$	280.00	248.89	285.60	297.14	297.14	297.60	316.00
	s	125.84	60.19	94.66	89.14	90.80	63.35	72.95
	se	44.49	20.06	29.93	33.69	34.32	28.33	25.79
Result of two Ss								
meaningful texts	n	14	14	14	14	14	14	14
	$\bar{X}$	210.29	259.43	332.00	325.14	300.57	309.14	318.29
	s	56.78	87.62	82.23	85.57	49.29	89.17	61.90
	se	15.18	23.42	21.98	22.87	13.17	23.83	16.54
0-order	n	14	14	14	14	14	14	14
	$\bar{X}$	364.57	322.29	392.00	325.71	374.86	349.14	397.14
	s	124.04	116.80	126.06	121.22	142.03	119.51	115.10
	se	33.15	31.22	33.69	32.40	37.96	31.94	30.76

and a normally spaced (RN for random normal) as well as an unusually spaced version of the 0-order approximation (RS for random spaced).

Differences are apparent for all measures comparing M and R versions except the angular extent of forward (4) and regressive (6) saccades. Row 8 shows words per fixation, i.e., the average number of words being accessible during a fixation that can be considered as a coarse measure of the size of the perception span. Although being somewhat artificial and somewhat unquestionable (McConkie & Rayner, 1976), this measure may at least have a heuristic function. As can be seen from row 8, words per fixation decreases from the left to the right, i.e., there is a clear facilitative effect of peripheral information processing in reading meaningful and normally spaced text (MN), but little facilitation is found in reading meaningful but unusually spaced text (MS). Reading random arrangements of words requires more than one fixation per word independent of the text material having unusually large spaces (RS) or not (RN). Our description of row 8 is confirmed by a Friedman test that yields that the differences between the summed ranks of words per fixation, i.e., the tendency of this ratio to decrease from the left to the right is highly significant (chi$_r^2$ = 36.97, $p < .001$). This is shown by subsequent Wilcoxon tests for individual comparisons in which all conditions differ significantly from one another (MN-MS: T = 0, $p < .005$; MS-RN: T = 10, $p < .01$; RN-RS: T = 0, $p < .005$).

The metric fixation time per word shown in row 9 takes about 150 msec less time to fixate a word contained in meaningful text (M versions) in comparison with a word embedded in randomly arranged text (R versions). In

TABLE 3
Means and Standard Deviations for 12 Subjects Having Read a
Normally Spaced Meaningful Text (See the Text Above)

		MN	MS	RN	RS
1 number of fixations	$\bar{X}$	38.15	48.23	68.31	75.38
	s	8.28	6.52	7.62	10.22
2 fixation durations (ms)	$\bar{X}$	212.56	209.19	273.99	271.09
	s	68.49	75.22	111.53	113.39
3 number of progressive saccades	$\bar{X}$	29.38	35.08	55.62	55.54
	s	7.63	5.12	7.33	7.31
4 size of progressive saccades (degree of visual angle)	$\bar{X}$	3.29	4.22	2.10	3.94
	s	1.39	1.70	.73	1.98
5 number of re-gressive saccades	$\bar{X}$	2.77	4.23	5.69	6.85
	s	2.28	3.37	3.30	4.85
6 size of regressive saccades (degree of visual angle)	$\bar{X}$	1.88	2.10	1.45	1.75
	s	.61	1.38	.61	1.04
7 number of words		54	48	63	60
8 words per fixation	$\bar{X}$	1.42	1.01	.92	.79
	s	.37	.12	.11	.10
9 fixation time per word (ms)	$\bar{X}$	150.18	211.75	299.15	340.16
	s	47.36	52.33	69.51	90.52

addition, fixation time on a word embedded in an unusually spaced text (S versions) is lengthened by about 50 msec compared to fixation time on a word contained in a normally spaced text (N versions). We again performed a Friedman test that shows that the differences between the summed ranks of fixation time per word (i.e., the tendency of this ratio to increase from the left to the right) is highly significant ($\text{chi}_r^2 = 35.86$, $p < .001$); subsequent comparisons among the conditions of interest (Wilcoxon tests) show that both the N and S versions and the M and R versions differ significantly (N–S: $T = 1$, $p < .005$; M–R: $T = 0$, $p < .005$). It seems likely that the 150 msec difference between the meaningful and randomly arranged texts is due to a word being contextually bound or not, while the 50 msec difference between the normally and unusually spaced texts is due to the additional requirements of programming saccades in reading texts with unusually big and permanently changing spaces between the words.

DISCUSSION

The question addressed in our experiment was whether there is a relationship between saccade size and fixation duration in reading. Concerning the amplitude of the following movement our result is quite clear: The varying amplitude of the subsequent saccade did not affect the fixation durations on the critical word. So far our result accords with Salthouse and Ellis (1980). With regard to amplitude of the prior movement, our results are not quite so clear: On the one hand there is a significant increase in fixation duration with the size of the preceding saccade ascending from 2.5° to 6.5°, but on the other hand this tendency is not found to continue. This is not consistent with the result of Salthouse and Ellis who found fixation duration to increase steadily with the prior movement amplitude ranging from 3° to 21°.

With regard to the 0–order approximations, our results are quite opposite those of Salthouse and Ellis. Our data do not show any relationship to the varying movement amplitudes, though reading context-free words was most similar to the vowel/no vowel decision task used by Salthouse and Ellis.

Of additional concern is the tendency of fixation duration on the critical word to increase with the prior movement amplitude ascending from 2.5° to 6.5°. This point is argued for by Salthouse & Ellis, taking up the notion of a "minimal pause time" as one component of fixation duration that had been earlier discussed by Arnold and Tinker (1939). This "minimal pause time," i.e., the minimal time required to stop and to restart the eyes, is considered to be some kind of a "physiological refractory period," which is influenced by the amplitude of the prior movement. Contrary to that, "stimulus processing" as the second component of fixation duration postulated by Salthouse and Ellis, assumed to be independent of the first, is not affected by the prior movement amplitude. The distinction of the two components on the basis of the prior movement amplitude is not made clear by the Salthouse and Ellis result: "the effect of the amplitude of the prior movement is assumed to be localized in one component, and yet when that component was isolated the effect was less than one-half of the magnitude evident when both components were present" (Salthouse & Ellis, 1980, p. 230). Accordingly, the effect of the prior movement amplitude should have also been apparent in our experiments—particularly because the mean fixation durations on the critical word are all shorter than the fixation durations on the target items Salthouse and Ellis observed in a comparable experiment, even though we did not expressly stress the "minimal pause time" component by instructing our subjects to fixate as briefly as possible.

An alternative explanation of the prior movement effect is suggested by a study of Mitrani, Yakimoff, and Mateeff (1970) who showed that the degree of saccadic suppression is dependent on the amplitude of saccadic eye movements. Arguing against an explanation in terms of saccadic suppression, Salthouse, Ellis, Diener, and Somberg (1981), presented an experiment in which subjects had to identify a target character displayed for 40 msec before, during, and/or after the fixation on the target position with a $10°$ saccade preceding as well as following. Independent of the target stimulus being presented in the first, middle, or last milliseconds of the fixation identification accuracy did not differ, i.e., there was no effect of (post- and/or pre-) saccadic suppression. Whatever relationship may exist between the prior movement effect and saccadic suppression, neither the saccadic suppression nor the refractory period explanations seems to be appropriate to our results. Neither seems able to account for the fact that there is no effect at all for the 0–order approximations as well as for the fact that there is no increase in fixation duration with the prior movement amplitude ascending from $6.5°$ to $8.5°$.

The explanation we suggest involves peripheral processing activities. Accordingly, in reading the random arrangements of words the opportunity to preprocess and/or anticipate the word in peripheral vision is restricted and every attempt to process turns out to be inefficient, i.e., time consuming. Thus, the eye movement pattern is adjusted in such a way that each word is fixated at least once, irrespective of text spacing. Errors in that adjustment as well as multiple fixations on words may account for the large data loss in our results. As there was no facilitation due to peripheral preprocessing, the critical word must be identified entirely during the fixation on it—independently of the size of the blank space preceding. Contrary to that, in reading the meaningful texts the subject is able to take advantage of the language constraints. Approaching a critical word that is controlled with regard to word length, word shape, syntactic function, etc., peripheral processing activities can be done successfully—provided that the blank space preceding is not too big. According to our data the critical distance is between 4.5° and 6.5°, i.e., beyond that amplitude of the preceding saccade, fixation duration on the critical word is no longer found to be facilitated by peripheral preprocessing.

Such an explanation in terms of peripheral processing activities is supported by Rayner, McConkie, and Ehrlich (1978). In one of their experiments subjects had to fixate a starting point, and as they did so a letter string appeared beginning 1°, 3°, or 5° to the right of the fixation point, respectively ending 1°, 3°, or 5° to the left of it. Thereupon the subject had to make a saccade to the stimulus pattern, which was replaced by the base word during the eye movement. It was the task of the subject to name the base word, and the naming latency was measured. For comparison with our experiments, the most interesting condition is the one in which the initially displayed letter string was identical with the base word. Under this condition there was a clear facilitative effect on naming time up to a distance of 3°, i.e., up to 3.75° reckoning in .75° for half the length of the base word. In our data the corresponding distance is between 4.5° and 6.5°. As suggested by McClelland and O'Regan (1981), the wider range of the facilitation effect in our reading task may be due to the subject being able to form linguistic expectations about the critical word that are based not only on peripheral visual cues, but also on syntactic and semantic constraints. However, this possibility remains to be tested in future experiments in which the transition probability between the preceding and the critical word will be varied.

In order not to be misunderstood: We are not able to reject the existence of the movement amplitude effect found by Salthouse and Ellis (1980), but we want to assert that there was no "movement amplitude effect" found in normal reading that could not be reduced to peripheral processing activities.

IV.4 Understanding Extended Discourse Through the Eyes: How and Why

Wayne L. Shebilske
University of Virginia

Dennis F. Fisher
U.S. Army Human Engineering Laboratory
Aberdeen Proving Ground, Maryland

How do people understand written discourse? As part of a group representing several disciplines and different research approaches we have addressed this question using many measures including eye movement recordings during reading of a 3,000 word passage. In this chapter we briefly explain why we feel it is important to observe eye movements given the objective and rationale of the larger research project. We describe how we solved methodological problems encountered when taking discontinuous eye movement records during reading of extended discourse.

Our purpose was not suited by traditional gross response measures like fixation duration and interfixation distance averaged over an entire passage, or by microanalysis of a few words or sentences at a time. We have therefore proposed new measures, which are firmly rooted in the first 80 years of eye movement research. Our goal is to relate these new methods to recent developments in reading research as underscored by comparing and contrasting them with those recently put forth by other investigators (e.g., Just & Carpenter, 1980).

OBJECTIVE AND RATIONALE

The last ten years have witnessed a growth of what Kintsch (1974) has called an "interactionist" theory of reading. In his view, the way in which a reader responds to a text plays as heavily in determining comprehension as does the way in which an author writes a text (cf. Estes & Shebilske, 1979; Iser, 1978). Interactionists typically analyze both the author's and the reader's contributions. They analyze what an author writes in terms of text structure by reducing text to a set of basic propositions and then define structure by the ways those propositions are organized into sentences and by their interdependency (e.g., Deese, 1980; Fredericksen, 1975a; Rumelhart, 1977; Kintsch & van Dijk, 1978). Most interactionists infer the reader's contribution by examining differences between the structure of text and the structure of paraphrastic recalls (Thorndyke, 1977; Rumelhart, 1977; Kintsch & van Dijk, 1978; Fredericksen, 1975b). The technique of measuring recall has been successful in supporting the interactionist view, but it has been limited by its inability to separate responses during recall from responses during reading (e.g., Fredericksen, 1975b; Levelt, 1978). Our group analyzes reading responses more directly by taking eye movement measures in conjunction with a battery of other tests including recalls.

Our research is motivated by the hope of helping the many high school and college students who have trouble learning from textbooks (Fisher & Peters, 1981; Shebilske, 1980). Eighty some years of eye movement research have yielded a precise and highly agreed upon description of reading eye movements (cf. Levy-Schoen & O'Regan, 1979), but researchers have been less successful at using those descriptions to improve reading instruction (Tinker, 1958). Efforts to train eye movements in reading clinics have failed due to an inadequate understanding of the relationship between eye movements and language processes (Shebilske, 1975). Since that relationship is now being further clarified (Rayner, 1983), the time is right for reconsidering classroom applications.

A major weakness of those who have trouble learning from textbooks is inadequate flexibility in their reading between various types of text (Gibson & Levin, 1975; Harris & Sipay, 1975; Rankin, 1974). A flexible reader is one who adapts reading rate and approach to fit situational, conceptual, and linguistic contexts. Situational context includes task demands, purpose, and presentation mode. Conceptual context includes concepts given earlier in a text and concepts in a reader's background knowledge. Linguistic context includes orthographic, syntactic, and semantic information (cf. Shebilske & Fisher, 1983). We have endeavored to show that flexibility with respect to these contexts is a compound of component strategies that are manifested in eye movement records not only between texts but within texts as well (cf. Shebilske & Fisher, 1981, 1983).

METHODOLOGICAL ISSUES

Our research combines factor-analytic and experimental approaches in a comprehensive analysis of how individual students modulate their rate and approach with respect to textual units that differ in their relationship to text structure. One variable, for instance, is the rated importance of units with respect to the author's main message. Our eye movement measures are used to analyze interrelationships between eye movements, text structure, subject factors, situational variables, and understanding. Others have used factor-analytic approaches (e.g., Davis, 1968), which have been criticized for isolating component skills that have little or no relevance outside of the taking of reading tests (cf. Spache & Spache, 1977). In contrast, we give typical classroom reading assignments that are more isomorphic to real world reading. Our assignments facilitated analysis of important components of reading behavior, but they also raise some sticky methodological issues. This paper reports progress on three of those issues:

1. Coming to grips with the lack of standardization in the measurement of fixations with TV-based monitoring systems.
2. Choosing a suitable unit for analyzing influences of higher-order language processes on eye movements.
3. Isolating and analyzing context effects.

Measuring Fixations

Psychophysiological characteristics of the oculomotor system constrain when and where readers can sample text. Readers get an impression of sweeping their eyes smoothly over a line of print while receiving a continuous view of text. The actual motor activity and visual input contrasts sharply with that impression. Readers move their eyes in a sequence of pauses and jumps. The pauses, which are called "fixations," are compelled by the oculomotor system to last for at least 85 msec (Lennerstrand, Bach-y-Rita, & Collins, 1975). More typically they range from about 100 msec to 400 msec during reading (Andriessen & de Voogd, 1973). The jumps, which are called "saccades," reach velocities as high as 175 degrees per second. Shebilske (1975) reviewed evidence that meaningful visual input is virtually wiped out during these rapid movements. He also described a miniexperiment that you can do to convince yourself that you cannot read during saccadic eye movements. One could say, then, that a reader is "functionally blind" during saccadic eye movements. Fixations patterns therefore reflect when, where, and for how long readers look at text.

Because of this discrete nature of visual input during reading, eye movement researchers must accurately measure fixations. It is not enough to build a device that will indicate eye positions from moment to moment. A system must also distinguish eye positions measured during saccadic movements from those measured during fixations. This distinction is relatively easy for systems that sample eye position 1,000 times per second (McConkie, Zola, Walverton & Burns, 1978), but it is more challenging for TV-based systems that sample at a rate of 60 times per second. Karsh and Breitenbach (this volume) demonstrated, for instance, that slight changes in computer algorithms that are used to define fixations in TV-based systems can result in dramatically different patterns of "fixations."

The raw data for Karsh and Breitenbach's demonstration was taken on the TV-based eye movement monitoring system at the Human Engineering Laboratory (HEL) while college students searched for target numbers. Every 1/60th of a second the HEL Oculometer specifies where the reader's eye is pointing in terms of vertical (X) and horizontal (Y) distances from the center of the reader's viewing screen. These X and Y coordinates make up the raw data points, which are stored on a magnetic tape for future off-line processing (For details of an earlier version of the Oculometer, see Lambert, Monty, & Hall, 1974). The data points are not all the same but rather are a small cluster of points, which is the unavoidable result of electronic jitter common to all video signal based systems. The dispersion of these data points is essentially a normal distribution. A bounded area that encompasses most of the distribution in the HEL Oculometer is presently designated as a square on the viewing screen that subtends slightly less than one degree visual angle at the eye. Any two or more points that fall within this "window of resolution" must be considered as one point whose position is given by the mean of that distribution. Karsh and Breitenbach describe a computer algorithm that defines "fixations" in terms of the mean of clusters of successive data points. They also showed the consequences of using the mean of *minimally* 2, 4, 6, or 8 successive points. With 2 point clusters, the resulting "fixation pattern" indicated a "fixation" on almost every word with many short "fixations" included in the pattern. As cluster size increased, the number of "fixations" decreased as did the number of very short "fixations." Karsh and Breitenbach also showed that size of the "window of resolution" is another criterion that has a drastic effect on how fixations are defined. Their demonstration raises the problem of how one can choose one set of criteria over another for use in computer algorithms that define fixations in data from TV-based systems.

A survey of recent literature made the choice of criteria all the more crucial. Our goal was to choose criteria that would allow us to compare our results with other published data. We found, however, that almost the entire range of criteria used in Karsh and Breitenbach's demonstration have been used in recently published eye movement experiments. For example,

Mandel (1979) used a criterion that corresponded to a minimum cluster size of eight, and Just and Carpenter (1980) used one that corresponded to a minimum cluster size of two or three. (Just and Carpenter did not state their criterion, but they reported that the total gaze time on one word was 50 msec in a record from one subject [page 330]. That gaze time could not be measured with a criterion greater than two or three successive samples taken at 16.7 msec intervals). We decided to turn to classical data for guidance.

The first 80 years of eye movement research have established a highly agreed upon description of reading eye movements, as mentioned earlier. This description should serve as a standard for evaluating computer-based systems. Although it is useful for researchers to describe their fixation defining algorithms in detail (e.g., Mandel, 1979; Karsh & Breitenbach, this volume), it is likely to be difficult to compare and contrast programs that differ in complex ways. We therefore propose that evaluation efforts should concentrate on the end products—the fixation patterns—instead of upon the programs themselves. Specifically, computer based systems should demonstrate that their data aligns with classical data in terms of fixation duration, interfixation distance, number of regressions, and other well established characteristics of reading eye movements (cf. McConkie, 1981, for similar suggestions).

Just and Carpenter (1980) did in fact compare their results with traditional data. They cited Buswell (1937), Dearborn (1906), Judd and Buswell (1922) in support of the fact that "when readers are given a text appropriate for their age level, they average 1.2 words per fixation. The words that are not always fixated tend to be short function words, like *the,* and *a*" (Just & Carpenter, 1980, p. 330). Based on this average, Just and Carpenter concluded that these early eye fixation studies indicate that readers fixate almost all content words. This appraisal corresponded to their own records. In one protocol of an individual subject (page 330), 76% of the words were fixated and every word that was skipped was a function word. In another composite record averaged across subjects (page 347), 98% of the words were fixated. Our own results also indicated that almost every word was fixated when we analyzed raw data with a minimum cluster size of two. One could combine these facts in an argument favoring a cluster size of two.

A closer examination lead us away from this criterion, however. Words per fixation, which is computed as a ratio of the total number of words divided by the total number of fixations, does not indicate the number of words fixated because readers fixate some words more than once. The consequences of referencing this statistic is the same with respect to all the traditional studies cited above. We have spelled out those consequences only for Judd and Buswell's (1922) data.

Figure 1 shows Judd and Buswell's (1922) plates 16 and 17 in which the word per fixation scores are 1.53 and 1.48 respectively. One can determine

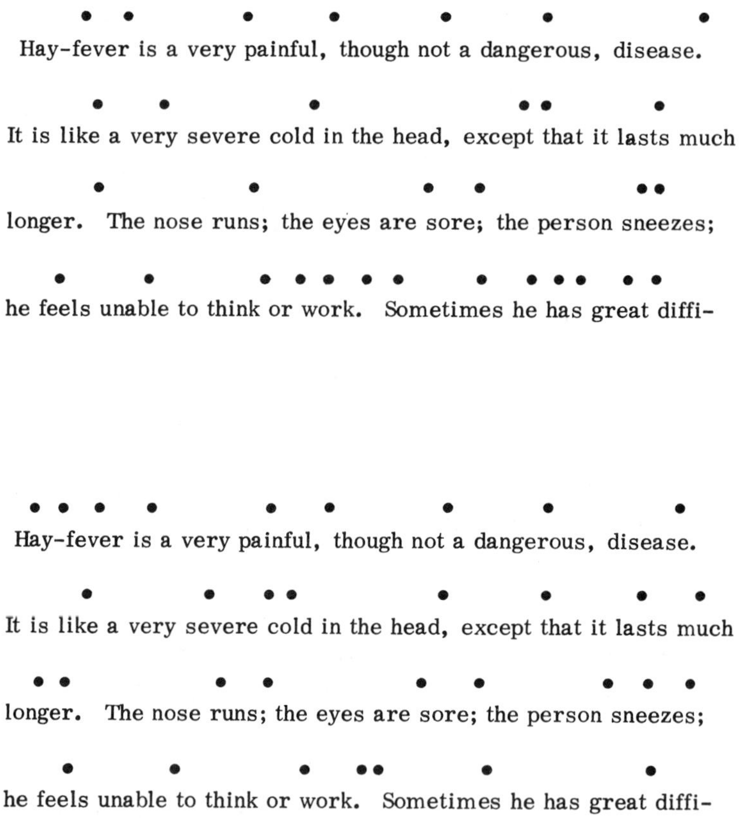

• •   •   •   •   •   •
Hay-fever is a very painful, though not a dangerous, disease.

   •   •   •   • •   •
It is like a very severe cold in the head, except that it lasts much

   •   •   •   •   • •
longer. The nose runs; the eyes are sore; the person sneezes;

  •   •   • • • •   •   • • •   • •
he feels unable to think or work. Sometimes he has great diffi-

 • • • •   •   •   •   •   •
Hay-fever is a very painful, though not a dangerous, disease.

     •   • • •   •   •   •   •
It is like a very severe cold in the head, except that it lasts much

 • •   •   •   •   •   •   •   •
longer. The nose runs; the eyes are sore; the person sneezes;

  •   •   •   • •   •   •
he feels unable to think or work. Sometimes he has great diffi-

FIG. 1.   Data adapted from Judd and Buswell (1922: Plates 16 and 17).
Each dot shows the position of a fixation.

how misleading the words per fixation statistic is by counting the actual
number of words fixated. The reader fixated 25 out of 49 words in the first
record (51%) and 27 out of 49 (55%) in the second. The reader fixated only
slightly more than half the words. Furthermore, many content words were
not fixated, which is consistent with Shebilske's (1975) findings that readers
skip content words as frequently as they skip function words in Judd and
Buswell's records.

While these results clearly show the inappropriateness of the word per fixation statistic, the records were taken with instructions unlike those used in
the studies under consideration. We therefore analyzed other records that
were taken on a variety of materials with more comparable instructions.
Table 1 shows the percentage of words fixated in 17 records from Judd and
Buswell (1922). Plates 16 and 17 came from a college student reading a

scientific text. Plate 16 was taken after the instruction "Read this paragraph through once silently. Read it very rapidly as you would read a newspaper article, just to find out what it is about." Plate 17 was produced immediately afterwards following the instructions "Now read it again more carefully. When you finish, you will be asked questions about it." Plates 10 and 12 are comparable to Plate 16; Plates 11 and 13 are comparable to Plate 17), except that Plates 10, 11, 12, and 13 were produced by sixth-graders. All other Plates were taken after instructions to read silently and carefully in preparation for answering questions, which were to follow. A fifth-grader produced Plates 3, 4, and 5 while reading paragraphs from a simple prose fiction, a geography text, and a textbook on rhetoric. Pupils in eleventh and twelfth grades produced Plates 33, 39, 45, 46, and 58 while reading a simple prose passage. Less than two-thirds of the words were fixated on eight of the records. Only four records show more than three-fourths of the words fixated, and no records show 85% or more of the words fixated.

In our experiment, the criterion of a minimal cluster size of two seems to overestimate the number of words fixated in comparison to classical eye movement data. Another inconceivable characteristic of the "fixation pattern" dictates against a minimal cluster size of two. Many of the "fixations" had durations between 34 and 85 msec, which as indicated earlier, is impossible given physiological constraints. The standard of other established eye movement data can also be used to reject the analysis. Table 2 shows that Judd and Buswell (1922) recorded 1 out of 388 fixations (0.3%) with a duration of less than 100 msec. Similarly, Tinker (1958) reported that *none* of his reader's fixations were less than 50 msec and only 1.7% were less than 100 msec. In contrast, nearly one quarter of the "fixations" were less than 100 msec when defined with a minimal cluster size of two.

TABLE 1
Proportion of Words Fixated During Silent Reading*

Plate Number	Number of Words	Proportion of Words Fixated	Plate Number	Number of Words	Proportion of Words Fixated
3	40	.60	33	44	.70
4	41	.76	39	34	.82
5	43	.72	45	44	.52
11	49	.81	46	44	.54
13	49	.73	58	44	.75
17	49	.55	54	40	.50
10	49	.63	55	40	.48
12	49	.81	57	40	.75
16	49	.51			

*Plate number refers to the numbers in Judd & Buswell (1922). See text for description.

TABLE 2
Proportion of Very Short Fixations During Silent Reading*

Plate Number	Number of Fixations	Fixations between 40 & 80 msec		Fixations between 80 & 100 msec	
		Number	Proportion	Number	Proportion
3	29	0	.000	0	.000
10&11	87	0	.000	2	.023
16&17	65	0	.000	2	.031
39	43	0	.000	1	.023
54	22	0	.000	1	.045
55	19	0	.000	1	.053
57	35	0	.000	0	.000
58	38	1	.026	0	.000
TOTAL	338	1	.003	7	.021

*Plate number refers to the numbers in Judd & Buswell (1922). Plates 4, 5, 12, 13, 33, 45, and 46 were excluded because of illegible data. See text for explanation.

The errors of overestimating number of words fixated and of underestimating fixation durations are related. Some of the raw data point are sampled while the eyes are making a saccadic jump over a word. Erroneous classifications occur with a minimal cluster of two. The program defines very short fixations in locations where the eyes are actually in the midst of saccades. We therefore reject the minimal cluster size of two criterion not only on the grounds that it does not align with traditional data, but also on the grounds that it does not meet the basic requirement of distinguishing fixations from saccades.

Larger minimal cluster criterions guard against classifying saccades as fixations. There is a danger of setting the criterion too high, however. The highest criterion of eight in Karsh and Breitenbach's sample is not the best, for instance. It misses too many fixations in comparison to lower criterion that provide adequate protection against classifying saccades as fixations. A program using a minimal cluster size of eight fails to detect all fixations that are less than 134 msec. Such a system would miss about 4% of the fixations observed by Andriessen and de Voogd (1973). In contrast, a minimal cluster size of six misses fixations that are less than 100 msec. Consequently, it would miss less than 2% of the fixations in Adriessen and de Voogd's data. At the same time, the criterion of a minimal cluster size of six, which the HEL system has employed for many years, fit other parameters of classical data quite well. For instance, in six records which were representative of eye movements during reading of a biology textbook, the average reading rate was 245 words per minute, the average duration of fixations was 255 msec, and the number of regressions was 14 per 100 words. (cf. Shebilske & Fisher, 1981, Table 4.) These values compare favorably with established norms for college students of 280 words per minute, reading rate, 240 msec fixation durations, and 15 regressions per 100 words (Taylor, Frackenpohl, & Pettee, 1960).

Our analysis leads us to stay with the criterion used for many years at HEL for defining fixations We are not satisfied, however, with the degree of standardization that is present today, and we are currently planning standardized tests that will hopefully improve the comparability of reading eye movement data across laboratories (cf. McConkie, 1981).

Choosing a Unit of Analysis

The decision about defining fixations in our raw data created another methodological problem. Our objective was to analyze eye movements over units of text that would reflect components of flexible reading in individuals, but no unit in current use fit our purpose. Since readers skip many content words while reading textbooks, we steered away from "gaze durations per word," which is becoming a popular unit of analysis (e.g., Just & Carpenter, 1980; Kliegl, Olson, & Davidson, 1983). Readers skip different words so that almost every word gets one "average gaze duration" when researchers average over subjects. It is unclear, however, how these averages relate to real time characteristics of any individual's reading behavior (cf. Shebilske & Fisher, 1981). We needed more global units that would enable us to measure each reader's processing time for almost every unit.

Levy-Schoen and O'Regan (1979) made an important distinction between local and global measures, which they define as follows:

> Local measures are made over a short time span and [are] taken in the vicinity of particular words of text . . . we expect them predominantly to reflect underlying processes that function over a short time span (p. 22).

> Global measures, on the other hand, are essentially combinations of these local measures taken over a long time span . . . [they] would be expected to reflect higher level cognitive processes, relying upon information gathered over a longer period of time (p. 22).

Traditional global measures consisting of parameters averaged over entire passages are available, but are clearly too gross with respect to our goal of measuring components of intra-passage flexibility.

Several global measures that are more appropriate have been proposed recently. Mandel (1979), for instance, subdivided text into segments corresponding to propositions in Kintsch's (1974) text grammar: This unit has yielded promising results, and it may become important in testing interactionists' theories. Carpenter and Just (1977) also pioneered a fruitful global unit. They measured "gaze duration" over whole sentences and showed that eye movements relate to important aspects of a text's thematic structure. For our purposes, however, we were concerned that propositions and sentences, which capture an author's units, may not capture the most relevant units to which readers respond when structuring an internal representation of text.

We decided to develop a new unit of analysis determined by responses of readers. We had a group of college students divide our passage according to the following instructions: "Now that you have read this passage, we would like you to go back through it and divide it into what we call "idea units." An idea unit encompasses a complete thought; and while idea units often coincide with sentences or are set off by punctuation, this is not always the case. More than one idea unit may occur in a single sentence; one idea unit may carry over from one sentence or paragraph to the next." Rotondo (1980) developed a single-linkage clustering algorithm which identified normative units in this data. (See Shebilske & Rotondo, 1981, for more details and for examples of units). These normative segments became our unit of analysis in eye movement studies on separate groups of readers. We quantified 18 characteristics of these units, and we observed the extent to which individual readers modulate their reading rate in words per minute for each unit with respect to the 18 characteristics.

Isolating and Analyzing Context Effects

The choice of a global unit created the additional problem of isolating various effects on eye movements. Global measures reflect combined influences of local processes operating over short time spans and higher-order processes operating over longer periods. Given different eye movement patterns for dissimilar global units, how does one isolate the effects of higher-order processes that integrate those units into a structured conceptual representation?

A key is in the fact that processes that integrate units should vary depending upon how the units are related to one another. One can capitalize on this key by performing a control experiment to determine whether or not an observed difference in eye movements for global units depends upon how the units are interrelated. Once different eye movement patterns are observed for unlike global units in a passage, separate groups of control subjects can read the same units in contexts that change the relationships between units. The results of this context manipulation will determine whether or not one has evidence of higher-order influences on eye movements.

If, on the one hand, an effect is stable when context changes, the original effect could in principal be explained by a combination of local influences.

For example, Mandel (1979) found more fixations per word and more regressions per word for propositions with higher levels in Kintsch's (1974) text grammar. Suppose that these effects were unaltered when the same text segments were read in a control that equated text-based levels. One might then argue that the original differences were caused by a combination of local effects. A reason for such local influences could be that authors might use less familiar words or more complicated syntax when they write propositions at higher levels. At any rate, the lack of interaction with context manipulations would leave open the possibility that local processes, such as word recognition, account entirely for the original effects.

If, on the other hand, an effect changes when a control context modifies the relationship between units, one has evidence for the influence of higher-order processes that integrate units. One of our studies on good readers provides an example (Shebilske & Fisher, 1981). We hypothesized that, for important meaning units, good readers allocate additional time and resources to those processes that integrate units into a conceptual representation. Perceived importance is a factor that can depend upon the relationship between units in the sense that the same idea can be important in one context and unimportant in another (cf. Karmiohl, 1981). We measured reading rates as a function of whether readers perceived a subset of units to be important or unimportant with respect to the main message of an excerpt from a biology textbook. The important ideas were read slower in their original context of the excerpt, but they were read at the same rate in a control context that was designed to equate relative importance. This context effect supported our hypothesis. Further analysis revealed that good readers slow down for important ideas by increasing their average fixation duration, and by increasing their regressions. It is doubtful that poor readers will employ the same flexible reading strategy (cf. Anderson, 1937; Olson, Kliegl, & Davidson, 1983).

In summary, local processes and higher-order processes can contribute to different eye movement patterns between dissimilar global measures. Manipulating context is a way to tease out higher-order influences. It is also a way to analyze components of flexible reading since flexiblity is defined in terms of modulations of reading behaviors with respect to context. Once context effects are isolated, they can be broken down by analyzing eye movement dynamics within global units.

APPLICATIONS

We are motivated, as mentioned earlier, by the hope of helping the many high school and college students who have trouble learning from textbooks. We are concentrating our research efforts on processes of appraising and assimilating text structure. In a study of over 1000 students from 7th grade, 10th grade, and college, we found that many students are deficient in assessment skills (See also Calfee & Curley, in preparation). They consistently disagreed with experts about the relative importance of ideas in a text (cf. Deese, 1980). The same study points to the assimilation of text structure as another critical factor. A surprising number of students agreed with expert assessments of text structure, but nevertheless failed to emphasize important ideas in a variety of recall tasks. They frequently recalled trivial information, and omitted important points even though they could discern relative importance when the text was in front of them. We believe that such students are deficient in assimilation skills that have traditionally gone under the name of "flexible" or "adaptive" reading. Resolution of the methodological issues that were taken up in this chapter will enable eye movement researchers to analyze individual differences in fundamental components of flexible reading strategies. Such analysis will hopefully pave the way for improved teaching of the advanced reading skills that students need in order to learn from textbooks (cf. Fisher & Peters, 1981).

ACKNOWLEDGMENTS

This project is a cooperative effort between investigators from the Department of Psychology and the McGuffey Reading center at the University of Virginia and from the Human Engineering Laboratory at Aberdeen Proving Ground, Maryland. The investigators in alphabetical order are: James Deese, Thomas H. Estes, Dennis F. Fisher, John A. Rotondo, Wayne L. Shebilske, and H. Elizabeth Wetmore. The work reported here was supported by Grant 00233 under the joint sponsorship of NSF and NIE.

IV.5

Processing of Sentences in Conditions of Aphasia as Assessed by Recording Eye Movements

Walter Huber
Department of Neurology
Technical University Aachen
German Federal Republic

Gerd Lüer
Uta Lass
Technical University Aachen
German Federal Republic

Central language disorders are characterized by specific and differential impairment of linguistic abilities. For example, in patients with Broca's aphasia the main symptoms are nonfluent, laborious speech, phonemic substitutions, and agrammatism, i.e. reduction of sentence structure (cf. e.g., Kerschensteiner, Poeck, Huber, Stachowiak, & Weniger, 1978). This particular pattern of aphasic symptoms most frequently corresponds with lesions of the frontal and central parts of the area supplied by the middle cerebral artery. Patients with Broca's aphasia have particular difficulties in handling the so-called function words, like articles, auxiliaries, prepositions, etc., and some of these patients neglect them totally. There is an ongoing controversy in the literature on precisely what the linguistic nature of the agrammatic deficit is and on whether it also occurs in both auditory and reading comprehension. In other words, it is a hitherto unresolved question whether this particular type of aphasic impairment affects linguistic processing in general or whether it is restricted to the articulatory output modality.

Most of the information about aphasic behavior is based on error analysis, which leads to rather indirect conclusions about the levels of processing that are specifically impaired in aphasia. An obvious advantage of the assessment of eye movements is the possibility of observing a more direct reflection of the linguistic processing that leads to a certain linguistic output. Our study attempts to define the relationship between linguistic output and the processing that precedes it when subjects are asked to search an array of written words for a sentence. As dependent variables we took frequency, time, and alteration of eye movements. We hypothesized that for normal controls the strengths of these variables would indicate both what is chosen for a solution and what is linguistically most favored. With aphasic subjects, however, we expected that the solution given would not necessarily be predicted by eye movement patterns. Aphasic reactions, unlike normal linguistic behavior, reflect difficulties of internal processing and difficulties that these patients have in linguistic output. Furthermore, the preceding internal processing of aphasic patients might also be different from that of the normal controls if their syntactic impairment can be attributed to a general or "central" language disorder.

The influence of three specific linguistic features on syntactic processing is controlled in this study. We know from psycholinguistic studies that normal comprehension may be determined by an actor-first-strategy (Bever, 1970). This means that a nominal phrase is most likely to be taken as the logical subject of a sentence if it can be interpreted as an actor. Recent neurolinguistic experiments (Heeschen, 1980) indicate that Broca's aphasics in particular rely on this strategy and that they have great difficulties in switching to other strategies. In constructing the items of our task, we made sure that the nominal elements allowed for an actor versus non-actor interpretation.

Another feature is the grammatical category of words. It is a classical issue in the aphasia literature that word category has a differential impact on the linguistic behavior of Broca's aphasics. Therefore, the stimulus words used in our task were strictly controlled with respect to the distribution of major and minor grammatical categories. We expected that the eye movements of Broca's aphasics would be more frequent and more extensive while scanning nouns and verbs in contrast to minor category words, like auxiliaries and participles, that function mainly as syntactic connectors.

Finally, it seemed to be an open question with respect to normal as well as to aphasic linguistic behavior whether in the assigned task the sentence structure would be conceptualized in a linear or in a hierarchical way. We expected that the varying degrees of syntactic binding among the constituents of the target sentence would be reflected by different values found for the eye movement variables.

METHODS

Subjects.   Included in the study were 17 students with a median age of 23 (range 20–32) and 9 aphasic patients with a median age of 51 (range 26–69). All aphasic subjects were out-patients receiving speech therapy. They were classified as having severe or moderate Broca's aphasia by means of the Aachener Aphasie Test (Huber, Poeck, Weniger, & Willmes, 1982). In all cases the etiology was vascular. Median duration of aphasia was 21 months (range 3–75). The lesions assessed by computer tomography were restricted to the frontal and central parts of the language area. The number of patients available was rather limited, as patients with corrected vision or with hemianopic deficits could of course not be considered. These additional selection criteria made it impossible to report at the present time on the behavior of patients with Wernicke's aphasia whose lesions typically involve the posterior part of the language area.

To make sure that the patients were familiar with the task, all of them were pretrained with a set of items whose critical linguistic features were different from those of the experimental items.

Material.   There was a total of four items. The first two were taken as "warm-up" items. Consequently, they were different in linguistic structure from the others. The linguistic structure of the experimental item is shown in Fig. 1. From the unordered array of sentence constituents the subject was asked to construct a sentence and was told that there is only one possible

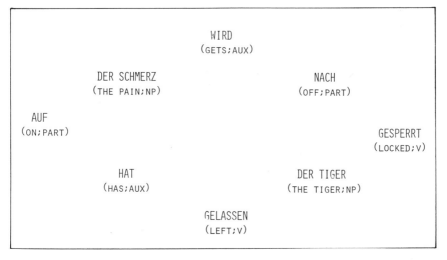

FIG. 1.   Linguistic structure of the experimental item.

solution. The target sentence is "Der Schmerz hat nachgelassen," translated word for word "The pain has off-left," meaning "The pain has gotten less." The remaining constituents do not allow for a correct alternative sentence because the verb particle "auf/on" is semantically inadequate. Only "ein/in" would lead to a correct second solution, namely "Der Tiger wird eingesperrt / The tiger gets in-locked." All further combinations of constituents of the target and the distractor sentences would also lead to linguistically inadequate solutions.

The two nominal phrases allow for contrasting actor versus non-actor interpretations. Only "the tiger" but not "the pain" can be taken as referring to a possible actor. The influence of content versus function words is controlled by having four constituents from the major syntactic categories, namely the two nominal phrases (NP) and the two verb participles (V), and four constituents from minor syntactic categories, namely the two auxiliaries (AUX) and the two verb particles (PART). The linguistic structure of both the target and the distractor sentences is illustrated in Fig. 2. The

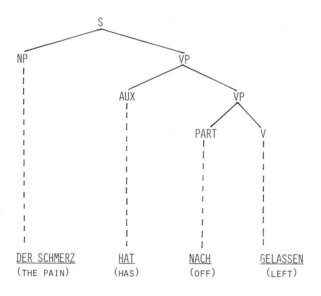

FIG. 2.   Linguistic structure of the sentence (S: sentence, NP: nominal phrase, VP: verbal phrase, AUX: auxiliary, PART: particle, V: verb).

constituents are ordered in a hierarchical way. Considering only single constituents, particle and verb would have the strongest binding. Furthermore, the binding between auxiliary and verb would be stronger than between nominal phrase and verb. However, if one assumes a linear structure, one would expect the strength of binding between constituents to decrease from left to right.

In order to control for possible preferences in the direction of gaze, we introduced a further item, which was linguistically parallel to the experimental item, except that the subject-NP of the target sentence had the interpretation of an actor. The linguistic structure of the experimental and the control item is shown in Fig. 3. Underlinings indicate the constituents to be selected for the correct solution. This design allowed for comparing eye movements toward the upper versus lower part, and toward the right versus left side of the screen. Upper/lower part was defined by constituent positions 7-8-1 versus 5-4-3, and right/left side by 1-2-3 versus 5-6-7. As we expected the actor/non-actor distinction to have the greatest influence on scanning, only the position of the actor-NP was systematically varied. A more extensive variation either by having a greater number of control items or by repeated presentations of the experimental item was dismissed, as neither stimuli nor task variables could have been kept comparable. In addition, a more extensive testing would have been too demanding for brain damaged patients.

Procedure. Before the multiple choice set was shown, the individual constituents were presented clockwise in circular order as indicated by the numbers in Fig. 3. The subject had to read them aloud or—with the aphasic subjects—the examiner read them aloud. By this procedure, we wanted to minimize the influence of word lengths, lexical familarity, reading difficulties, etc. All stimuli were presented on slides and the duration of projections was determined by the subjects themselves. The subjects were told to push a button when they felt sure about the correct solution. The aphasic subjects could give the solution either verbally or by pointing. The whole test, including calibration of eye movements of the individual subject, lasted about 30-40 minutes.

The subject was seated about 190 cm away from the screen (100 × 75 cm) with his head fixed. Viewed from this position, the midpoints of the eight constituents were separated from one another by a visual angle of 6°. Thus, during fixation of one constituent, adjacent constituents were out of focus. One gaze was defined as an uninterrupted sequence of fixations upon the same constituent position, defined as an ellipse (22.5 × 14.3 cm) around the constituent. The stimuli words were written in capital letters with a height of 2 cm.

The eye movements were measured by tracking the corneal reflection center with respect to the pupil center via a video camera (cf. Young &

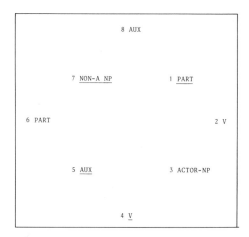

FIG. 3.   Linguistic structure of the experimental (right) and the control item (left).

Sheena, 1975). The x and y coordinates were calculated every 40 msec. The coordinates were recorded and monitored by computer (system DEBIC 80).

RESULTS

Table 1 gives the mean time and the range of times needed for reading the individual constituents of the experimental item and for constructing the sentence from the multiple choice set of constituents as well as the linguistic quality of answers given. All of the students, but none of the aphasic pa-

TABLE 1
Time for Reading and Constructing

| | | Presentation of Stimuli | | |
		Individual Reading	*Multiple Choice Constructing*	*Linguistic Adequacy of Solution Given*
STUDENTS N = 17	MDN	0.16 sec	5.2 sec	all correct
	RANGE	(0.11-0.27)	(1.1- 17.4)	
APHASICS N = 9	MDN	0.26 sec	114.0 sec	all erroneous
	RANGE	(0.13-0.44)	(18.4-239.2)	3x on target sentence 2x on distractor sentence 2x blending of both 2x no reaction

tients, found the correct solution. There is a marked difference between the two groups only with respect to time for constructing. Comparing students to aphasics, we have a proportion of about 1:22 in constructing the sentence, but only about 1:1.6 in reading the individual constituents.

Following specific hypotheses concerning the differential influence of linguistic features on the eye movement behavior of aphasic patients versus students, we compared the frequency and duration values of each individual patient with the median values of the control group. Statistical evaluation made use of the binomial test (one-tailed) with an alpha-level of 2%. The null-hypothesis was rejected only if no more than one of the nine aphasic patients showed values in the opposite direction.

Actor Phrase.   In Table 2 the values for gaze frequency and gaze duration are separately summed up for all the constituents of the target and the distractor sentences. Both frequency and duration in processing the target sentence are lower in the aphasics' than in the students' group. On statistical evaluation, the directed hypothesis was accepted.

The high values for the distractor sentence in the aphasic group were mainly determined by the priority given to processing the nominal phrase that could be interpreted as an actor (cf. Table 3). As expected, all aphasic subjects looked more frequently and longer at the actor than at the non-actor phrase. The students, however, showed a different pattern of processing. Like the aphasics, they looked more frequently at the actor phrase, but their gaze durations were longer with respect to the non-actor phrase. Furthermore, the priorities given to the actor phrase were greater in the

TABLE 2
Processing of Target Versus Distractor Sentences

| | Gaze Frequency (Percentages) | | Gaze Duration (Percentages) | |
	Target Sentence	Distractor Sentence	Target Sentence	Distractor Sentence
	MDN	MDN	MDN	MDN
Students	55.6	44.4	69.4	30.6
N = 17				
Aphasics				
Subj. 1	38.6	61.4	33.0	67.0
2	41.9	58.1	30.9	69.1
3	45.8	54.2	29.3	70.7
4	49.4	50.6	44.5	55.5
5	52.0	48.0	51.4	48.6
6	29.6	70.4	11.6	88.4
7	40.7	59.3	41.0	59.0
8	51.5	48.5	56.4	43.6
9	47.1	52.9	42.3	57.7

TABLE 3
The Influence of Actor Interpretation

| | Gaze Frequency (Percentages) | | Gaze Duration (Percentages) | |
	Non-Actor (Target)	Actor (Distractor)	Non-Actor (Target)	Actor (Distractor)
Students N = 17	MDN[1] 10.8	MDN[1] 16.7	MDN[2] 13.9	MDN[1] 9.5
Aphasics Subj. 1	8.2	29.2	11.2	20.2
2	5.4	30.2	6.5	36.4
3	10.4	16.7	8.3	27.1
4	5.6	28.9	3.9	35.4
5	8.6	22.3	6.5	21.8
6	1.9	33.3	0.6	63.1
7	4.8	30.3	4.3	26.5
8	12.1	30.3	23.8	26.7
9	10.6	27.1	14.4	33.3

directed hypothesis   [1]accepted   [2]not accepted (binominal test, one-tailed, $\alpha = 2\%$)

aphasics' than in the students' group. This was the case for both gaze variables and was sustained by statistical evaluation.

Word Category.   Next, we analyzed the influence of major versus minor word category, or content versus function words. Table 4 shows that students did not behave differently with respect to word category. The aphasics, however, attended more to constituents that contained content words, and they did so with higher gaze frequency and duration than the students. On applying the binominal test, the directed hypothesis was again accepted.

Sentence Structure.   In Table 5 frequencies and durations are summed up for constituents of the same category. The values are presented in the order: nominal phrase (NP)—auxiliary (AUX)—particle (PART)—verb (V), which represents the correct syntactic structure of both the target and the distractor sentences. The values found for the students decrease from left to right, indicating a linear and not a hierarchical conceptualization of sentence structure. In the aphasic group, we again found a different distribution. Nominal phrase and verb are the two categories which are longest and most frequently looked at.

Parallel differences were found when we analyzed gaze alterations. In Table 6, the gaze alterations between each pair of categories in both directions are summed up. With the students, the data show that pairs of constit-

TABLE 4
The Influence of Word Category

	Gaze Frequency (Percentages)		Gaze Duration (Percentages)	
	Major Category *(Content Words)* *NP + V*	*Minor Category* *(Function Words)* *AUX + PART*	*Major Category* *(Content Words)* *NP + V*	*Minor Category* *(Function Words)* *AUX + PART*
	MDN	MDN	MDN	MDN
Students N = 17	50.0	50.0	51.7	48.3
Aphasics				
Subj. 1	67.3	32.7	77.3	22.7
2	69.0	31.0	76.0	24.0
3	54.2	45.8	59.4	40.6
4	63.9	36.1	70.1	29.9
5	49.1	50.9	45.2	54.8
6	63.0	37.0	85.9	14.1
7	67.6	32.4	66.3	33.7
8	66.7	33.3	73.3	26.7
9	69.4	30.6	79.9	20.1

TABLE 5
Processing of Sentence Structure

	Gaze Frequency (Percentages)				Gaze Duration (Percentages)			
	NP	AUX	PART	V	NP	AUX	PART	V
MDN	MDN	MDN	MDN	MDN	MDN	MDN	MDN	
Students	30.0	30.0	22.2	12.5	28.0	25.0	23.1	14.3
N = 17								
Aphasics								
Subj. 1	37.4	21.1	11.7	29.8	31.3	14.2	8.5	46.0
2	35.7	15.5	15.5	33.3	42.9	15.3	8.7	33.1
3	27.1	25.0	20.8	27.1	35.4	18.3	22.3	24.0
4	34.4	19.4	16.7	29.5	39.3	17.8	12.1	30.8
5	30.8	14.3	36.6	18.3	28.2	9.5	45.3	17.0
6	35.2	9.2	27.8	27.8	63.7	1.6	12.5	22.2
7	35.2	12.4	20.0	32.4	30.8	12.4	21.3	35.5
8	42.4	24.2	9.1	24.2	50.5	21.8	4.9	22.8
9	37.6	16.5	14.1	31.8	47.7	10.5	9.5	32.3

uents were more intensively processed if they included elements that are relatively close to the initial position of the sentence. However, with the aphasic subjects, alterations between those constituents that carry most of the semantic information, namely between nominal phrase and verb, either far exceeded all other pairs or were among the most intensively processed ones. Furthermore, the frequences of alterations between these two constituents were significantly higher in the predicted direction in the aphasics' than in the students' group.

The mean percentages for gaze frequency and duration are given in Table 7 with respect to constituents represented either on the right versus left side or on the upper versus lower part of the screen (cf. Fig. 3). Both groups scanned the constituents of each item more often and longer in the lower than in the upper part of the screen. No left/right preference was found for the control item. But with the experimental item, the aphasic subjects showed a right preference, whereas the students tended to have a left preference.

This differential distribution between the groups seems, however, to be conditioned by the position of the actor phrase and by the priority with which it was processed by each of the groups. In Fig. 4, the frequency and duration values of the two items are compared for the two groups. The differences between the two groups in the experimental item are determined by the linguistic contrast between actor and non-actor interpretation that differentiates between distractor-NP and target-NP. The position of the distracting actor-NP is on the lower right side of the screen; the target-NP is on the upper left side. In the control item, however, the target-NP is marked as actor and is presented on the lower left side (cf. Fig. 3). Correspondingly,

TABLE 6
Gaze Alterations Between Two Constituent Categories (Percentages)

	NP→AUX	NP→PART	NP→V	AUX→PART	AUX→V	PART→V
Students N = 17	MDN 21.1	MDN 13.0	MDN 13.2	MDN 13.4	MDN 2.0	MDN 0
Aphasics Subj. 1	18.8	6.5	45.3	12.9	10.6	2.9
2	7.8	11.7	46.9	10.9	10.2	8.6
3	12.8	17.0	19.2	12.8	23.4	12.8
4	18.4	12.3	35.8	7.8	11.2	10.1
5	6.9	28.7	16.7	19.5	2.3	17.8
6	7.6	26.4	35.9	9.4	1.9	17.0
7	11.8	9.7	47.2	9.7	3.5	14.6
8	31.3	9.4	37.5	9.4	6.3	0
9	14.3	9.5	40.5	7.1	11.9	11.9

TABLE 7
Influence of Gaze Direction

I gaze frequency (mean percentages)

		screen position			screen position		
		left	right	diff. (r-l)	upper	lower	diff. (l-u)
experimental	students	50.0	50.0	0	34.5	65.5	+31.0
item	aphasics	34.7	65.3	+30.6	24.3	75.7	+51.4
control	students	51.8	48.2	− 3.6	37.5	62.5	+25.0
item	aphasics	51.6	48.4	− 3.2	36.8	63.2	+24.4

II gaze duration (mean percentages)

		left	right	diff. (r-l)	upper	lower	diff. (l-u)
experimental	students	60.3	39.7	− 30.6	41.7	58.3	+16.6
item	aphasics	27.5	72.5	+45.0	28.9	71.1	+42.2
control	students	49.0	51.0	+ 2.0	28.6	71.4	+42.8
item	aphasics	54.8	45.2	− 9.6	29.0	71.0	+42.0

we have in Table 7 a differential distribution between the two groups with respect to position for the experimental item only, but not for the control item.

DISCUSSION

Eye movements of aphasic patients and controls were recorded via a video camera while the subjects were scanning an unordered circular array of sentence constituents. The subjects had to determine those constituents that can be combined into a well-formed sentence. Before this sentence construction task, the constituents were presented individually in order to control for reading capacity.

As expected, the aphasic subjects had more difficulties than the students in finding a sentence. This is reflected both in their erroneous answers and in the time they needed for construction, which was greater for each aphasic individual than for each of the students. These difficulties of the aphasics cannot be explained by difficulties in visual encoding of the single constituents, as the differences between the two groups were much less pronounced in reading.

In the control group, priority was clearly given to processing the target sentence, as their higher percentages for duration as well as for frequency of gaze indicate. In other words, the assessment of eye movements during processing of the sentence predicts the linguistic output. Among the aphasics this was not the case and there was no clear correlation with their answers. One explanation for this differential distribution can be based on the aphasic subjects' processing of the actor phrase, which belonged to the distractor sentence. It seems that the aphasics relied primarily on a solution that integrated the actor phrase rather than switch to an alternative linguistic strategy as the normals did.

This interpretation became more plausible when we analyzed the processing of single sentence constituents. The linguistic structure of the target and the distractor sentences was completely parallel, except for the nominal phrase (NP) when taken as subject. Only the NP that belonged to the distractor sentence could be interpreted as an actor. Analyzing only those data for the two NPs, the two groups showed differential distributions. Aphasics gave priority to the actor-NP with respect to both gaze variables, frequency and duration. The normal controls looked more frequently at the actor-NP, but longer at the target-NP. This pattern, indeed, suggests that the controls, like the aphasics, applied an actor-first-strategy, as reflected by gaze frequency, but the controls gave up this strategy when they began to conceptualize the target sentence. This, furthermore, suggests that gaze duration depends more directly on the processing of the output than does gaze frequency.

Another linguistic feature that was systematically controlled in this study was word category. Both the target and the distractor sentences included two major and two minor constituents. Major constituents contain content words, whereas minor constituents are made of function words. The aphasic subjects were clinically classified as patients with Broca's aphasia. Their spontaneous speech output was characterized by agrammatic ut-

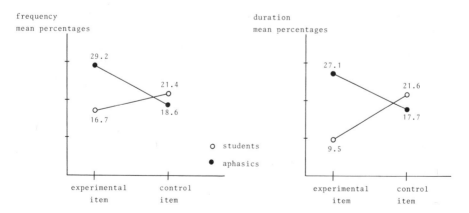

FIG. 4.   Influence of the actor phrase in the experimental and control items.

terances, which typically consist of sequences of content words only. Therefore, we were particularly interested in whether function versus content words would also be differentially affected in their eye movement behavior. This was indeed the case, as all aphasic subjects except one scanned major constituents longer and more frequently than minor constituents. The mean difference was 33.4% for frequency and 46.6% for duration. No clearcut mean differences were found in the control group or in one patient who did not fit the aphasic general pattern.

When analyzing the influence of sentence structure, we found that controls processed constituents near the beginning of the sentence more intensively than those toward the end. This makes a linear, rather than hierarchical, conceptualization of the sentence structure quite plausible, at least as far as receptive selection processes are concerned. Linear conceptualization implies that the choice of sentence constituents becomes linguistically more restricted as more constituents are chosen. Therefore, the intensity of processing will gradually decrease in a multiple choice task like ours.

For the aphasic patients the data do not suggest a similar linear conceptualization of sentence structure. The processing of the sentence structure seems to have been semantically based, i.e., the aphasic patients relied primarily on those constituents that contain content words. This became quite apparent when alterations of gaze for pairs of constituents were analyzed. Compared to the median performance of the controls, each of the aphasic subjects looked more frequently between the two major constituents than did the controls. This finding for the aphasics is incompatible with a linear conceptualization of the sentence structure as, according to German syntax, the two major constituents, namely subject-NP and verb participle, have to be in the initial and in the final position, respectively, in the sentences we used. For both the controls and the aphasics, the variable gaze alteration reflects strategies of syntactic processing very much in the same way as the variables gaze frequency and duration.

With regard to the linguistic status of aphasic symptoms, our study indicates that agrammatism is a general linguistic deficit that is not limited to the speech output, but also affects receptive selection processes in a sentence construction task.

ACKNOWLEDGMENTS

We would like to thank Professor Dr. Klaus Poeck, director of the Neurology Department, RWTH Aachen, for his support and Hans-Willi Schroiff for his help in running the experiment.

V REFERENCES

Acker, W., & Toone, B. Attention, eye tracking and schizophrenia. *British Journal of Social and Clinical Psychology,* 1978, *17,* 173–181.

Algayer, H., & Heller, D. Funktionsanalyse eines Systems zur Registrierung der Augenbewegungen beim Lesen. *Psychologische Beiträge* 1978, *20,* 331–344.

Allum, J. H. J., Tole, R. J., & Weiss, A. D. MITNYS II: A digital program for on-line analysis of nystagmus. *IEEE Transactions,* 1975, BME-22, 196–202.

Ammons, R. B., Ulrich, P., & Ammons, C. H. Voluntary control of perception of depth in a two-dimensional drawing. *Proceedings of the Montana Academy of Science,* 1959, *19,* 160–168.

Anderson, I. H. Studies in the eye-movements of good and poor readers. *Psychological Monographs,* 1937, *48,* 1–35.

Andriessen, J. J., & de Voogd, A. H. Analysis of eye movement patterns in silent reading. *I.P.O. Annual Progress Report,* 1973, *8,* 29–34.

Antes, J. R. The time course of picture viewing. *Journal of Experimental Psychology,* 1974, *103,* 62–70.

Antes, J. R., & Penland, J. G. Picture context effects on eye movement patterns. In D. F. Fisher, R. A. Monty, & J. W. Senders (Eds.), *Eye movements: Cognition and visual perception.* Hillsdale, NJ: Lawrence Erlbaum Associates, 1981.

Anzaldi, E., & Mira, E. An interactive program for the analysis of ENG tracings. *Acta Otolaryngologica,* 1975, *80,* 120–127.

Armstrong, P., & Wastie, M. L. *X-ray diagnosis,* London: Blackwell, 1981.

Arnold, D. C., & Tinker, M. A. The fixational pause of the eyes. *Journal of Experimental Psychology,* 1939, *25,* 271–280.

Bach-y-Rita, P., Collins, C. C., & Hyde, J. E. *The control of eye movements.* New York: Academic Press, 1971.

Bahill, A. T., Adler, D., & Stark, L. Most naturally occurring human saccades have magnitudes of 15 degrees or less. *Investigative Ophthalmology,* 1975, *14,* 468–469.

Bahill, A. T., Clark, M. R., & Stark, L. Dynamic overshoot in saccadic eye movement is caused by neurological control signal reversals. *Experimental Neurology,* 1975, *48,* 107–122.

Bahill, A. T., Iandolo, M. J., & Troost, B. T. Smooth pursuit eye movements in response to unpredictable target waveforms. *Vision Research,* 1980, *20,* 923–931.

Bakan, P., & Shotland, R. L. Lateral eye movements, reading speed, and visual attention. *Psychonomic Science,* 1969, *15,* 93–94.

Baker, R., & Berthoz, A. (Eds.) *Control of gaze by brainstem neurons.* Amsterdam: Elsevier, 1977.

Baker, M. A., & Loeb, M. Implications of measurement of eye fixations for a psychophysics of form perception. *Perception & Psychophysics,* 1973, *13,* 185–192.

Baloh, R. W., Honrubia, V., & Sill, A. W. Eye-Tracking and Optokinetic nystagmus. Results of quantitative testing in patients with well-defined nervous system lesions. *Annals of Otology Rhinology,* 1977, *86,* 108.

Baloh, R. W., Konrad, H. R., Sills, A. W., & Honrubia, V. The saccade velocity test. *Neurology,* 1975, *25,* 1071–1076. (a)

Baloh, R. W., Kumley, W. E., & Honrubia, V. Algorithm for analyses of saccadic eye movements using a digital computer. *Aviation Space Environmental Medicine,* 1976, *47,* 523–527.

Baloh, R. W., Sills, A. W., Kumley, W. E., & Honrubia, V. Quantitative measurement of saccade amplitude, duration and velocity. *Neurology,* 1975, *25,* 1065–1070. (b)

Baloh, R. W., Yee, R. D., & Honrubia, V. Internuclear ophthalmoplegia. I. Saccades and dissociated nystagmus. *Archives of Neurology,* 1978, *35,* 484–489.

Barlow, H. B. Slippage of contact lenses and other artifacts in relation to fading and regeneration of supposedly stable retinal images. *Quarterly Journal of Experimental Psychology,* 1963, *15,* 36–51.

Bartz, A. G. Peripheral detection and central task complexity. *Human Factors,* 1976, *18,* 63–70.

Becker, W. The control of eye movements in the saccadic system. *Bibliotheca Ophthalmologica* 1972, *82,* 233–243.

Becker, W., & Fuchs, A. F. Further properties of the human saccadic system: Eye movements and correction saccades with and without fixation points. *Vision Research,* 1969, *9,* 1247–1258.

Becker, W., & Fuchs, A. (Eds.) *Progress in oculomotor research.* Amsterdam: Elsevier, 1981.

Becker, W., & Jürgens, R. An analysis of the saccadic system by means of double step-stimuli. *Vision Research,* 1979, *19,* 967–983.

Bellamy, L. J., & Courtney, A. J. Development of a search task for the measurement of peripheral visual acuity. *Ergonomics,* 1981, *24,* 497–509.

Bever, T. G. The cognitive basis for linguistic structures. In J. R. Hayes (Ed.), *Cognition and the development of language.* New York: Wiley, 1970.

Biederman, I. Perceiving real-world scenes. *Science,* 1972, *177,* 77–80.

Biederman, I., Glass, A. L., & Stacy, E. W. Searching for objects in real world scenes. *Journal of Experimental Psychology,* 1973, *97,* 22–27.

Biederman, I., Rabinowitz, J. C., Glass, A. L., & Stacy, E. W. On the information extracted from a glance at a scene. *Journal of Experimental Psychology,* 1974, *103,* 597–600.

Boghen, D., Troost, B. T., Daroff, R. B., Dell'Osso, L. F., & Birkett, J. E. Velocity characteristics of normal human saccades. *Investigative Ophthalmology,* 1974, *13,* 619–623.

Bouis, D., Baude, P., & Vossius G. An improved non-contact type ophthalmograph. *Proceedings of the 28th ACEMB Conference,* New Orleans, LA, 1975, 323.

Bouis, D., & Vossius, G. Adaptives PI-verhalten der Kontrolle der Komtinuierlichen Augenfolgebewegung, *Biomedizinische Technik,* 1978, *23,* 146–147.

Bouma, H. Interaction effects in parafoveal letter recognition. *Nature,* 1970, *226,* 177–178.

Bouma, H. Visual search and reading: Eye movements and functional visual field: A tutorial review. In J. Requin (Ed.), *Attention and performance VIII.* Hillsdale, NJ: Lawrence Erlbaum Associates, 1978.

Bouma, H. Visual interference in the parafoveal recognition of initial and final letters of words. *Vision Research,* 1973, *13,* 767-782.

Bouma, H., & de Voogd, A. H. On the control of eye saccades in reading. *Vision Research,* 1974, *14,* 271.

Bretland, P. M. *Essentials of Radiology.* London: Butterworths, 1978.

Brewster, D. On the optical illusion of the conversion of cameos into intaglios, and of intaglios into cameos, with an account of other analoguous phenomena. *Edinburgh Journal of Science,* 1826, *4,* 99-108.

Brigham, F. R. *Visuelle Zielentdeckung.* Institut für Unfallforschung des TÜV Rheinland e.V., Abschlussbericht, Köln, 1979.

Brown, B., & Monk, Th. The effect of local target surround and whole background constraint on visual search times. *Human Factors,* 1975, *17,* 81-88.

Buchsbaum, M., Pfefferbaum, A., & Stillman, R. Individual differences in eye movement patterns. *Perception & Psychophysics,* 1972, *35,* 895-901.

Buizza, A., Schmid, R., Zanibelli, A., Mira, E., & Semplici, P. Quantification of vestibular nystagmus by an interactive computer program. *Otorhinolarynology,* 1978, *40,* 147-159.

Buswell, G. T. How adults read. *Supplementary educational monographs* (45). Chicago, IL: University of Chicago, 1937.

Cabiati, C., & Pastormerlo, M. *Un sistema per 1 'analisi automatica dei movimenti saccadici degli occhi.* Thesis, University of Pavia, Italy, 1979.

Calfee, R., & Curley, R. Structures of prose in the content areas. In J. Flood (Ed.), *Understanding reading comprehension,* in preparation.

Campbell, F. W., & Robson, J. C. Application of Fourier analysis to the visibility of grating. *Journal of Physiology,* 1968, *197, 551-566.*

Carmody, D. P., Nodine, C. F., & Kundel, H. L. Global and segmented search for lung nodules of different edge gradients. *Investigative Radiology,* 1980, *15,* 224-253.

Carpenter, R. H. S. *Movements of the eyes.* London: Pion Ltd., 1977.

Carpenter, P. A., & Just, M. A. Reading comprehension as eyes see it. In M. A. Just & P. A. Carpenter (Eds.), *Cognitive processes in comprehension.* Hillsdale, NJ: Lawrence Erlbaum Associates, 1977.

Cavicchio, R. A. *Parametric adjustment of saccadic eye movements.* Unpublished Ph.D. Dissertation, Tufts University, 1975.

Cegalis, J. A., & Sweeney, J. A. Eye movements in schizophrenia: A quantitative analysis. *Biological Psychiatry,* 1979, *14,* 13-26.

Chastain, G., & Burnham, C. A. The first glimpse determines the perception of an ambiguous figure. *Perception & Psychophysics,* 1975, *17,* 221-224.

Chiang, C. A theory of ambiguous pattern perception. *Bulletin of Mathematical Psychology,* 1976, *38,* 497-504.

Claparède, E. La genèse de l'hypothèse. *Archives de Psychologie,* 1933, *24,* 2-155.

Clare, J. N. Recognition as an extension to the detection process. In J. N. Clare & M. A. Sinclair (Eds.), *Search and the human observer.* London: Taylor & Francis, 1979.

Coles, P. R., Sigman, M., & Chessell, K. Scanning strategies of children and adults. In Butterworth, G. (Ed.), *The child's representation of the world.* New York: Plenum Press, 1977.

Collewijn, H. The normal range of horizontal eye movements in the rabbit. *Experimental Neurology,* 1970, *28,* 132-143.

Cook, G. *Control systems study of the saccadic eye-movement mechanism.* Sc. D. Thesis, M.I.T., Cambridge, MA, 1965.

Couch, F. H., & Fox, J. C. Photographic study of ocular movements in mental disease. *Archives of Neurology and Psychiatry,* 1934, *31,* 556-578.

Cowey, A. The basis of a method of perimetry with monkeys. *Quarterly Journal of Experimental Psychology,* 1963, *15,* 81-90.

Davis, F. R. Research in comprehension in reading. *Reading Research Quarterly,* 1968, *3,* 499–544.

Day, M. E. An eye-movement phenomenon relating to attention, thought, and anxiety. *Perceptual and Motor Skills,* 1964, *19.* 443–446.

De Jong, D., & Melvill Jones, G. Akinesia, hypokinesia and bradykinesia in the oculomotor system of patients with Parkinson's disease. *Experimental Neurology,* 1971, *32,* 58–68.

Dearborn, W. *The psychology of reading,* (Columbia University contributions to philosophy and psychology). New York: Science Press, 1906.

Deese, J. Text structure, strategies, and comprehension in learning from textbooks. In J. Robinson (Ed.), *Research in science education: New questions, new directions.* Boulder, CO: BSCS, 1980.

Dewey, J. *How we think.* Second edition. Boston: Heath, 1933.

Dichgans, J., & Bizzi, E. (Eds.). *Central control of eye movements and motion perception.* Basel: Karger, 1972.

Dick, G. L. Computer analysis of rapid eye movement. *Computer Programs in Biomedicine,* 1978, *8,* 29–34.

Didday, R. L., & Arbib, M. A. Eye movements and visual perception: A 'two visual system' model. *International Journal of Man-Machine Studies,* 1975, *7,* 547–569.

Diefendorf, A. R., & Dodge, R. An experimental study of the ocular reactions of the insane from photographic records. *Brain,* 1908, *31,* 451–489.

Ditchburn, R. W. *Eye movements and visual perception. Oxford: Clarendon Press, 1973.*

Easter, S. S. The time course of saccadic eye movements in goldfish. *Vision Research,* 1975, *15,* 405–409.

Edwards, D. C., & Goolkasian, P. A. Peripheral vision location and kinds of complex processing. *Journal of Experimental Psychology,* 1974, *102,* 244–249.

Ellis, S. R., & Stark, L. Eye movements during the viewing of Necker cubes. *Perception,* 1978, *7,* 575–581.

Engel, F. L. Visual conspicuity, directed attention and retinal locus. *Vision Research,* 1971, *11,* 563–576.

Engel, F. L. *Visual conspicuity as an external determinant of eye movements and selective attention.* Doctoral dissertation, TH Eindhoven, 1976.

Engel, F. L. Visual conspicuity, visual search and fixation tendencies of the eye. *Vision Research,* 1977, *17,* 95–108.

Enoch, J. M. Effect of the size of a complex display upon visual search. *Journal of the Optical Society of America,* 1959, *49,* 280–286.

Erickson, R. A. Visual search performance in a moving structured field. *Journal of the Optical Society of America,* 1964, *54,* 399–405.

Estes, T. H., & Shebilske, W. L. Comprehension: Of what the reader sees of what the author says. In M. L. Kamil & S. J. Moe (Eds.), *Twenty-ninth Yearbook of the National Reading Conference,* 1980, 99–104.

Evans, C. R., & Marsden, R. P. A study of the effect of perfect retinal stabilization on some well-known visual illusions, using the after-image as a method of compensation for eye movements. *Scandinavian Journal of Psychology,* 1966, *23,* 242–248.

Evinger, L. C., & Fuchs, A. F. Saccadic, smooth pursuit and optokinetic eye movements of the trained cat. *Journal of Physiology* (London), 1978, *285,* 209–229.

Falmagne, R. Construction of a hypothesis testing model for concept identification. *Journal of Mathematical Psychology,* 1970, *7,* 60–96.

Farrel, R. J., & Anderson, C. D. *The effect of display field size on image interpretation performance.* Document D 180-19056-1, The Boeing Company, Seattle, Washington, 1975.

Findlay, J. M. A simple apparatus for recording microsaccades during visual fixation. *Quarterly Journal of Experimental Psychology,* 1974, *26,* 167–170.

Findlay, J. M. Local and global influences on saccadic eye movements. In D. F. Fisher, R. A.

Monty, & J. W. Senders (Eds.), *Eye movements: Cognition and visual perception.* Hillsdale, NJ: Lawrence Erlbaum Associates, 1981. (a)

Findlay, J. M. Visual information processing for saccadic eye movements. In A. Hein & M. Jeannerod (Eds.), *Spatially coordinated behavior.* New York: Springer, 1981. (b)

Findlay, J. M. Global processing for saccadic eye movements. *Vision Research,* in press.

Fisher, D. F., & Peters, C. W. *Comprehension and the competent reader.* New York: Praeger Publishers, 1981.

Fisher, D. F., Monty, R. A., & Senders, J. W. (Eds.) *Eye movements: Cognition and visual perception.* Hillsdale, NJ: Lawrence Erlbaum Associates, 1981.

Flagg, B. N. *Children and television: Effects of stimulus repetition on eye activity.* Unpublished doctoral dissertation, Harvard University, 1977.

Flamm, L. E., & Bergum, B. O. Reversible perspective figures and eye movements. *Perceptual and Motor Skills,* 1977, *44,* 1015-1019.

Flekkoy, K. Neurophysiological aspects of distractability in schizophrenics. *Acta Psychiatrica Scandinavica,* 1980, *61,* 461-472.

Flugel, J. C. The influence of attention in illusions of reversible perspective. *British Journal of Psychology,* 1913, *5,* 357-397.

Foos, P. W., Smith, K. H, Sabol, M. A., & Mynatt, B. T. Constructive processes in simple linear order problems. *Journal of Experimental Psychology: Human Learning and Memory,* 1976, *2,* 759-766.

Frase, L. T. A structural analysis of the knowledge that results from thinking about text. *Journal of Educational Psychology Monograph,* 1969, *60,* (6, Part 2).

Frase, L. T. Influence of sentence order and higher level text processing upon reproductive and productive memory. *American Educational Research Journal,* 1970, *7,* 307-319.

Fredericksen, C. H. Acquisition of semantic information from discourse: Effects of repeated exposures. *Journal of Verbal Learning and Verbal Behavior,* 1975, *14,* 153-169. (a)

Fredericksen, C. H. Representing logical and semantic structures of knowledge acquired from discourse. *Cognitive Psychology,* 1975, *1,* 371-458. (b)

Friedman, A., & Liebelt, L. S. On the time course of viewing pictures with a view towards remembering. In D. F. Fisher, R. A. Monty, & J. W. Senders (Eds.), *Eye movements: Cognition and visual perception.* Hillsdale, NJ: Lawrence Erlbaum Associates, 1981.

Fröschl, T., Heller, D., & Müller, H. *Zur Präzision der Augenbewegungen beim Lesen.* Forschungsbericht des Psychologischen Instituts der Universität Würzburg, 1980.

Fuchs, A. F. Saccadic and smooth pursuit eye movements in the monkey. *Journal of Physiology* (London), 1967, *191,* 609-631.

Fuchs, A. F. The saccadic system. In P. Bach-y-Rita, C. C. Collins, & J. E. Hyde (Eds.), *The control of eye movements.* New York: Academic Press, 1971, 343-362.

Gale, A. G. *The role of eye movements in figure perception.* Unpublished doctoral thesis, University of Durham, Durham, 1980.

Gale, A. G., Johnson, F., & Worthington, B. S. On-line real time analysis of eye movements. *Journal of the Physiological Society,* 1978, *276,* 23P.

Gale, A. G., Johnson, F., & Worthington, B. S. Psychology and radiology. In D. J. Oborne, M. M. Gruneberg, & J. R. Eiser (Eds.), *Research in psychology and medicine,* Vol. 1. London: Academic Press, 1979.

Gale, A. G., Johnson, F., & Worthington, B. S. Research in medical image perception—a microprocessor application. In J. P. Paul, M. M. Jordan, & M. W. Ferguson-Pell (Eds.), *Computing in medicine.* London: Macmillans, 1982.

Garland, L. H. Studies in the accuracy of diagnostic procedures. *American Journal of Roentgenology,* 1959, *82,* 25-28.

Geibelmann, H., & Tropf, H. *Some applications of the fast image analysis system S.A.M.* Submitted to: IMEKO '82, Berlin (West), May 24-28, 1982.

Geissler, H. G., Puffe, M., & Scheidereiter, U. Memory codes and processing: Strategies in complex classification tasks. In H. G. Geissler (Ed.), *Modern trends in psychophysics*. Amsterdam: North Holland Publishing Company, 1982.

George, R. W. The signficance of the fluctuations experienced in observing ambiguous figures and in binocular rivalry. *Journal of General Psychology*, 1936, *15*, 39–61.

Gibson, E. J., & Levin, H. *The psychology of reading*. Cambridge, MA: MIT Press, 1975.

Glen, J. S. Ocular movements in reversibility of perspective. *Journal of General Psychology*, 1940, *23*, 243–281.

Gould, J. D. Looking at pictures. In R. A. Monty & J. W. Senders (Eds.), *Eye movements and psychological processes*. Hillsdale, NJ: Lawrence Erlbaum Associates, 1976.

Gould, J. D., & Dill, A. B. Eye movement parameters and pattern discrimination. *Perception & Psychophysics*, 1969, *6*, 311–320.

Griggs, R. A. Recognition memory for deducible information. *Memory and Cognition*, 1976, *4*, 643–647.

Groner, R. Methodische und psychologische Probleme bei der Messung und Interpretation von Augenbewegungen. *Psychologische Rundschau*, 1975, *26*, 76–80.

Groner, R. *Hypothesen im Denkprozess. Grundlagen einer verallgemeinerten Theorie auf der Basis elementarer Informationsverarbeitung*. Bern, Stuttgart & Wien: Huber, 1978.

Groner, R., & Fraisse, P. (Eds.) *Cognition and eye movements*. Amsterdam & Berlin: North Holland & Deutscher Verlag der Wissenschaften (joint edition), 1982.

Groner, R., & Groner, M. Towards a hypothetico-deductive theory of cognitive activity. In R. Groner & P. Fraisse (Eds.), *Cognition and eye movements*. Amsterdam & Berlin: North Holland & Deutscher Verlag der Wissenschaften (joint edition), 1982.

Groner, R., Kaufmann, F., Bischof, W. F., & Hirsbrunner, H. Das Berner System zur Analyse von Blickrichtung und Pupillengrösse. *Forschungsberichte aus dem Psychologischen Institut der Universitat Bern*, 1974–2.

Guiss, L. W., & Kuenstler, P. A retrospective view of survey photofluorograms of persons with lung cancer. *Cancer*, 1960, *13*, 91–95.

Hagen, M. A. Picture perception: Toward a theoretical model. *Psychological Bulletin*, 1974, *81*, 471–497.

Harris, A. J., & Sipay, E. R. *How to increase reading ability: A guide to developmental and remedial methods* (6th ed.). New York: David McKay Company, Inc., 1975.

Hartje, W., Steinhauser, D., & Kerschensteiner, M. Diagnostic value of saccadic pursuit eye movement in screening for organic cerebral dysfunction. *Journal of Neurology*, 1978, *217*, 253–260.

Hartline, H. K. Intensity and duration in the excitation of single photo-receptor units. *J. Cellular and Comparative Physiology*, 1934, *5*, 229–247.

Heeschen, C. Strategies of decoding actor-object-relations by aphasic patients. *Cortex*, 1980, *16*, 5–19.

Heller, D. Under das Elektrookulogramm beim Lesen. Dissertation Universität Erlangen-Nürnberg, Erlangen, 1976.

Heller, D. Eye movements in reading. In R. Groner & P. Fraisse (Eds.), *Cognition and eye movements*. Amsterdam: North-Holland, 1982.

Heller, D., Moos, M., & Stahl, H. *Ein Vergleich zweier psychophysischer Methoden mit Hilfe von Augenbewgungen beim Streckenmitteln*. Forschungsbericht 1979 des Psychologischen Instituts der Universität Würzburg. Würzburg, 1980. (ISBN 3-9800392-0-X)

Henriksson, N. G., Pyykko, I., Schalen, L., & Wennmo, L. Velocity patterns of rapid eye movements. *Acta Otolaryngologica*, 1980, *89*, 504–512.

Henriksson, N. G., Hindfelt, B., Pyykko, I., & Schalen, L. Rapid eye movements reflecting neurological disorders. *Clinical Otolaryngology*, 1981, *6*, 111–119.

Herberts, G., Abrahamsson, S., Einarsson, S., Hofmann, H., & Linder, P. Computer analysis of electronystagmographic data. *Acta Otolaryngologica*, 1968, *65*, 200–208.

Hochberg, J. In the mind's eye. In R. N. Haber (Ed.), *Contemporary theory and research in visual perception*. New York: Holt, Rhinehart & Winston, 1968.

Hochberg, J. Attention, organization and consciousness. In D. C. Mostosky (Ed.), *Attention: Contemporary theory and analysis.* New York: Appleton-Century Crofts, 1970. (a)

Hochberg, J. Components of literacy: Speculations and exploratory research. In H. Levin & J. W. Williams (Eds.), *Basic studies on reading.* New York: Basic Books, 1970. (b)

Holcomb, J. M., Holcomb, H. H., & De La Pena, A. Selective attention and eye movements while viewing reversible figures. *Perceptual and Motor Skills,* 1977, *44,* 639–644.

Holzman, P. S., Kringlen, E., Levy, D. L., & Haberman, S. J. Deviant eye tracking in twins discordant for psychosis. A replication. *Archives of General Psychiatry,* 1980, *37,* 627–631.

Holzman, P. S., & Levy, D. L. Smooth pursuit eye movements and functional psychoses; a review. *Schizophrenia Bulletin,* 1977, *3,* 15–27.

Holzman, P. S., Proctor, L. R., & Hughes, D. W. Eye-tracking patterns in schizophrenia. *Science,* 1973, *181,* 179–181.

Holzman, P. S., Proctor, L. R., Levy, D. L., Yasillo, N. J., Meltzer, H. Y., & Hurt, S. W. Eye-tracking dysfunctions in schizophrenic patients and their relatives. *Archives of General Psychiatry,* 1974, *31,* 143–151.

Howarth, C. I., & Bloomfield, J. R. Towards a theory of visual search. AGARD Conference Proceedings, No. 41. London, 1968.

Huber, W., Poeck, K., Weniger, D., & Willmes, K. *Der aachener aphasie test.* Göttingen: Hogrefe, 1982.

Huttenlocher, J. Constructing spatial images: A strategy in reasoning. *Psychological Review,* 1968, *75,* 550–560.

Huygen, P. L. M. Nystagmometry: The art of measuring nystagmus parameters by digital signal processing. *Otorhinolarynology,* 1979, *41,* 206–220.

Hyde, J. Some characteristics of voluntary ocular movements in the horizontal plane. *American Journal of Ophthalmology,* 1959, *48,* 85–94.

Ikeda, M., & Takeuchi, T. Influence of foveal load on the functional visual field. *Perceptual & Psychophysics,* 1975, *18,* 255–260.

Intraub, H. Presentation rate and the representation of briefly glimpsed pictures in memory. *Journal of Experimental Psychology: Human Learning and Memory,* 1980, *6,* 1–12.

Intraub, H. Identification and processing of briefly glimpsed visual scenes. In D. F. Fisher, R. A. Monty, & J. W. Senders (Eds.), *Eye movements: Cognition and visual perception.* Hillsdale, NJ: Lawrence Erlbaum Associates, 1981.

Iser, W. *The act of reading: A theory of aesthetic response.* Baltimore: Johns Hopkins University Press, 1978.

Johnson, F. Gale, A. G., & Worthington, B. S. Microprocessor equipment to analyze eye movements during radiograph scanning. Proceedings of the I.E.R.E. conference *Microprocessors in Automation and Control,* 1978, *41,* 93–96.

Johnson-Laird, P. M. The three term series problem. *Cognition,* 1972, *1,* 57–82.

Judd, C. H., & Buswell, G. T. Silent reading: A study of the various types. *Supplementary Educational Monographs* (23). Chicago, IL: University of Chicago Press, 1922.

Julesz, B. *Foundation of cyclopean perception.* Chicago: The University of Chicago Press, 1971.

Jürgens, R., & Becker, W. Is there a linear addition of saccades and pursuit movements? In G. Lennerstrand & P. Bach-y-Rita (Eds.), *Basic Mechanisms of ocular motility and their clinical implications.* Oxford: Pergamon Press, 1975.

Just, M. A., & Carpenter, P. A. Eye fixations and cognitive processes. *Cognitive Psychology,* 1976, *8,* 441–480.

Just, M. A., & Carpenter, P. A. A theory of reading: From eye fixations to comprehension. *Psychological Review,* 1980, *87,* 329–354.

Kapoula, Z. A., O'Regan, K. J., & Levy-Schoen, A. Etude de la régulation des durées de fixation dans une tâche de lecture simplifiée. *Psychologie Française,* 1980, *26,* 102–103.

Karmiohl, C. M. *Behavioral vs. formal procedures of text analysis:* Discourse style, task demands, and reading strategies. Unpublished Masters Thesis, University of Virginia, 1981.

Kästner, A., & Wirth, W. Die Bestimmung der Aufmerksamkeitsverteilung innerhalb des Sehfeldes mit Hilfe von Reaktionsversuchen. *Psychologische Studien,* 1908, *3,* 361-392, 1909, *4,* 139-200.

Kaufmann, J. L., & Bullinger, A. Exploration oculaire en situation de règle dépendante. (Quelques faits de sondage sur des aspects cognitifs dans le controle du système oculomoteur.) *Cahiers de Psychologie,* 1980, *23,* 3-22.

Kawabata, N., Yamagami, K., & Noaki, M. Visual fixation points and depth perception. *Vision Research,* 1978, *18,* 853-854.

Kendall, G. M., Darby, S. C., Harris, S. V., & Rae, S. *A frequency survey of radiological examinations carried out in National Health Service Hospitals in Great Britain in 1977 for diagnostic purposes.* NRPB-R104, Harwell, National Radiological Protection Board, 1980.

Kennedy, J. M. *A psychology of picture perception.* San Francisco: Jossey-Bass, 1974.

Kerschensteiner, M., Poeck, K., Huber, W., Stachowiak, F. J., & Weniger, D. Die Broca-Aphasie. *Journal of Neurology,* 1978, *217,* 223-242.

Kintsch, W. *The representation of meaning in memory.* Hillsdale, NJ: Lawrence Erlbaum Associates, 1974.

Kintsch, W., & van Dijk, T. A. Toward a model of text comprehension and production. *Psychological Review,* 1978, *85,* 363-394.

Kirkham, T. H., & Kamin, D. F. Slow saccadic eye movements in Wilson's disease. *Journal of Neurology, Neurosurgery and Psychiatry,* 1974, *37,* 191-194.

Kliegl, R., Olson, R. K., & Davidson, B. J. Perceptual and psycholinguistic factors in reading. In K. Rayner (Ed.), *Eye movements in reading: Perceptual and linguistic aspects.* New York: Academic Press, 1983.

Kommerell, G. *Augenbewegungsstörungen.* München: Bergmann, 1978.

Korn, A. Visual search: Relation between detection performance and visual field size. *Proceedings of the First European Annual Conference on Human Decision Making and Manual Control.* Delft University, May, 1981, 27-34.

Körner, F. H. Non-visual control of human saccadic eye movements. In G. Lennerstrand, & P. Bach-y-Rita (Eds.), *Basic mechanisms of ocular motility and their clinical implications.* Oxford: Pergamon Press, 1975, 565-569.

Kornetsky, C. The use of a simple test of attention as a measure of drug effects in schizophrenic patients. *Psychopharmacologia* (Berlin), 1972, *24,* 99-106.

Kowler, E., & Steinman, R. M. The effect of expectations on slow oculomotor control—I. Periodic target steps. *Vision Research,* 1979, *19,* 619-652.

Kraiss, K. F., & Knäuper, A. Prediction of visual search performance based on visual lobe area measurements. *Proceedings of the European Annual Conference on Human Decision and Manual Control.* Delft: University of Technology, 1981.

Krause, W. Eye fixations and three-term series problems, or: Is there evidence for task-independent information units? In R. Groner & P. Fraisse (Eds.), *Cognition and eye movements.* Amsterdam & Berlin: North Holland & Deutscher Verlag der Wissenschaften (joint edition), 1982.

Kreel, L. *Outline of radiology.* London: Heinemann, 1971.

Krendel, E. S., & Wodinsky, J. Search in an unstructured visual field. *Journal of the Optical Society of America,* 1960, *50,* 562-568.

Kries, V. J., & Auerbach, F. Die Zeitdauer einfachster psychischer Vorgänge. *Archiv für Physiologie,* 1877, 297-378.

Kries, V. J., & Hall, G. S. Uber die Abhängigkeit der Reaktionszeiten vom Ort des Reizes. *Archiv für Physiologie,* 1879, Supplement, S. 6 ff.

Kuechenmeister, C. A., Linton, P. H., Mueller, T. V., & White, H. B. Eye tracking in relation to age, sex, and illness. *Archives of General Psychiatry,* 1977, *34,* 578-579.

Kundel, H. L. Visual sampling and estimates of the location of information on chest films. *Investigative Radiology,* 1974, *9,* 87-93.

Kundel, H. L., & La Follette, P. S. Visual search patterns and experience with radiological images. *Radiology,* 1972, *103,* 523-528.

Kundel, H. L., Nodine, C. F., & Carmody, D. Visual scanning, pattern recognition and decision making in pulmonary nodule detection. *Investigative Radiology,* 1978, *13,* 175-181.

Kundel, H. L., & Revesz, G. Lesion conspicuity, structured noise and film reader error. *American Journal of Roentgenology,* 1976, *126,* 1233-1238.

Kundel, H. L., & Wright, D. J. The influence of prior knowledge on visual search strategies during the viewing of chest radiographs. *Radiology,* 1969, *93,* 315-320.

Lambert, R. H., Monty, R. A., & Hall, R. J. High speed data processing and unobtrusive monitoring of eye movements. *Behavioral Research Methods and Instrumentation,* 1974, *6,* 525-530.

Leeper, R. A study of a neglected portion of the field of learning—the development of sensory organization. *Journal of Genetic Psychology,* 1935, *46,* 41-74.

Lehmann, D., Meles, H. P., & Mir, Z. Average multichannel EEG potential fields evoked from upper and lower hemiretina latency differences. *Electorencephalography and Clinical Neurophysiology,* 1977, *43,* 725-731.

Lehmann, D., & Skrandis, W. Multichannel evoked potential fields show different properties of the human upper and lower hemiretina systems. *Experimental Brain Research,* 1979, *35,* 151-159.

Lennerstrand, G., Bach-Y-Rita, P., & Collins, C. C. (Eds.) *Basic mechanisms of ocular motility and their clinical implications.* London: Pergamon Press, 1975.

Leonhard, K. *The classification of endogenous psychoses* (5th ed.). New York: Irvington Publishers, 1979. (Originally published as: *Aufteilung der endogenen Psychosen,* 1957.)

Levelt, W. J. M. A survey of studies in sentence perception: 1970-1976. In W. J. M. Levelt & G. B. Flores d'Arcais (Eds.), *Studies in the perception of language.* New York: Wiley, 1978.

Levin, S., Lipton, R. B., & Holzman, P. S. Pursuit eye movements in psychopathology: Effects of target characteristics. *Biological Psychiatry,* 1981, *16,* 255-267.

Levy-Schoen, A. Flexible and/or rigid control of oculomotor scanning behavior. In D. F. Fisher, R. A. Monty, & J. W. Senders (Eds.), *Eye movements: Cognition and visual perception.* Hillsdale, NJ: Lawrence Erlbaum Associates, 1981.

Levy-Schoen, A., & O'Regan, K. The control of eye movements in reading. In P. A. Kolers, M. E. Wrolstad, & H. Bouma (Eds.), *Processing of visible language,* Volume 1. New York: Plenum Press, 1979.

Levy-Schoen, A., & Rigaut-Renard, C. Préperception ou activation motrice au cors du TR oculomoteur? In J. Requin (Ed.), *Functions anticipatrices du systemè nerveux et processus psychologique.* Paris: Edition C.N.R.S., 1980.

Lindsey, D. T., Holzman, P. S., Haberman, S., & Yasillo, N. J. Smooth-pursuit eye movements: A comparison of two measurement techniques for studying schizophrenia. *Journal of Abnormal Psychology,* 1978, *87,* 491-496.

Littman, D., & Becklen, R. Selective looking with minimal eye movements. *Perception and Psychophysics,* 1976, *20,* 77-79.

Llewellyn-Thomas, E. Movements of the eye. *Scientific American,* 1968, *219,* 89-95.

Llewellyn-Thomas, E. Search behaviour. *Radiologic Clinics of North America,* 1969, *7,* 403-417.

Llewellyn-Thomas, E., & Lansdowne, E. L. Visual search patterns of radiologists in training. *Radiology,* 1963, *81,* 288-292.

Loeb, J. Ueber die optische Inversion ebener linearzeichnungen bei ein-äugiger Betrachtung. *Pflügers Archiv,* 1887, *40,* 274-282.

Loftus, G. R. Eye fixations and recognition memory for pictures. *Cognitive Psychology,* 1972, *3,* 525-551.

Loftus, G. R. On-line eye movement recorders: The good the bad, and the ugly. *Behavioral Research Methods and Instrumentation,* 1979, *11,* 188-191.

Loftus, G. R. Tachistoscopic simulation of eye fixations on pictures. *Journal of Experi-*

mental Psychology: Human Learning and Memory, 1981, *7,* 369–376.

Loftus, G. R., & Kallman, H. J. Encoding and use of detail information in picture recognition. *Journal of Experimental Psychology: Human Perception and Performance,* 1978, *4,* 565–572.

Lovie, A. D., & Lovie, P. The effect of a horizontally structured field and target brightness on visual search and detection time. *Ergonomics,* 1968, *11,* 359–367.

Mackworth, N. H. Visual noise causes tunnel vision. *Psychonomic Science,* 1965, *3,* 67–68.

Mackworth, N. H. Stimulus density limits the useful field of views. In R. A. Monty & J. W. Senders (Eds.), *Eye movements and psychological processes.* Hillsdale, NJ: Lawrence Erlbaum Associates, 1976, 307–321.

Mackworth, N. H., & Morandi, A. J. The gaze selects informative details within pictures. *Perception & Psychophysics,* 1967, *2,* 547–552.

Magnussen, S. Reversibility of perspective in normal and stabilized viewing. *Scandinavian Journal of Psychology,* 1970, *11,* 153–156.

Mandel, T. S. Eye movement research on the propositional structure of short texts. *Behavior Research Methods & Instrumentation,* 1979, *11,* 180–187.

Mandler, J. M., & Parker, R. E. Memory for descriptive and spatial information in complex pictures. *Journal of Experimental Psychology: Human Learning & Memory,* 1976, *2,* 38–48.

Matin, L. A possible hybrid mechanism for modification of visual direction associated with eye movements: the paralyzed eye experiment reconsidered. *Perception,* 1976, *5,* 233–239.

May, H. J. Oculomotor pursuit in schizophrenia. *Archives of General Psychiatry,* 1979, *36,* 827.

Mayer, E., Bullinger, A., & Kaufmann, J. L. Motricité oculaire et cognition dans une tache spatiale. *Archives de Psychologie,* 1979, *XLVII* (183), 309–320.

McClelland, J. L., & O'Regan, K. Expectations increase the benefit derived from parafoveal visual information in reading words aloud. *Journal of Experimental Psychology: Human Perception and Performance,* 1981, *7,* 634–644.

McConkie, G. W. On the role and control of eye movements in reading. In P. A. Kolers, M. E. Wrolstad, & H. Bouma (Eds.), *Processing of visible language, Vol. 1.* New York, London: Plenum Press, 1979.

McConkie, G. W. Evaluating and reporting data quality in eye movement research. *Behavior Research Methods & Instrumentation,* 1981, *13,* 97–106.

McConkie, G. W., & Rayner, K. The span of the effective stimulus during a fixation in reading. *Perception and Psychophysics,* 1975, *17,* 578–586.

McConkie, G. W., & Rayner, K. Identifying the span of the effective stimulus in reading: Literature review and theories of reading. In H. Singer & R. B. Ruddell (Eds.), *Theoretical models and processes of reading.* Newark, DE: International Reading Association, 1976.

McConkie, G. W., Zola, D., Wolverton, G. S., & Burns, D. D. Eye movement contingent display control in studying reading. *Behavior Research Methods and Instrumentation,* 1978, *10,* 154–166.

McLaughlin, S. C. Parametric adjustment in saccadic eye movements. *Perception and Psychophysics,* 1967, *2,* 359–362.

Megaw, E. D., & Richardson, J. Target uncertainty and visual scanning strategies. *Human Factors,* 1979, *21,* 302–315.

Meiers Art Judgment Test, Bureau of Educational Research and Service, University of Iowa, Iowa City, 1940.

Meiers Aesthetic Perception Test, Bureau of Educational Research and Service, University of Iowa, Iowa City, 1962.

Merchant, J. *Laboratory oculometer.* NASA CR-1422, Honeywell, Inc. Radiation Center, Lexington, MA, 1969.

Merrill, E. G., & Stark, L. Optokinetic nystagmus: Double stripe experiment. *Quarterly Progress Report Research Laboratory of Electronics M.I.T.*, 1963, *70*, 357-359.

Meschan, I. *Synopsis of analysis of roentgen signs in general radiology.* Philadelphia: Saunders, 1976.

Michaels, D. L., & Tole, J. R. A microprocessor-based instrument for nystagmus analysis. *Proceedings of the IEEE*, 1977, *65*, 730-735.

Michard, A., Tetard, C., & Levy-Schoen, A. Attente du signal et temps de reaction. *L'Année Psychologique*, 1974, *74*, 387-402.

Michel, W. F., & Halliday, A. M. Differences between the occipital distribution of upper and lower field pattern-evoked responses in man. *Brain Research*, 1971, *32*, 311-324.

Miller, G. A., & Selfridge, J. A. Verbal context and the recall of meaningful material. *American Journal of Psychology*, 1950, *63*, 176-185.

Millward, R. B., & Wickens, I. D. Concept identification models. In D. H. Krantz, R. C. Atkinson, R. D. Luce, & P. Suppes (Eds.), *Learning, memory and thinking. Contemporary developments in mathematical psychology*, (Vol. 1). San Francisco: Freeman, 1974.

Mitrani, L., Yakimoff, N., & Mateeff, St. Dependence of visual suppression on the angular size of voluntary saccadic eye movements. *Vision Research*, 1970, *10*, 411-415.

Monty, R. A. An advanced eye movement measuring and recording system. *American Psychologist*, 1975, *30*, 331-335.

Monty, R. A., & Senders, J. W. (Eds.) *Eye movements and psychological processes.* Hillsdale, NJ: Lawrence Erlbaum Associates, 1976.

Moyer, R. S. Comparing objects in memory: Evidence suggesting an internal psychologics. *Perception and Psychophysics*, 1973, *13*, 180-184.

Mutschler, H. *Operator performance in real time, air-to-ground reconnaissance missions under task-loading conditions.* AGARD-CPP 266/267, 1979, S. 17.1-17.10.

Neisser, U. Decision-time without reaction-time: Experiments in visual scanning. *American Journal of Psychology*, 1963, *76*, 376-385.

Neisser, U. Visual search. *Scientific American*, 1964, *210*, 94-102.

Neisser, U. *Cognitive psychology.* New York: Appleton, 1967.

Neisser, U. *Cognition and reality.* San Francisco: W. H. Freeman, 1976.

Nelson, W. W., & Loftus, G. R. The functional field of view during picture viewing. *Journal of Experimental Psychology: Human Learning and Memory*, 1980, *6*, 391-399.

Newell, A., & Simon, H. A. *Human problem solving.* Englewood Cliffs, New Jersey: Prentice Hall, 1972.

Newman, N., Gay, A. J., Stroud, M. H., & Brooks, J. Defective rapid eye movements in progressive supranuclear palsy. *Brain*, 1970, *93*, 775-784.

Ni, M. D. A minicomputer program for automatic saccade detection and linear analysis of eye movement system using sine wave stimulus. *Computer Programs in Biomedicine*, 1980, *12*, 27-41.

Nickerson, R. S. Short-term memory for complex meaningful visual configurations: A demonstration of capacity. *Canadian Journal of Psychology*, 1965, *19*, 155-160.

Nodine, C. F., & Fisher, D. F. *Perception and pictorial representation.* New York: Praeger, 1979.

Norman, D. A., & Rumelhart, D. E. *Explorations in cognition.* San Francisco: Freeman, 1975.

Noton, D., & Stark, L. Eye movements and visual perception. *Scientific American*, 1971, *224*, 35-43. (a)

Noton, D., & Stark, L. Scanpaths in saccadic eye movements while viewing and recognizing patterns. *Vision Research*, 1971, *11*, 929-942. (b)

Noton, D., & Stark, L. Scanpaths in eye movements during pattern perception. *Science*, 1971, *171*, 308-311. (c)

O'Regan, K. Moment to moment control of eye saccades as a function of textual parameters in reading. In P. A. Kolers, M. W. Wroldstad, & H. Bouma (Eds.), *Processing of visible language.* New York: Plenum Press, 1979. (a)

O'Regan, K. Saccade size control in reading: Evidence for the linquistic control hypothesis. *Perception and Psychophysics,* 1979, *25,* 501–509. (b)

O'Regan, J. K. A better horizontal eye movement calibration method: smooth pursuit and zero drift. *Behavior Research Methods and Instrumentation,* 1978, *10,* 393–397.

Olson, R. K., Kliegl, R., & Davidson, B. J. Individual differences in reading processes and eye movements. In K. Rayner (Ed.), *Eye movements in reading: Perceptual and linguistic aspects.* New York: Academic Press, 1983.

Oster, Ph. J., & Stern, J. A. Measurement of eye movements. Electrooculography. In J. Martin & P. H. Venables (Eds.), *Techniques in psychophysiology.* New York: Wiley, 1980.

Pailhous, J. L'analyse de taches complexes par les mouvements oculaires. *L'Année Psychologique,* 1970, *70,* 487–504.

Pailhous, J., & Bullinger, A. The role of interiorisation of material properties of informa- tion acquiring devices in exploratory activities. *Communication and Cognition,* 1978, *11,* 209–234.

Parker, R. F. Picture processing during recognition. *Journal of Experimental Psychology: Human Perception and Performance,* 1978, *4,* 284–293.

Perenin, M. T., & Prablanc, C. Anomalies des saccades oculaires dans un cas d'heredo- degenerescence spino-cerebelleuse. *Revue E.E.G.,* 1974, *4,* 489–494.

Pheiffer, C. H., Eure, S. B., & Hamilton, C. B. Reversible figures and eye movements. *American Journal of Psychology,* 1956, *69,* 452–455.

Pivik, R. T. Target velocity and smooth pursuit eye movements in psychiatric patients. *Psychiatric Research Reports,* 1979, *1,* 313–323.

Pollack, R., & Spence, D. Subjective pictorial information in visual search. *Perception and Psychophysics,* 1968, *3,* 41–44.

Pollatsek, A., Bolozky, S., Well, A. D., & Rayner, K. Asymmetries in the perceptual span for Israeli readers. *Brain and Language,* 1981, *14,* 174–180.

Potter, M. C. Meaning in visual search. *Science,* 1975, *187,* 965–966.

Potter, M. C. Short-term conceptual memory for pictures. *Journal of Experimental Psychology: Human Learning and Memory,* 1976, *2,* 509–522.

Potts, G. R. The role of inference in memory for real and artificial information. In R. Revlin & R. E. Mayer (Eds.), *Human reasoning.* New York: Wiley, 1978.

Potts, G. R. Information processing strategies used in the encoding of linear orderings. *Journal of Verbal Learning and Verbal Behavior,* 1972, *11,* 727–740.

Prinz, W., & Kehrer, L. Recording detection distances in continuous visual search. In R. Groner & P. Fraisse (Eds.), *Cognition and eye movements.* Amsterdam: North-Holland, 1982.

Pritchard, R. M. Visual illusion viewed as stabilized retinal images. *Quarterly Journal of Experimental Psychology,* 1958, 10, 77–81.

Pritchard, R. M. Stabilized images on the retina. *Scientific American,* 1961, *204,* 72–78.

Pritchard, R. M., Heron, W., & Hebb, D. O. Visual perception approached by the method of stabilized images. *Canadian Journal of Psychology,* 1960, *14,* 67–77.

Rankin, E. F. The measurement of reading flexibility: Problems and perspective. *Reading information series: Where do we go?* International Reading Association, 1974.

Rayner, K. The perceptual span and peripheral cues in reading. *Cognitive Psychology,* 1975, *7,* 65–81.

Rayner, K. *Eye movements in reading: Perceptual and linguistic aspects.* New York: Academic Press, 1983.

Rayner, K., & McConkie, G. W. What guides a reader's eye movements? *Vision Research,* 1976, *16,* 829–837.

Rayner, K., McConkie, G. W., & Ehrlich, S. Eye movements and integrating information across fixations. *Journal of Experimental Psychology: Human Perception and Performance,* 1978, *4,* 529-544.

Rayner, K., Well, A. D., & Pollatsek, A. Asymmetry of the effective visual field in reading. *Perception & Psychophysics,* 1980, *27,* 537-544.

Restle, F. The selection of strategies in cue learning. *Psychological Review,* 1962, *69,* 329-343.

Riebel, F. A. Use of the eyes in x-ray diagnosis. *Radiology,* 1958, *70,* 252-258.

Robinson, D. A. Models of the saccadic eye movement control system. *Kybernetik,* 1973, *14,* 71-83.

Robinson, D. A. The mechanics of human saccadic eye movements. *Journal of Physiology* (London), 1964, *174,* 245-264.

Rotondo, J. A. Clustering analysis of subjective partitions of text. Paper presented at the National Reading Conference, December, 1980.

Rumelhart, D. E. Understanding and summarizing brief stories. In D. LaBerge & S. J. Samuels (Eds.), *Basic processes in reading: Perception and comprehension.* Hillsdale, NJ: Lawrence Erlbaum Associates, 1977.

Rushton, W. A. H. Visual pigments in man. Liverpool: Liverpool University Press, 1962.

Saida, S., & Ikeda, M. Useful visual field size for pattern perception. *Perception & Psychophysics,* 1979, *25,* 119-125.

Sakano, N. The role of eye movements in various forms of perception. *Psychologia* (Kyata), 1963, *6,* 215-227.

Salthouse, T. A., & Ellis, C. L. Determinants of eye-fixation duration. *American Journal of Psychology,* 1980, *93,* 207-234.

Salthouse, T. A., Ellis, C. L., Diener, D. C., & Somberg, B. L. Stimulus processing during eye fixations. *Journal of Experimental Psychology: Human Perception and Performance,* 1981, *7,* 611-623.

Sanders, A. F. Some aspects of the selective process in the functional visual field. *Ergonomics,* 1970, *13,* 101-117.

Savitzky, A., & Golay, M. J. E. Smoothing and differentiation of data by simplified least squares procedures. *Analytical Chemistry,* 1964, *36,* 1627-1638.

Schick, F. V., & Radke, H. A method for semi-automatic analysis of eye movements. In J. Moraal & K. F. Kraiss (Eds.), *Manned system and design.* New York, London: Plenum Press, 1981.

Schilder, P., Pasik, P., & Pasik, T. On-line analysis of optokinetic nystagmus by small general purpose digital computer. *Acta Otolaryngologica,* 1973, *76,* 443-449.

Schmid, R. Techical problems in stimulation, recording and analysis of eye movements. In R. Schmid & D. Zambarbieri (Eds.), *Eye movement analysis in neurlogical diagnosis.* Report of Center of Bioengineering, University of Pavia, Italy, 1981, 199-231.

Schmid, R., & Zambarbieri, D. *Eye movement analysis in neurological diagnosis.* Report of Center of Bioengineering, University of Pavia, Italy, 1981.

Schneider, W., & Shiffrin, R. M. Controlled and automatic human information processing: I. Detection, search and attention. *Psychological Review,* 1977, *84,* 1-66.

Senders, J. W., Fisher, D. F., & Monty, R. A. (Eds.) *Eye movements and the higher psychological functions.* Hillsdale, NJ: Lawrence Erlbaum Associates, 1978.

Shackel, B. Eye movement recording by electro-oculography. In P. H. Venables & I. Martin (Eds.), *A manual of psychophysiological methods.* Amsterdam: North-Holland Publishing, 1967.

Shagass, C., Amadeo, M., & Overton, D. A. Eye-tracking performance in psychiatric patients. *Biological Psychiatry,* 1974, *9,* 245-260.

Shagass, C., Roemer, R. A., & Amadeo, M. Eye-tracking performance and engagement of attention. *Archives of General Psychiatry,* 1976, *33,* 121-125.

Shannon, C. E. The mathematical theory of communication. *Bell System Technical Journal,* 1948, *27,* 379–423.

Shebilske, W. L. Reading eye movements from an information-processing point of view. In D. W. Massaro (Ed.), *Understanding language: An information-processing analysis of speech perception, reading and psycholinguistics.* New York: Academic Press, 1975.

Shebilske, W. L. Structuring an internal representation of text: A basis for literacy. In P. A. Kolers, M. E. Wrolstad, & H. Bouma (Eds.), *Processing of visual language,* Volume 2. New York: Plenum Press, 1980.

Shebilske, W. L., & Fisher, D. F. Eye movements reveal components of flexible reading strategies. In M. L. Kamil (Ed.), *31st Yearbook of the National Reading Conference.* Clemson, SC, 1981.

Shebilske, W. L., & Fisher, D. F. Eye movements and context effects during reading of extended discourse. In K. Rayner (Ed.), *Eye movements in reading: Perceptual and linguistic aspects.* New York: Academic Press, 1983.

Shebilske, W. L., & Rotondo, J. A. Typographical and spatial cues that facilitate learning from textbooks. *Visible Language,* 1981, *15,* 41–54.

Shiffrin, R. M., & Schneider, W. Controlled and automatic human information processing: II. Perceptual learning, automatic attending and a general theory. *Psychological Review,* 1977, *84,* 127–190.

Sigman, M., & Coles, P. Visual scanning during pattern recognition in children and adults. *Journal of Experimental Child Psychology,* 1980, *30,* 265–276.

Sills, A. W., Honrubia, V., & Kumley, W. E. Algorithm for the multi-parameter analysis of nystagmus using a digital computer. *Aviation Space Environmental Medicine,* 1975, *46,* 934–942.

Simon, G. *X-ray diagnosis for clinical students and practitioners,* (Second Edition). London: Butterworths, 1967.

Sisson, E. D. Eye movements and the Schroder stair figure. *American Journal of Psychology,* 1935, *47,* 309–311.

Slater, A. M., & Findlay, J. M. The corneal reflection technique and the visual preference method: Sources of error. *Journal of Experimental Child Psychology,* 1975, *20,* 240–247.

Snyder, H. L., & Taylor, D. F. *Computerized analysis of eye movements during static display visual search.* Aerospace Medical Research Laboratory Report No. AMRL–TR–79–91, Ohio, 1976.

Spache, G., & Spache, E. *Reading in the elementary school.* Boston: Allyn & Bacon, 1977.

Spitz, H. H. Scanpaths and pattern recognition. *Science,* 1971, *173,* 753.

Spooner, J. W., Sakala, S. M., & Baloh, R. W. Effect of aging on eye tracking. *Archives of Neurology,* 1980, *37,* 575–576.

Standing, L. Learning 10,000 pictures. *Quarterly Journal of Experimental Psychology,* 1973, *25,* 207–222.

Standing, L., Conezio, J., & Haber, R. N. Perception and memory for pictures: Single-trial learning of 2560 visual stimuli. *Psychonomic Science,* 1970, *19,* 73–74.

Stark, L., & Ellis, S. R. Scan paths revisited: Cognitive models direct active looking. In D. F. Fisher, R. A. Monty, & J. W. Senders (Eds.), *Eye movements: Cognition and visual perception.* Hillsdale, NJ: Lawrence Erlbaum Associates, 1981.

Starr, A. A disorder of rapid eye movements in Huntington's Chorea. *Brain,* 1967, *90,* 545–564.

Sternberg, S. The discovery of processing stages: Extension of Donders' method. In W. G. Koster (Ed.), *Attention and performance II, and Acta Psychologica,* 1969, *30,* 276–315.

Stryker, M., & Blakemore, C. Saccadic and disjunctive eye movements in cats. *Vision Research,* 1972, *12,* 2005–2013.

Sung, C. K. *Entwurf und Aufbau eines Bildmustergenerators in Fernsehnorm.* Diplomarbeit 1980, Institut für Prozessbtechnik u. Prozessbleittechnik, TU Karlsruhe in Zusammenarbeit mit dem Fraunhofer-Institut für Informations- und Datenverarbeitung, Karlsruhe.

Suppes, P., Cohen, M., Laddaga, R., Anliker, J., & Floyd, R. Research on eye movements in arithmetic performance. In R. Groner & P. Fraisse (Eds.), *Cognition and eye movements.* Amsterdam & Berlin: North Holland & Deutscher Verlag der Wissenschaften (joint edition), 1982.

Sutton, D. *A textbook of radiology and imaging* (3rd ed.). Edinburgh: Churchill Livingston, 1980.

Swets, J. A. Attention. *Annual Review of Psychology,* 1970, *21,* 339–366.

Taylor, S. E., Frackenpohl, H., & Pettee, J. L. Grade level norms for the components of the fundamental reading skill. *EDL Information and Research Bulletin,* No. 3. Huntington, NY: Educational Developmental Laboratories, 1960.

Thorndyke, P. W. Cognitive structures in comprehension and memory of narrative discourse. *Cognitive Psychology,* 1977, *9,* 77–110.

Tinker, M. A. Recent studies of eye movements in reading. *Psychological Bulletin,* 1958, *55,* 215–231.

Tole, J. R., & Young, L. R. MITNYS: a hybrid program for on-line analysis of nystagmus. *Aerospace Medicine,* 1971, *42,* 508–511.

Townsend, C. A., & Fry, G. A. Automatic scanning of aerial photographs. In A. Morris & E. P. Horne (Eds.), *Visual search techniques.* Washington, National Academy of Sciences, 1960.

Trevarthen, C. B. Two mechanisms of vision in primates. *Psychologische Forschung,* 1968, *31,* 299–337.

Troost, B. T., Daroff, R. B., & Dell'Osso, L. F. Eye tracking patterns in schizophrenia. *Science,* 1974, *184,* 1202–1203.

Troost, B. T., Weber, R. B., & Daroff, R. B. Hemispheric control of eye movements. I. Quantitative analysis of refixation saccades in a hemispherectomy patient. *Archives of Neurology,* 1972, *27,* 441–448.

Troost, B. T, Weber, R. B., & Daroff, R. B. Hypometric saccades. *American Journal of Ophthalmology,* 1974, *78,* 1002–1005.

Tuddenham, W. J. Visual search, image organization and reader error in Roentgen diagnosis. *Radiology,* 1962, *78,* 694–704.

Tuddenham, W. J., & Calvert, W. P. Visual search patterns in Roentgen diagnosis. *Radiology,* 1961, *76,* 255–256.

Vidal-Madjar, A., & Levy-Schoen, A. *Can we talk of irreducible ocular reaction time?* Paper given at the IIIrd European Conference on Visual Perception, Brighton, 1980.

Voss, M. Narrowing of the visual field as indicator of mental work load? In J. Moraal & K. F. Kraiss (Eds.), *Manned systems design: Methods, equipment, and applications.* New York: Plenum Press, 1981.

Vossius, G. Adaptive control of saccadic eye movements. *Bibliotheca Ophthalmologica,* 1972, *82,* 244–250.

Vossius, G., & Werner, G. The functional control of the eye tracking system and its digital stimulation. IFAC IVth Congress, 1969. Warsaw, Poland.

Walker-Smith, G., Gale, A. G., & Findlay, J. M. Eye movement strategies involved in face perception. *Perception,* 1977, *6,* 313–326.

Wallin, J. E. W. The duration of attention, reversible perspectives and the refractory phase of the reflex arc. *Journal of Philosophical Psychology and Scientific Methods,* 1910, *7,* 33–38.

Westheimer, G. Mechanism of saccadic eye movements. *American Journal of Ophthalmology,* 1954, *52,* 710–724.

Widdel, H., & Kaster, J. Eye movement measurement in assessment and training of visual performance. In J. Moraal & K. F. Kraiss (Eds.), *Manned systems design: Methods, equipment, and applications.* New York: Plenum Press, 1981, pp. 251–270.

Wieland, B. A., & Mefferd, R. B. Individual differences in Necker cube reversal rates and perspective dominance. *Perceptual & Motor Skills,* 1967, *24,* 923–930.

Wildberger, H. Visual evoked potentials: Expected and unexpected influences by visual field defects. In A. Huber & D. Klein (Eds.), *Neurogenetics and Neuro-Ophthalmology.* Amsterdam: North Holland/Elsevier, 1981.

Wirth, W. Die Klarheitsgrade der Regionen des Sehfeldes bei verschiedenen Verteilungen der Aufmerksamkeit. *Psychologische Studien,* 1907, *2,* 30-88.

Wirth, W. *Die experimentelle Analyse der Bewusstseinsphänomene.* Braunschweig: Vieweg, 1908.

Wirth, W. die Reaktionszeiten. In A. Bethe, G. von Bergmann, E. Embden, & A. Ellinger (Hrsg.), *Handbuch der normalen und pathologischen Physiologie,* Bd. X. Berlin: Springer, 1927.

Wolfe, J. W., Engelken, E. J., Olson, J. W., & Allen, J. P. Cross-power spectral density analysis of pursuit tracking. Evaluation of central and peripheral pathology. *Annals of Otology Rhinology and Laryngology,* 1978, *87,* 837-844.

Wright, F. W. *The radiological diagnosis of lung and mediastinal tumours.* London, Butterworths: 1973.

Wyman, D., & Steinman, R. M. Small step tracking: Implications for the Oculomotor "dead zone." Vision Research, 1973, *13,* 2165-2172.

Yarbus, A. L. *Eye movements and vision.* New York: Plenum Press, 1967.

Yerushalmy, J. The statistical assessment of the variability in observer perception and description of roentgenographic pulmonary shadows. *Radiologic Clinics of North America,* 1969, *1,* 381-390.

Young, L. R., Forster, J. B., & Van Houtte, N. *A revised stochastic sampled data model for eye tracking movements.* Fourth annual NASA University Conference on Manual Control, NASA, sp. 192, Springfield, MA, 1968.

Young, L. R., & Sheena, D. Survey of eye movement recording methods. *Behavioral Research Methods and Instrumentation,* 1975, *7,* 397-429.

Zahn, T. P., Rosenthal, D., & Shakow, D. Reaction time in schizophrenic and normal subjects in relation to the sequence of series of regular preparatory intervals. *Journal of Abnormal Social Psychology,* 1961, *63,* 161.

Zee, D. S., Optican, L. M., Cook, J. D., Robinson, D. A., & King Engel, W. Slow saccades in spinocerebellar degeneration. *Archives of Neurology,* 1976, *33,* 243-251.

Zimmer, A. Einige Ursachen der Inversionen mehrdeutiger stereometrischer Konturenzeichnungen. *Zeitschrift für Z. Sinnesphysiologie,* 1913, *47,* 106-158.

Zinchenko, V. P., & Vergiles, N. Y. Formation of visual images. Studies of stabilized retinal images. B. Haigh (Trans.) New York, New York Consultants Bureau, 1972.

Zusne, L., & Michels, K. M. Nonrepresentational shapes and eye movements. *Perceptual & Motor Skills,* 1964, *18,* 11-20.

Author Index

Subject Index